Contemporary Surgical Clerkships

Series Editor

Adam E. M. Eltorai, Marlborough, USA

This series of specialty-specific books will serve as high-yield, quick-reference reviews specifically for the numerous third- and fourth-year medical students rotating on surgical clerkships. Edited by experts in the field, each book includes concise review content from a senior resident or fellow and an established academic physician. Students can read the text from cover to cover to gain a general foundation of knowledge that can be built upon when they begin their rotation, or they can use specific chapters to review a subspecialty before starting a new rotation or seeing a patient with a subspecialty attending.

These books will be the ideal, on-the-spot references for medical students and practitioners seeking fast facts on diagnosis and management. Their bullet-pointed format, including user-friendly figures, tables and algorithms, make them the perfect quick-reference. Their content breadth covers the most commonly encountered problems in practice, focusing on the fundamental principles of diagnosis and management. Carry them in your white coat for convenient access to the answers you need, when you need them.

Jason Roostaeian • Michael Delong
Nirbhay S. Jain
Editors

Plastic Surgery Clerkship

A Guide for Senior Medical Students

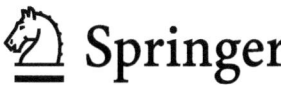

Editors
Jason Roostaeian
Clinical Professor, Division of
Plastic Surgery
UCLA Medical Center
Los Angeles, CA, USA

Michael Delong
Assistant Professor-in-Residence, Division
of Plastic Surgery
UCLA Medical Center
Los Angeles, CA, USA

Nirbhay S. Jain
PGY-6 Resident, Division of Plastic Surgery
UCLA Medical Center
Los Angeles, CA, USA

ISSN 2730-941X ISSN 2730-9428 (electronic)
Contemporary Surgical Clerkships
ISBN 978-3-031-99097-7 ISBN 978-3-031-99098-4 (eBook)
https://doi.org/10.1007/978-3-031-99098-4

© The Editor(s) (if applicable) and The Author(s), under exclusive license to Springer Nature Switzerland AG 2025

This work is subject to copyright. All rights are solely and exclusively licensed by the Publisher, whether the whole or part of the material is concerned, specifically the rights of translation, reprinting, reuse of illustrations, recitation, broadcasting, reproduction on microfilms or in any other physical way, and transmission or information storage and retrieval, electronic adaptation, computer software, or by similar or dissimilar methodology now known or hereafter developed.
The use of general descriptive names, registered names, trademarks, service marks, etc. in this publication does not imply, even in the absence of a specific statement, that such names are exempt from the relevant protective laws and regulations and therefore free for general use.
The publisher, the authors and the editors are safe to assume that the advice and information in this book are believed to be true and accurate at the date of publication. Neither the publisher nor the authors or the editors give a warranty, expressed or implied, with respect to the material contained herein or for any errors or omissions that may have been made. The publisher remains neutral with regard to jurisdictional claims in published maps and institutional affiliations.

This Springer imprint is published by the registered company Springer Nature Switzerland AG
The registered company address is: Gewerbestrasse 11, 6330 Cham, Switzerland

If disposing of this product, please recycle the paper.

Contents

1	**Fundamentals of Plastic Surgery**............................... Jacquelynn P. Tran and Yara Samman	1
2	**Wound Healing and Scar Formation** .... Nirbhay S. Jain	13
3	**Flaps and Grafts** .... Annalisa Lopez	23
4	**Tissue Expansion**... Annalisa Lopez	35
5	**Microsurgery**... Edward H. Nahabet	39
6	**Transplantation Biology and Vascularized Composite Allotransplantation**... Jasmine Lee, Kshipra Hemal, and Allyson R. Alfonso	49
7	**Local Anesthesia** .... Jacquelynn P. Tran and Yara Samman	55
8	**Lasers in Plastic Surgery** .... Andi J. Cummins	61
9	**Skin Lesions: Benign and Malignant** .... Evelyn Reed	71
10	**Burn**... Katherine J. Choi and Christopher H. Pham	85
11	**Pressure Ulcers** .... Yara Samman and Jacquelynn T. Lee	93
12	**Head and Neck Anatomy/Function**........................... Alice Yu, Josh Hwang, and Kristen Echanique	101

13	**Cleft Lip and Palate**	119
	Brendan J. Cronin	
14	**Velopharyngeal Dysfunction**	137
	Brendan J. Cronin	
15	**Craniofacial Microsomia**	147
	Brendan J. Cronin	
16	**Congenital Melanocytic Nevi**	155
	Brendan J. Cronin	
17	**Vascular Malformations**	161
	Shervin Etemad	
18	**Craniosynostosis**	169
	Sumun Khetpal	
19	**Orthognathic Surgery**	175
	Mia Joseph	
20	**Facial Clefts and Hypertelorism**	187
	Brendan J. Cronin	
21	**Ear Reconstruction and Otoplasty**	197
	Brendan J. Cronin	
22	**Nasal Reconstruction**	209
	Sumun Khetpal and Nirbhay S. Jain	
23	**Scalp Reconstruction**	215
	Jack D. Sudduth and Jessica L. Marquez	
24	**Eyelid Reconstruction**	225
	Zachary Dezeeuw	
25	**Lip Reconstruction**	235
	Emily L. Geisler	
26	**Facial Fractures**	243
	Brendan J. Cronin	
27	**Head and Neck Tumors**	261
	Kshipra Hemal, Allyson R. Alfonso, and Jasmine Lee	
28	**Complex Head and Neck Reconstruction**	267
	Alexandre J. Bourcier and Edward H. Nahabet	
29	**Facial Paralysis**	281
	Shervin Etemad	
30	**Breast Anatomy**	289
	Shamit Prabhu	

31	**Gynecomastia** Laurel D. Ormiston and Kaylee B. Scott	293
32	**Breast Reduction** Katherine J. Choi	299
33	**Breast Implants, Augmentation, and Mastopexy** Michael W. Wells and Irene A. Chang	305
34	**Prosthetic-Based Breast Reconstruction** Harsh Patel	313
35	**Autologous Breast Reconstruction** Corbin Muetterties	319
36	**Abdominoplasty and Body Contouring** Alexis L. Boson	327
37	**Liposuction** Patrick R. Keller	337
38	**Facial Analysis** Sean Saadat	345
39	**Nonsurgical Facial Rejuvenation** Emily L. Geisler	351
40	**Face and Neck Lift** Edward H. Nahabet	359
41	**Rhinoplasty** Sean Saadat	369
42	**Blepharoplasty** Edward H. Nahabet	379
43	**Brow Lift** Irene A. Chang and Michael W. Wells	387
44	**Botox/Filler** Kaylee B. Scott and Laurel D. Ormiston	397
45	**Brazilian Butt Lift** Patrick R. Keller	409
46	**Hand Anatomy, Function, and Exam** Nirbhay S. Jain	419
47	**Hand Infections** Nirbhay S. Jain	433
48	**Compression Neuropathies** Nirbhay S. Jain	441

49	**Nerve Transfers, Repairs, and Complex Amputation** . . . . Nirbhay S. Jain	451
50	**Brachial Plexus** . . . . Nirbhay S. Jain	457
51	**Hand Fractures** . . . . Nirbhay S. Jain	463
52	**Wrist Fractures** . . . . Nirbhay S. Jain	469
53	**Hand Tendon Injuries** . . . . Nirbhay S. Jain	477
54	**Tendon Transfers** . . . . Nirbhay S. Jain	485
55	**Ligament Injuries** . . . . Nirbhay S. Jain	489
56	**Digital Replantation and Revascularization** . . . . Corbin Muetterties	495
57	**Thumb Reconstruction** . . . . Udayan Betarbet	503
58	**Dupuytren's Disease** . . . . Meaghan L. Barr	511
59	**Hand Tumors** . . . . Udayan Betarbet	515
60	**Vascular Injuries of the Hand** . . . . Nirbhay S. Jain	531
61	**Congenital Hand** . . . . Nirbhay S. Jain	537
62	**Rheumatoid Arthritis** . . . . Meaghan L. Barr	547
63	**Osteoarthritis** . . . . Carter J. Boyd and Jonathan M. Bekisz	555
64	**Chest Reconstruction** . . . . Harsh Patel	563
65	**Abdominal Wall Reconstruction** . . . . Erika Samlowski	567

66	**Lower Extremity Reconstruction**	577
	Harsh Patel	
67	**Perineal Reconstruction**	583
	Andi J. Cummins	
68	**Lymphedema**	593
	Irene A. Chang and Michael W. Wells	
69	**Gender Affirming Surgery**	603
	Alexis L. Boson	
Index		611

Chapter 1
Fundamentals of Plastic Surgery

Jacquelynn P. Tran and Yara Samman

Plastic Surgery: Overview and Scope of Practice

- The plastic in plastic surgery does not refer to synthetic materials:
  - Plastic comes from the Greek root *plastikos*, which means to mold or to change.
  - Plastic surgery has been around since the 600s BC, making it one of the oldest disciplines in medicine.
  - Plastic surgery was first used to describe the field in the 1800s, before silicone implants were invented.
- Plastic surgery has one of the most diverse scopes of practice in the field of surgery:
  - Plastic surgeons are unique in that they operate on patients from neonates to the elderly and in every region of the body with all types of surgeries:
    - Wound coverage and reconstruction using the patient's own tissue following trauma or tumor extirpation.
    - Hand surgery: fractures, soft tissue reconstruction, peripheral nerve decompression, brachial plexus injuries, tendon repair, revascularization or replantation of traumatically amputated digits and hand.
    - Pediatric plastic surgery: craniofacial anomalies, cleft lip and palate, craniosynostosis, congenital hand and feet anomalies, vascular malformations.
    - Adult craniofacial surgery, including fractures, orthognathic surgery, and cranioplasty.

J. P. Tran (✉) · Y. Samman
University of Texas Medical Branch Division of Plastic Surgery, Galveston, TX, USA
e-mail: jptran@utmb.edu; ybsamman@utmb.edu

- Aesthetic surgery from head to toe.
- Care of the burn patient in both acute and reconstructive phases.
- Gender Affirmation surgery, including feminization and masculinization.
- Composite tissue allotransplantation: also known as vascularized composite allograft (VCA), which is the transfer of a functional unit of non-organ human tissue from one human to another. This functional unit can include the skin, muscle, tendon, bone, blood vessels, and nerves. Successfully documented VCAs include the face, hand, and penis [1–3].
  – Only a small part of plastic surgery is cosmetic surgery.
- Plastic surgery is a principle-based discipline, not disease-based:
  – Purest form of anatomic application in surgery
- Many surgical procedures adopted by other fields can be traced back to plastic surgery:
  – Head and neck reconstructions now performed by ENT surgeons were mainly developed by plastic surgeons.
  – Abdominal wall reconstruction performed by general surgeons.
  – Organ allotransplantation (Dr. Joseph Murray, father of the kidney transplant, was trained as a plastic surgeon).

Most Commonly Performed Procedures

- According to the American Society of Plastic Surgeons statistics report [4]:
  – Top 5 cosmetic surgical procedures, 15.6 million reported in 2020 (total count in 2020):
    (i) Rhinoplasty (352,555)
    (ii) Eyelid surgery (325,112)
    (iii) Facelift (234,374)
    (iv) Liposuction (211,067)
    (v) Breast augmentation (193,073)
  – Top 5 reconstructive procedures, 6.8 million reported in 2020 (total count in 2020):
    (i) Tumor excision (5.2 million)
    (ii) Laceration repair (386,710)
    (iii) Maxillofacial surgery (256,085)
    (iv) Scar revision (263,643)
    (v) Hand surgery (206,928)

Reconstructive Ladder of Plastic Surgery

- Commonly referenced paradigm that systematically organizes reconstructive options by complexity [5].
- Reconstruction should be performed by evaluating options from least to most complex to see which accomplishes goals of form and function:

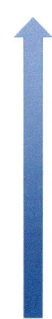

- Free flap
- Pedicle flaps
- Tissue expansion
- Local flaps
- Dermal matrices
- Skin graft
- Negative pressure wound therapy
- Closure by secondary intention
- Primary closure

Key Principles of Plastic Surgery

- *Preserve form and function.*
    - The primary goal of reconstructive surgery is to provide wound coverage for traumatic or surgically created wound, restore function, and improve quality of life.
    - Form determines function; providing an appropriate form will allow for improved function.
    - Replace like with like tissue when possible:
        - Examples:
            (i) Fibula bone free flap for mandible reconstruction following tumor extirpation
            (ii) Nose reshaping with cartilage graft from the nasal septum, ear, or rib

(iii) Palmaris longus tendon graft for tendon reconstruction and ligament reconstruction [6]
(iv) Full-thickness eyelid skin defects covered with full-thickness skin graft from adjacent region for the best skin color, quality, and texture match, such as the postauricular or supraclavicular regions
(v) Using tissue expander to increase hair-bearing skin for burn alopecia reconstruction [7]

- *Always have a backup plan, measure twice, and cut once.*
  - Consider the reconstructive ladder for each case.
  - Do not burn lifeboats:
    (i) When planning a surgery, build in contingencies in case the plan fails.
    (ii) Examples:
      - When doing a free flap for a hand, take it from the contralateral side so the ipsilateral groin is available for a pedicled flap.
- *Address modifiable risk factors.*
  - Factors associated with poor wound healing:
    - Malnutrition
    - Corticosteroid use
    - Obesity
    - Uncontrolled diabetes mellitus
    - Nicotine-containing products
    - Uncontrolled or unresolved infection
    - Untreated peripheral vascular disease
    - Adequate wound bed preparation
  - Assess perioperative risk:
    - Baseline functional status
    - History of cardiopulmonary disease and need for cardiac risk assessment
    - Venothrombotic risk assessment

Wound Closure and Sutures

- *Types of Closure*
  - *Primary closure*
    - Skin edges are re-approximated surgically using suture or staples upon presentation.
    - Principles of primary closure:

- Use atraumatic technique to minimize damage to skin edge; avoid pinching the skin with forceps or hemostat.
- Thorough washout and debridement of any contamination; freshen wound edge as needed:
  - Good blood flow means good healing.
- Tension-free closure; approximate but do not strangulate tissue.
- Avoid primary closure in infected wound beds.

- *Secondary intention closure*
  - Wound is allowed to heal through the development of granulation tissue and daily dressing changes.
  - Treatment for wound dehiscence without any exposed vital structures (muscle, tendon, vessels, nerves, bone).
  - Preferred choice for infected or contaminated wound beds and animal bites
- *Delayed primary closure (tertiary closure)*
  - Contaminated wounds upon presentation are left open for observation or surgically debrided and closed primarily at a later date when the wound bed is clean.

Closure Methods

- *Suture*
  - Suture choices include:
    - Absorbable vs nonabsorbable
    - Synthetic vs. natural
    - Monofilament vs. polyfilament
  - Preferred option for tissue under tension.
  - Achieves wound edge eversion.
  - Avoid prolonged suture retention; timeframe for removal varies by region:
    - Face: 5–7 days
    - Trunk: 7–10 days
    - Extremity: 10–14 days
- *Stainless steel staples*
  - Good option for scalp and other hair-bearing regions
  - Nonreactive, quick, epidermal re-approximation not as precise as suture, requires removal
  - Less ischemic so may be good in compromised tissue, though prone to worse scarring

- Not well tolerated in pediatric population
- *Skin adhesives*
  - If used as a method of closure, wound edge must be free of tension.
  - *Cyanoacrylate glue such as Ethicon DERMABOND®*: may be used in conjunction with sutures as the final layer of skin closure or as a water-tight dressing.
  - *Surgical tapes such as 3M Steri-Strips™*: similar to cyanoacrylate glue, may be used in conjunction with suture.
  - Typically, in plastic surgery, these are adjuncts to sutures to prevent contamination, not meant to replace them.
- *Common Primary Closure Techniques* (Fig. 1.1)
  - *Simple interrupted*: The needle enters the tissue at 90 degrees through the same depth and distance from either wound edge in a superficial to deep fashion. The knot is tied on top of the tissue closed.
  - *Simple running*: The stitch is started the same way as a simple interrupted closure; however, the suture is not cut and continues to "run" through the skin for the length of the laceration similar to a baseball stitch.
  - *Running subcuticular/intracuticular*: The needle weaves through the dermal-epidermal junction without leaving any marks on the skin. This method is the preferred final skin closure method for surgical incisions. The wound edge must not be under tension to achieve edge-to-edge approximation and an aes-

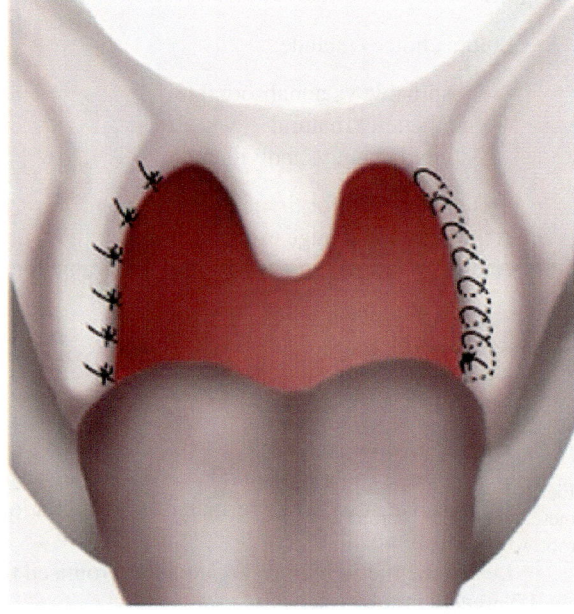

Fig. 1.1 Examples of interrupted suture technique (left side) and running suture (right side)

thetically acceptable scar. Unresolved wound edge tension may result in dehiscence or widened/hypertrophic scar (Figs. 1.2, 1.3 and 1.4).
- *Horizontal/vertical mattress*: Preferred choice for wounds under tension and glabrous skin of the hand and feet. The horizontal mattress configuration leads to more tissue ischemia compared to vertical mattress (Fig. 1.5).
- *Deep dermal suture*: Begin by entering the skin on one aspect from the deep side and exiting at the dermal-epidermal junction and then entering the skin at the dermal-epidermal junction across and exiting deep. This allows for the knot to be buried under the skin.
- *Classic plastic surgery closure for the skin*: 3-0 Monocryl suture for deep dermal stitches and 4-0 Monocryl suture for running subcuticular.

- *Sutures and Needles* (Fig. 1.6)
  - *Needle point configurations*

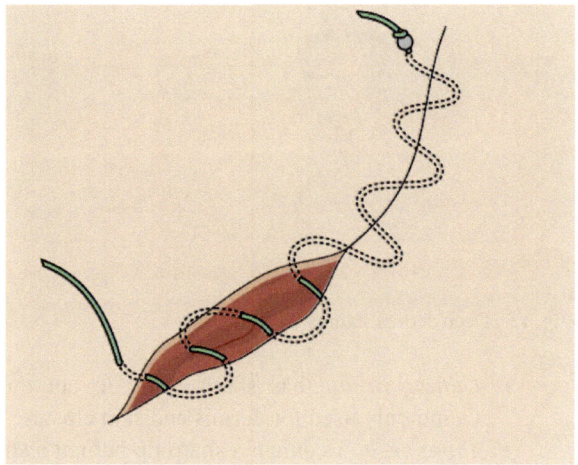

Fig. 1.2 Running subcuticular suture technique

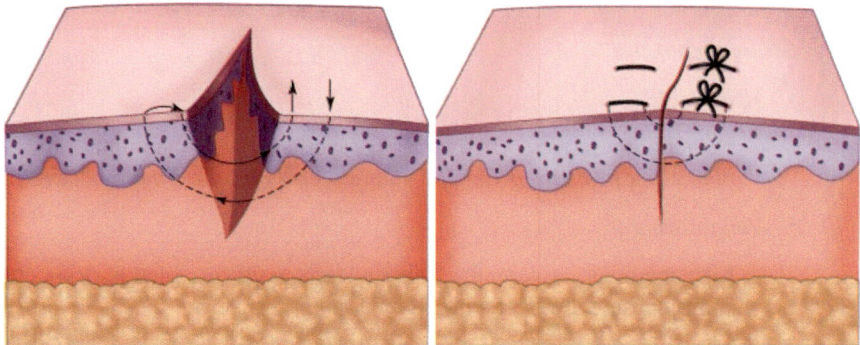

Fig. 1.3 Vertical mattress suture technique

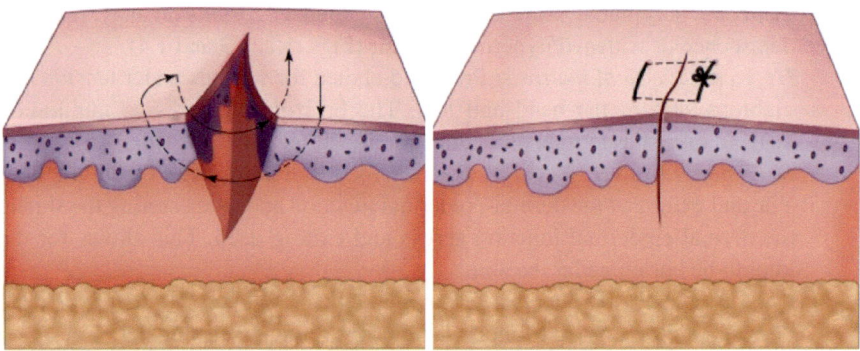

Fig. 1.4 Horizontal mattress suture technique

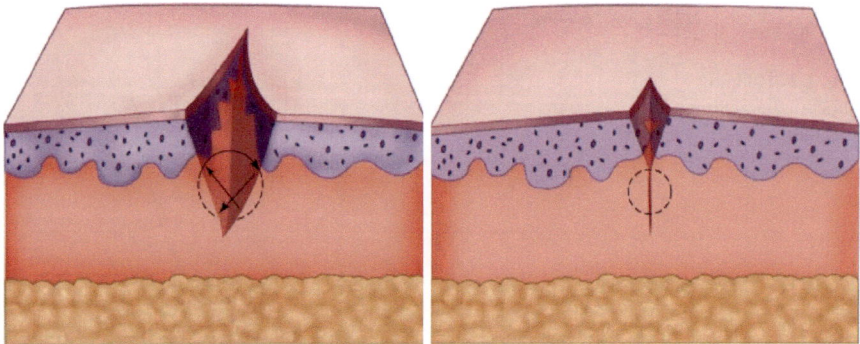

Fig. 1.5 Deep dermal sutures

- *Cutting needle* has sharp edges to cut through and penetrate tissue. Commonly used for dermis and skin closure
- *Taper needles* contain a sharp tip but not a sharp edge along the length of the needle. Requires more pushing as the tissue spreads around the needle. Commonly used to repair mucosa, fascia, muscle, and tendon

– *Suture Material*

- *Absorbable*
  - Degradation process via *hydrolysis* (synthetic suture, minimal inflammation) or *proteolysis* (natural suture such as gut, enzyme-mediated)
- *Nonabsorbable*
  - Like any other implant, the body undergoes cell-mediated reaction and forms capsule around the foreign body
- *Monofilament*

1 Fundamentals of Plastic Surgery

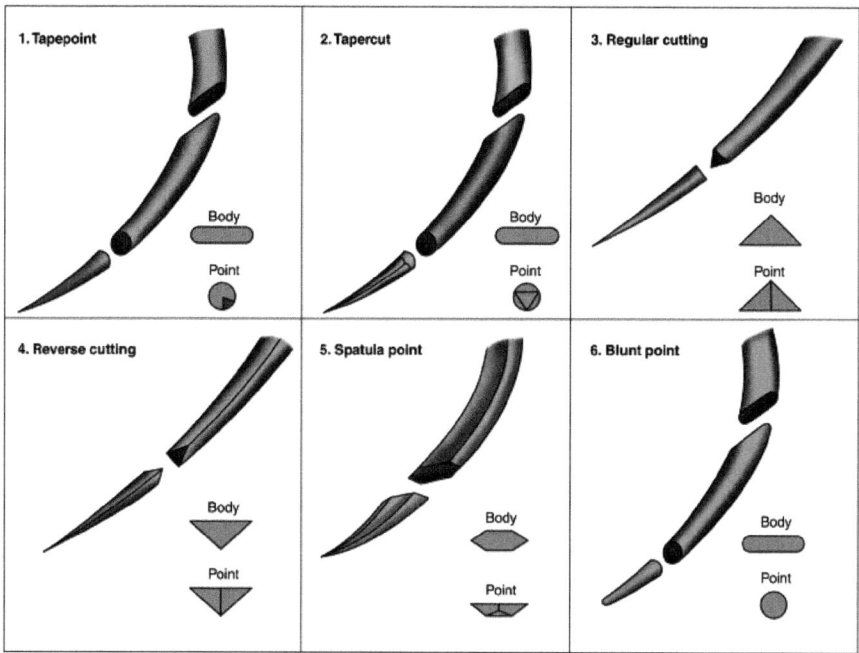

Fig. 1.6 Suture needle types

- Less tissue reactivity and infection risk, travels through tissue with less friction
- Weaker than polyfilament
- *Polyfilament (braided)*
  - Stronger, braided, more tissue reactivity though can carry bacteria
- *Commonly used sutures*

	Location	Length	Filament
Fast gut	Skin (face)	<1 week	Monofilament
Plain gut	Skin (face)	1–2 weeks	Monofilament
Chromic gut	Skin (hands), mucosa, muscle	4 weeks	Monofilament
Monocryl	Skin	4 weeks	Monofilament
Vicryl	Fascia, mucosa, muscle, vascular ties	4–6 weeks	Polyfilament
Polydioxanone (PDS)	Fascia	6–8 weeks	Monofilament
Silk	Vascular ties	Permanent	Polyfilament
Ethibond	Tendon	Permanent	Polyfilament
Nylon	Skin, tendon, vascular anastomosis	Permanent	Monofilament
Prolene	Skin, Fascia, tendon, vascular anastomosis	Permanent	Monofilament

Plastic Surgery Clerkship Pearls

The Three As of Surgery: Be Affable, Available, and Able
- *Always try to help.*
  - Try to anticipate what will be needed on rounds or in the operating room via observation and communicating with the team.
  - Have wound care and dressing change supplies ready for the patient.
- *Have a positive attitude.*
  - We understand not everyone is interested in surgery. Your attitude is key to success. If you are distant and disinterested, it makes it very hard to engage and educate.

Operating Room Etiquette and Expectations
- Read about the surgical cases for the upcoming day along with the patient's medical and surgical history.
  - What are the indications for surgery for this particular patient?
  - Review pertinent anatomy for the area.
- Commonly asked questions relate to anatomy, indications for surgery, complications of surgery, and alternative treatments.
- *Come early.*
  - Introduce yourself to the patient, resident, and faculty. Introduce yourself to the scrub tech, nurse, and anesthesia team.
  - Give your gloves and gown to scrub tech before the start of the case.
- *Lend a hand.*
  - Help move patients to and from the OR table and stretcher.
  - Help position patients.
- *Anticipate and participate.*
  - There is no task too small to do.
  - Once the nurse is about to prep the patient (clean the surgical field), it is time to scrub – medical students should be either the first or the last person scrubbed. The goal is to minimize interruptions in the normal OR workflow. If you wait too long, the scrub tech will be busy draping and trying to get the case started.
  - Hold the retractor that is placed in the operative field. Ask the surgeon if you can assist in retracting. Suction if you aren't holding a retractor.
  - Cut suture: long ~1 cm, short ~ 2–3 mm. On top of the knot: slide scissors down directly on top of the knot, and cut without leaving any tails.
  - Practice suturing and knot tying, but understand that excellent surgical skill is not a replacement for a good attitude and good knowledge.
  - Do not demand to do suture during surgery.

References

1. Pomahac B, Papay F, Bueno EM, Bernard S, Diaz-Siso JR, Siemionow M. Donor facial composite allograft recovery operation: Cleveland and Boston experiences. Plast Reconstruct Surg. 2012;129(3)
2. Momeni A, Chang B, Levin LS. Technology and vascularized composite allotransplantation (VCA) – lessons learned from the first bilateral pediatric hand transplant. J Mater Sci Mater Med. 2016;27
3. Cetrulo CL Jr, Li K, Salinas HM, Treiser MD, Schol I, Barrisford GW, et al. Penis Transplantation First US Experience. Ann Surg. 2018;267(5)
4. American Society of Plastic Surgeons. 2020 Plastic Surgery Statistics Report [Internet]. ASPS National Clearinghouse of Plastic Surgery Procedural Statistics. 2020 [cited 2022 Jun 23]. Available from: https://www.plasticsurgery.org/documents/News/Statistics/2020/plastic-surgery-statistics-full-report-2020.pdf
5. Janis JE, Kwon RK, Attinger CE. The new reconstructive ladder: Modifications to the traditional model. Plast Reconstruct Surg. 2011;127(SUPPL. 1 S)
6. Lee KH, Jo YH, Kim SJ, Choi WS, Lee CH, Kim JH. clinical results of autogenous palmaris longus tendon graft for ruptures of multiple extensors in rheumatoid hands. J Hand Surg. 2018;43(10)
7. McCauley RL. Tissue expansion reconstruction of the scalp. Semin Plast Surg. 2005;19(02)

Chapter 2
Wound Healing and Scar Formation

Nirbhay S. Jain

Tissue Anatomy and Structure [1]

- Critical structures are typically made up of collagen:
  - Type I collagen: skin, tendon, scar, bone
    - Typical collagen ratio in the skin is 4:1 of type I/type III.
  - Type II: cartilage
  - Type III: blood vessels
  - Type IV: basement membrane
  - Cross-linking of cartilage depends on vitamin C and hydroxylation of proline
    - Loss of vitamin C causes collagen weakness and bleeding of mucosal membranes—known as scurvy.
- Skin
  - Ectodermal, five main layers in the epidermis (from deep to superficial; see Fig. 2.1):
    - Stratum basale (melanin)
    - Stratum spinosum
    - Stratum granulosum
    - Stratum lucidum
    - Stratum corneum (acellular)
  - Deep is the dermis with looser papillary and denser reticular

---

N. S. Jain (✉)
Division of Plastic Surgery, Department of Surgery, University of California, Los Angeles, Los Angeles, CA, USA
e-mail: nsjain@mednet.ucla.edu

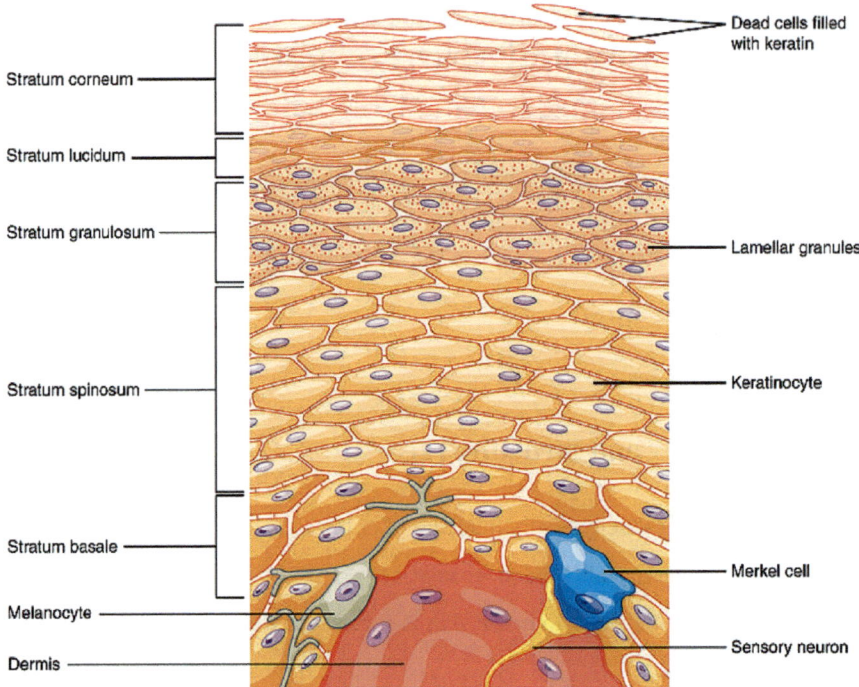

Fig. 2.1 Layers of the skin from superficial to deep

- Muscle
    - Mesodermal, made up of sarcomeres organized in fibers, fascicles, and then bundles forming muscles
- Bone
    - Mesodermal (except the skull—neural crest).
    - Cortical bone is the main portion; cancellous bone makes up less.
- Nerve
    - Typically dealing with peripheral nerves, made up of axons organized into fascicles and then nerves

Principles of Wound Healing of the Skin and Soft Tissue

- Typical wound healing is done by either primary intention (bringing edges of wound together) or secondary intention (allowing wound to heal on its own).
- Phases of wound healing:

- Inflammatory
  - Vasoconstriction and coagulation driven by platelets.
  - Vasodilation allows transmigration of neutrophils (dominates at 24 h) and then macrophages (dominates at 2–3 days) to release cytokines to attract fibroblasts.
  - Neutrophils are not necessary for wound healing, but macrophages are.
- Proliferative stage
  - Driven by fibroblasts, which dominate from day 3 to 14.
  - Keratinocytes begin to migrate in due to loss of contact inhibition.
  - Collagen deposition.
  - Neovascularization.
- Remodeling phase
  - Driven by matrix metalloproteinases and myofibroblasts
  - 5% of strength by 1 week, 30% at 3 weeks, 80% at end

– Epithelialization occurs in approximately 24 h:
- Mobilization due to loss of contact inhibition.
- Cells migrate across and divide and differentiate.

– Wound healing in each type of tissue is broadly the same; however, some specifics do exist:
- Muscles
  - Goes through destructive phase over the first week (analogous to inflammatory)
  - Transitions to repair over several weeks and then remodeling
- Bone
  - Primary bone healing typically requires rigid fixation.
  - Secondary bone healing from casts requires callus formation and immobilization.
  - Types of healing:
    - Osteoconductive: Donor bone acts as a framework for bone healing.
    - Osteoinduction: Donor substance (BMP) induces differentiation of local bone to form new bone.
    - Osteogenesis: Formation of new bone from the donor bone (vascularized bone or cancellous graft).
- Tendon
  - Tendon grafts act similar to osteoconductive bone: acts as a scaffold.
- Cartilage

- Tissue itself is avascular and cannot heal well.
- Superficial cartilage cannot heal; full thickness can through ingrowth of fibrous tissue.
- Nerve
  - Distal to injury, axons degenerate via Wallerian degeneration.
  - Axonal regrowth occurs proximally with growth cones and neurotrophic factors.
  - Growth occurs at approximately 1 mm/day, need to reinnervate muscle by about 1 year before irreversible atrophy of neuromuscular junction occurs.

Failures in Healing

- Dehiscence occurs most commonly at 1 week after injury, as remodeling begins with residual inflammation:
  - Associated factors include poor technique, malnutrition, smoking, hematoma, infection, and seroma.
- Chronic wound failure:
  - Failure of wound integrity after 3 months.
  - Worsened with diabetes, venous stasis, ischemic tissue loss, and pressure sores.
  - Long-term wounds may develop squamous cell cancer (Marjolin's ulcer), biopsy long-standing nonhealing wounds.
  - Derangements include increased MMPs.
  - Associated with poor vitamin intake (C, B6, folate, E), diabetes, smoking, low zinc, and steroids.
  - Anemia does not impair wound healing.
- Bone failure:
  - Delayed union or nonunion
  - Associated with poor health of the patient, low vitamin D, poor reduction, complex fractures, infection, delay in treatment
- Tendon failure:
  - If immobilized too long, get adhesions and weak repair.
  - If overused, then can tear tendon.
- Nerve pathology:
  - Neuromas and failure of axonal regeneration
  - Can also get inappropriate healing

2 Wound Healing and Scar Formation

Principles of Scarring

- Visible scar is in *all* full-thickness skin injuries; the goal is to minimize scarring.
  - Better scars if:
    - Older
    - Lighter skin
    - Controlled surgical incision, not trauma
    - Scar placed parallel to tension lines
    - Proper surgical techniques:
      - Minimize trauma to skin edges.
      - Evert skin.
      - Minimal tension on closure.
      - Appropriate suture choice and removal.
      - Appropriate opposition of the skin edges.
- Scars go through visible changes; most become red and inflamed and fade by 1 year.
- Can limit scarring through limited sun exposure (scars do not tan as well as surrounding skin), silicone sheets (modulate hydration to moisten scars), and scar massage to break up thicker connective tissue:
  - All other scar supplements do not have proven scarring benefits.

Pathologic Scarring (see Table 2.1)

- Hypertrophic scarring (Fig. 2.2)
  - Raised, erythematous, pruritic
  - Within border of wound
  - Most common with traumatic injury

Table 2.1 Comparison of keloids and hypertrophic scars

	Keloid	Hypertrophic scar
Collagen type dominant	I	III
Myofibroblast activity	Low	High
Fibroblast activity	High	Low
Blood vessel density	Low	High
Time to presentation after injury	Short	Long
Natural regression	Never	Often
Extent	Beyond wound	Within wound
Collagen organization	No	Yes

Fig. 2.2 Hypertrophic scarring

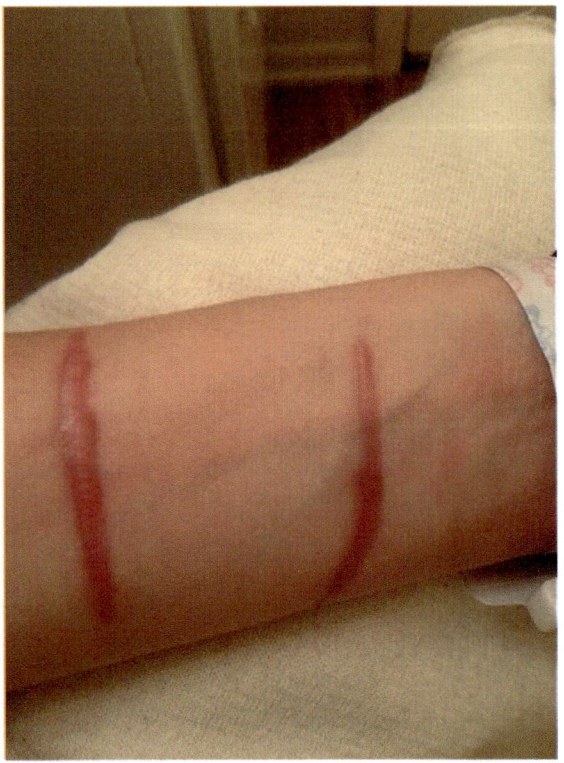

- More seen with tensioned closures and darker skin
- Occurs approximately 2 months after injury, worsens, and then may regress
- Has myofibroblast and excess collagen III, organized collagen presentation
- Manage with:
  - Pressure garments
  - Silicone sheeting
  - Steroid injections
  - Excision and scar release
- Keloids (Fig. 2.3)
  - Enlarging mass beyond the boundary of the wound
  - Increased fibroblast and collagen I, disorganized collagen presentation
  - Decreased myofibroblast and blood vessels
  - Associated with genetics, darker skin, age, and hormones and particular anatomic locations (chest, neck, jawline, ear)
  - Will never regress on own
  - Manage with:
    - Pressure garments

Fig. 2.3 Keloids

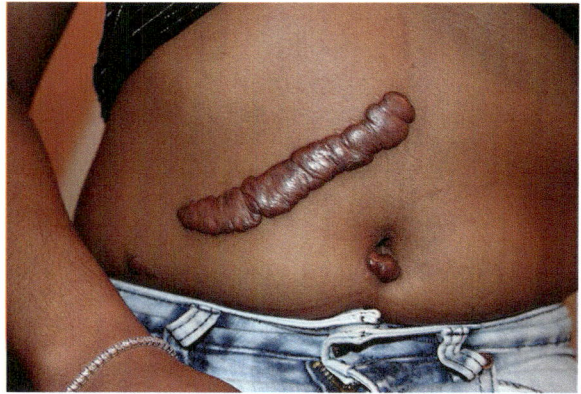

- Silicone sheets
- Steroids (good for itching, bad for getting rid of keloids)
- Surgical excision:
  - Need excellent technique and minimal tension closure
  - Often pair with radiation therapy to minimize recurrence

Principles of Wound Care

- Wounds can be classified in many ways:
  - Duration (acute v chronic)
  - Traumatic vs atraumatic
  - Contaminated or clean
  - Size and exposure
- In evaluating wounds, need to evaluate in context of the entire body:
  - Ischemic injury
  - Gross infection
  - Hypoxia or concomitant health issues
  - Radiation and edema
  - Neurovascular exam
- Specific physical exam characteristics of wounds:
  - Local radiation and edema
  - Color and perfusion
  - Induration and fluid collections
  - Hemorrhage
  - Contaminant
  - Foreign bodies

- Other wounds
- Location and etiology
- Depth and exposed structures
- Granulation, fibrinous exudate, odor
- Tracts and tunnels

– Key labs and imaging:
  - CBC, prealbumin.
  - ESR and CRP are nonspecific.
  - Imaging of affected areas with XR or CT as appropriate.
  - ABI is good for vasculature.
  - Biopsy and culture if concern for contaminant or cancer (Marjolin's ulcer).

– Managing wounds:
  - Wounds should be cleaned with debridement if concern for contamination to reduce bioburden and turn chronic wounds to acute wounds to promote healing:
    – Can be done with surgery, enzymes (collagenase), mechanical (VERSAJET), and autolytic (body debridement)
  - Appropriate dressings protect wounds, keep them clean, and promote granulation:
    – Nonocclusive dressings
      - Wet to dry: Basic dressing allows for mechanical debridement.
        – Critical to allow dressing to dry to have contaminant stick to the gauze to debride
      - Wet to wet: Do over structures that need moisture (tendon, bones, nerves, vessels).
    – Semiocclusive dressings
      - Allow air, not liquids, to pass through (Tegaderm).
      - Do not use if contaminated.
    – Occlusive dressings
      - Hydrogels and hydrocolloids.
      - Highly absorbant.
      - Alginate is a form with silver, which is antibacterial.
    – Negative pressure wound therapy: the wound vac
      - Reduces edema and removes exudate.
      - Useful in exudative wounds.
      - Do not use on infected tissues, cancer, and neurovascular structures.

Managing and Optimizing Surgical Wounds

- Surgical wounds are classified as
  - Clean
  - Clean-contaminated (respiratory or GU procedures)
  - Contaminated: grossly infected tissue but not purulent
  - Dirty: all others
- Principles of Incision placement
  - Understand which areas are prone to scarring (shoulder, sternum) and which heal better (eyelid, hand dorsum).
  - Bevel to avoid hair follicles in hair-bearing areas.
  - Design incisions along the line of resting tension (see Fig. 2.4).
- Longitudinal in the extremity, transverse in the trunk
- Use appropriate technique:
  - Incision made perpendicular to the skin with equal thickness dermis on both sides without bevel.

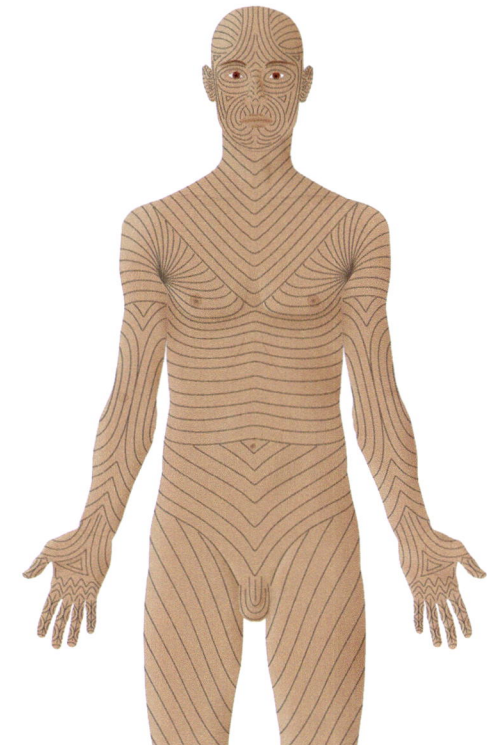

Fig. 2.4 Resting lines of skin tension

- Clean surgical field.
- Avoid excess trauma to the skin (use hooks, not pinching).
- Tension-free closure with wound edge eversion and appropriate opposition of skin edges.
- Sutures that do not leave marks.
- Appropriate removal of sutures.

Reference

1. Broughton G, Janes JE, Attinger CE. The basic science of wound healing. Plast Reconstruct Surg. 2006;117:12–34.

Chapter 3
Flaps and Grafts

Annalisa Lopez

Grafts vs Flaps: Key Concepts [2–4]

Vascular supply transfer is a critical factor in distinguishing the difference between a graft and a flap. A graft relies solely on the recipient site's blood supply through passive diffusion of oxygen and nutrients, while a flap is perfused by its own blood supply.

Grafts must therefore be placed on vascular beds. Grafts are also less durable than flaps and should be avoided in areas that require robust tissue. However, flaps are more technically challenging. Indications for flap placement include:

- Exposed bone without periosteum
- Exposed tendon without paratenon
- Exposed major vessel
- Exposed major nerve
- Pressure-bearing area
- Cosmetic or functional benefit

Grafts [1–3]

A skin graft is a great method of supplying the epidermis and dermis to a defect that cannot be closed primarily.

A. Lopez (✉)
Division of Plastic Surgery, The University of Texas Medical Branch, Galveston, TX, USA
e-mail: annlopez@utmb.edu

Primary Contracture: Immediate contraction of graft upon harvesting a graft, mediated in skin grafts by elastin. The thicker the graft, the more primary contracture.

Secondary Contracture: Delayed contraction of a graft after healing is complete, mediated in skin grafts by myofibroblasts, inhibited by dermis. The thinner the graft, the more secondary contracture.

Type of skin grafts include:

- Autografts: skin taken from patient and placed on the same patient (e.g., skin taken from a patient's thigh onto their forearm)
- Allograft: skin from another human donor, typically cadaveric
- Xenograft: skin from an animal (e.g. pig skin)

Skin grafts are stratified as follows:

- Split-thickness skin graft (STSG)
    - Composition—epidermis and partial dermis:
        - Donor site heals by itself with dressings, resulting in a patch scar.
    - Applications: burns, fasciotomy sites, non-extensive cancer resections
    - Thickness: typically harvested in 1000ths of an inch, from ~10/1000 to ~20/1000
    - Advantages:
        - Can be meshed to improve surface area and may lead to decreased risk of graft failure due to seroma or hematoma
        - Can provide better contour as compared to FTSG
        - Less primary contracture (less dermis = less elastin composition = less primary contracture)
    - Disadvantages:
        - Decreased cosmesis due to "waffled" or "fish skinned" appearance if meshed to increase surface area
        - More secondary contracture (thought to be attributed to myofibroblasts) as compared to FTSG which limits the ability to be placed over flexural surfaces:
            - Thicker grafts have less secondary contracture.
    - Contracture: Secondary contracture > primary contracture.
- Full-thickness skin graft (FTSG)
    - Composition—epidermis and full thickness of the dermis:
        - Donor site is closed primarily, healing as a linear scar.

Table 3.1 Comparison of split-thickness skin graft and full-thickness skin graft

	Split	Full
Thickness	Partial dermis	Full-thickness dermis
Metabolic demand	Lower	Higher
Locations	Used for general body	Used for the face, eyes, hands, joints
Harvest site	Heals in on own, scars but can be reharvested	Closed primarily, cannot be reharvested
Cosmetics	Often poor	Improved
Dominant contracture	Secondary	Primary
Hair/subcutaneous structures	Takes on recipient site	Takes on donor site

- Applications: Ear reconstruction, eyelid reconstruction, hand and joint reconstruction.
- Contracture: Primary contracture > secondary contracture (Table 3.1).

- Composite grafts
  - Composition: composed of two or more types of tissue, for example, the skin and cartilage
  - Advantages: Better at improving contour
  - Disadvantages: Have higher risk of failure due to higher metabolic demand
  - Applications: Ear and eyelid reconstruction

- Other grafts
  - Bone, cartilage, tendon, nerve, and vessel grafts are often used:
    - Bone grafts are typically osteoconductive in nature (see Chap. 2).
    - Cartilage grafts are subject to warping.
    - Other grafts serve mainly as matrix for scar (tendon) or conduits for tissues to grow through (nerve, vessel).

Stages of skin graft take the following:

1. Imbibition
   (a) This involves the absorption of oxygen and nutrients by the graft from the wound bed (recipient bed), and fibrin layer adherence occurs to secure the graft.
   (b) Time frame: 24–48 h.

2. Inosculation
   (a) This involves the beginning of vascularization of the graft from the wound bed where capillary beds from the graft and the donor site (wound bed) begin aligning with one another and connections are starting to be established.
3. Revascularization
   (a) Complete vascularization of the graft

Flaps

As detailed above, flaps are reliant on their own blood supply. This can be random pattern (without an isolated vessel), axial/pedicled (with an isolated vessel), or free (with a vessel disconnected and reconnected with microsurgery). Additionally, flaps can be classified by their tissue composition, being fasciocutaneous, myocutaneous, muscle, osseous, osteocutaneous, or any combination thereof.

- **Theories for Flap Vascularization** [5–7]
  - *Angiosome theory*: Any section of tissue can be divided into three-dimensional blocks in which each segment of the skin and underlying tissue is supplied by specific arteries and veins, which are known as angiosomes.
    - There are theorized to be 40 angiosomes which are all interconnected with anastomotic arteries or collateral "choke" vessels.
  - *Fasciocutaneous plexus*: Any section of tissue is supplied by a network of vascular plexuses derived from fascial layers in the following order from superficial to deep: cutaneous, fasciocutaneous, adipofascial, septocutaneous, and musculocutaneous flaps.
- **Random Pattern Local Flaps** [8–12]
  - Random pattern flaps depend on the surrounding tissue to provide vascularity to the flap:
    - Flaps should be made at a ratio of 3:1 to 4:1 at maximum, with the length along the axis of perfusion being greater than the width.
    - Often, the tip of the flap can become ischemic, resulting in wound breakdown.
    - Local flaps can be inset for coverage and then divided at a later date, for example, groin flap or forehead flap.
  - *Advancement flaps*: Tissue undermined and locally advanced in a unidirectional fashion:

Fig. 3.1 Angiosomes of the foot

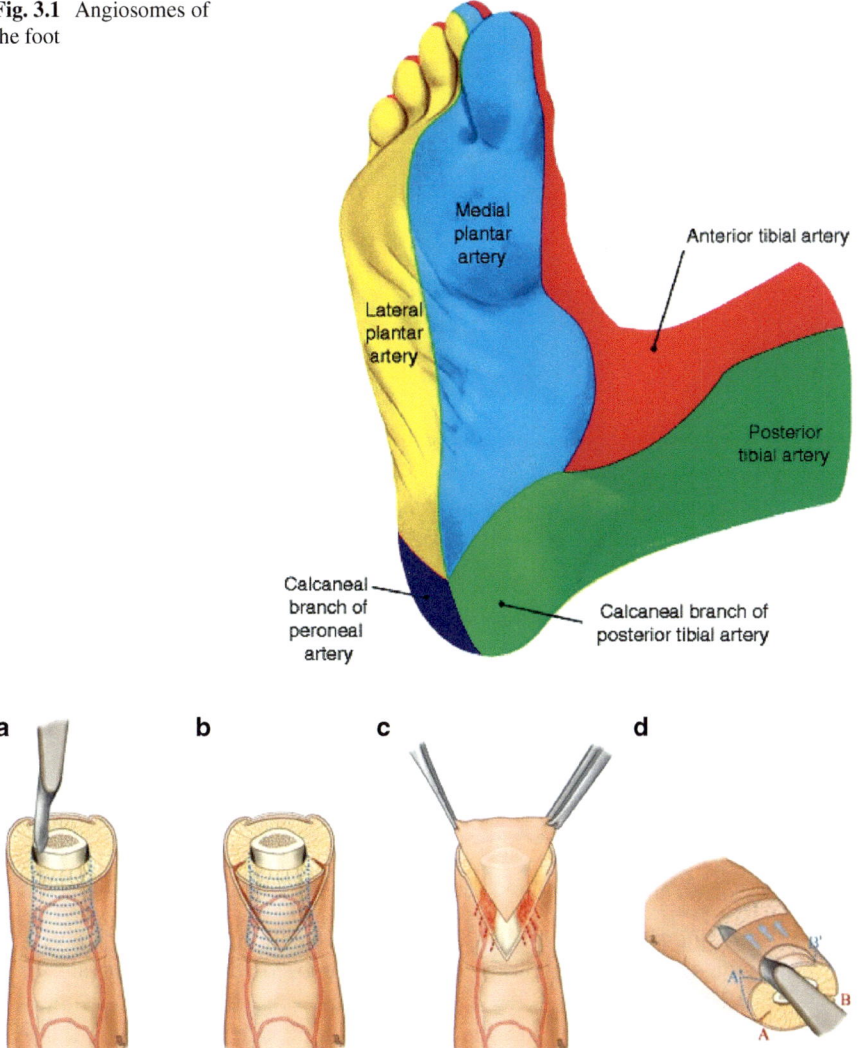

Fig. 3.2 Example of advancement V-Y flap for fingertip coverage

- *For example, V-Y flap, single advancement (finger reconstruction), double advancement, Burow's wedge flap (Figs. 3.1 and 3.2).*

– *Rotational flaps*: A semicircular flap rotated around a determined pivot point to allow for rotation of the tissue into deficit; of note, this creates a smaller triangular standing cone deficit which can then be grafted.

- *For example, scalp reconstruction after Mohs surgery (Fig. 3.3)*

Fig. 3.3 Rotational flap design

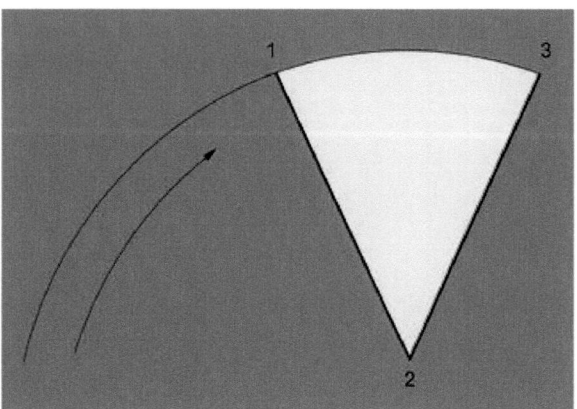

- *Transposition flap*: Flaps that are rotated laterally in order to close an adjacent soft tissue deficit; of note, these can be unilobed or bilobed flaps.
  - *For example, nasal tip or scalp reconstruction*
  - *Z-plasty*: a form of transposition flap that can be used to increase vertical length along an incision or scar
    - Application: This technique can be used to lengthen scars along flexural surfaces to increase range of motion, for instance, cases of scar contracture along the axilla, antecubital fossa, or fingers (Table 3.2 and Fig. 3.4).
- **Axial Flaps**
  - Flaps with an isolated blood vessel can be pedicled or free:
    - *Free flap*: a flap in which the vascular pedicle will be freely transferred with the overlying tissue to be anastomosed to a recipient site (e.g., DIEP flap)
    - *Pedicled flap*: a flap in which the vascular pedicle will remain attached to underlying transposed tissue, for example, latissimus for breast reconstruction
  - Can be done as a "normal" or "reverse" flap:
    - "Normal" flaps are done off the direction of flow of an artery.
    - "Reverse" flaps rely on retrograde flow and depend on collateral circulation distally (Fig. 3.5).

3 Flaps and Grafts

Table 3.2 Anticipated length gain based on angle of the Z-plasty

Angle of Z-plasty	% Vertical limb gain
30 degrees	25% gain
45 degrees	50% gain
60 degrees	75% gain
75 degrees	100% gain
90 degrees	120% gain

Of note, W-plasty and M-plasty are similar techniques to assist with relaxing skin tension along preexisting scars to assist with either allowing for greater motion or to assist with breaking up the scar for aesthetic purposes

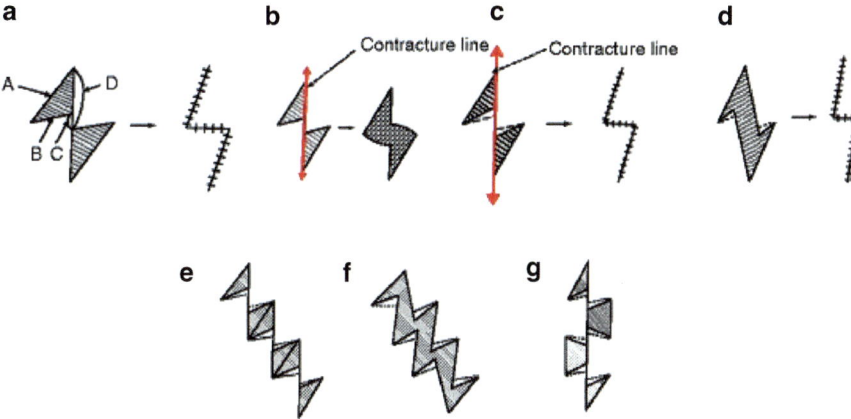

Fig. 3.4 Z-plasty and W-plasty configurations

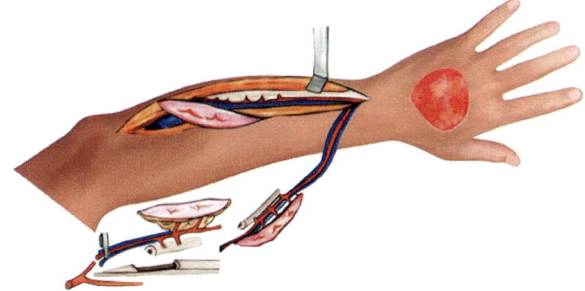

Fig. 3.5 Osteocutaneous pedicle flap

- Pedicled flaps can be done as full flaps or perforator flaps:
    - Full flaps are taken without dissection of branches off the pedicle.
    - Perforator flaps are taken off of specific branches that penetrate the superficial tissue to supply the subcutaneous tissue, which allows for muscle- and fascial-sparing flaps, but are more technically challenging:
        - Perforators are classified as direct, septocutaneous, and myocutaneous.
- Free flaps are pedicled flaps where the pedicle has been disconnected and reconnected to recipient vessels with microsurgery.
- **Common Flap Types**
    - A detailed list of flaps will be mentioned in each section:
        - It is left up to the reader to look up pertinent surgical details as an exercise.
        - Common workhorse flaps are listed below with their classification and vessel:
            - Latissimus dorsi: type V, thoracodorsal, intercostal perforators
            - Gastrocnemius: type I, medial sural
            - Anterolateral thigh: septocutaneous or myocutaneous, descending lateral circumflex
            - Gracilis: type II, SFA, medial circumflex femoral
            - Rectus abdominis: III, DIE, SEA
            - DIEP: myocutaneous, DIE
            - RFFF: myocutaneous, radial artery
    - *Mathes and Nahai classification for pedicled and free muscular flaps* [13, 14] (Table 3.3)
- **Adjunctive Maneuvers for Flaps** [15–20]
    - *Delayed flap*:
        - Used to improve the perfusion to a flap before transfer.
        - A flap that is initially partially excised with exception of the vascular pedicle. This allows for partial disruption of the blood supply of the flap while allowing the vascular pedicle to remain intact—this encourages dilation of choke vessels as well as hypertrophy and hyperplasia of blood vessels.
        - The flap may then be completely excised at a later date.
        - For example, during DIEP flap reconstruction, the DIEP flap will be partially dissected at the time of mastectomy with the pedicle left intact (*usually wrapped with nonstick gauze*). The superficial aspect flap will then be secured back into place with staples or sutures. The patient is then be taken

3 Flaps and Grafts

Table 3.3 Mathes and Nahai classification system for muscle flaps

Type	Vascular supply	Flap examples
I	Single dominant vascular pedicle	Gastrocnemius Tensor fascia lata
II	A dominant and minor vascular pedicles	Gracilis Trapezius
III	Two dominant vascular pedicles	Rectus abdominis Gluteus maximus
IV	Multiple segmental vascular pedicles	Sartorius
V	Single dominant vascular pedicle with additional second segmental pedicles	Latissimus dorsi Pectoralis major

  back for surgery at a later time, and the pedicle will be transected and anastomosed.
 – *Prelaminated flap*: A flap in which additional tissue (e.g., cartilage) is incorporated into the original flap; this is usually based on a preexisting axial flap.
 – *Prefabricated flap*: The transfer of a vascular pedicle onto a site of desired donor tissue. This allows for vascularization of the planned flap prior to transfer. This can be performed through microvascular anastomosis or local tissue transfer. After a 6–8-week period to allow for vascularization, the flap will then completely be transferred with the pedicle to the recipient site.
 – *Flap inset and division*:
   • Inset refers to placing a flap at the location of treatment. Often, for pedicled flaps, the pedicle can be divided after neoangiogenesis at the site of inset occurs robustly enough that the flap will survive without the pedicle intact. This typically happens at 3–4 weeks after inset.
 – *Supercharging*:
   • Flaps with inadequate blood flow for a single pedicle may have a second pedicle anastomosed.
 – *Indocyanine green angiography*:
   • Allows for visualization of inflow of flap to assess vascularity.
• **Flap Monitoring and Aftercare**
 – Depends on flap used and institutional practices.

- Typically comprised of vascular checks via Doppler of anastomosis, evaluation of capillary refill to assess venous congestion, and potentially near-infrared spectroscopy (ViOptix).
- Typically, failures occur within the first 24 hours and are more commonly venous than arterial.

References

1. Ratner D. Skin grafting: from here to there. Dermatol Clin. 1998;16(1):75–90.
2. Andreassi A, Bilenchi R, Biagioli M, D'Aniello C. Classification and pathophysiology of skin grafts. Clin Dermatol. 2005;23(4):332–7.
3. Hallock GG, Morris SF. Skin grafts and local flaps. Plast Reconstr Surg. 2011;127(1):5e–22e.
4. Hill SM, Thornton JF. Total and near-total nasal reconstruction. In: Atlas of operative maxillofacial trauma surgery. London: Springer; 2020. p. 571–82.
5. Alexandrescu V, Söderström M, Venermo M. Angiosome theory: fact or fiction? Scand J Surg. 2012;101(2):125–31.
6. Taylor GI, Palmer JH. The vascular territories (angiosomes) of the body: experimental study and clinical applications. Br J Plast Surg. 1987;40(2):113–41.
7. Nakajima H, Fujino T, Adachi S. A new concept of vascular supply to the skin and classification of skin flaps according to their vascularization. Ann Plast Surg. 1986;16:1–19.
8. Shockley WW. Scar revision techniques: z-plasty, w-plasty, and geometric broken line closure. Facial Plast Surg Clin. 2011;19(3):455–63.
9. Salam GA, Amin JP. The basic Z-plasty. Am Fam Physician. 2003;67(11):2329–32.
10. Goutos I, Yousif AH, Ogawa R. W-plasty in scar revision: geometrical considerations and suggestions for site-specific design modifications. Plast Reconstr Surg Glob Open. 2019;7(4):e2179.
11. Krishnan R, Garman M, Nunez-Gussman J, Orengo I. Advancement flaps: a basic theme with many variations. Dermatologic Surg. 2005;31:986–94.
12. LoPiccolo MC. Rotation flaps—principles and locations. Dermatologic Surg. 2015;41:S247–54.
13. Wagner IJ. Classification of the vascular anatomy of muscles: experimental and clinical correlation. In: 50 Studies every plastic surgeon should know, vol. 14. CRC Press; 2014. p. 27.
14. Geddes CR, Morris SF, Neligan PC. Perforator flaps: evolution, classification, and applications. Ann Plast Surg. 2003;50(1):90–9.
15. Mehta A, Goldman JJ. Axial flaps. In: StatPearls [Internet]. Treasure Island: StatPearls Publishing; 2020.
16. Sloan GM, Reinisch JF. Flap physiology and the prediction of flap viability. Hand Clin. 1985;1(4):609–19.
17. Laporta R, Longo B, Sorotos M, Pagnoni M, Santanelli di Pompeo F. Breast reconstruction with delayed fat-graft-augmented DIEP flap in patients with insufficient donor-site volume. Aesth Plast Surg. 2015;39(3):339–49.
18. Pribaz JJ, Weiss DD, Mulliken JB, Eriksson E. Prelaminated free flap reconstruction of complex central facial defects. Plast Reconstr Surg. 1999;104(2):357–65.

19. Pribaz JJ, Fine N, Orgill DP. Flap prefabrication in the head and neck: a 10-year experience. Plast Reconstr Surg. 1999;103(3):808–20.
20. Gunnarsson GL, Jackson IT, Westvik TS, Thomsen JB. The freestyle pedicle perforator flap: a new favorite for the reconstruction of moderate-sized defects of the torso and extremities. Eur J Plast Surg. 2015;38(1):31–6.

Chapter 4
Tissue Expansion

Annalisa Lopez

Physiology [4–9]

- Tissue expansion works by modification of tissue structure, both mechanically and biologically:
  - Mechanical Creep.
    - Physiologic changes at the cellular level from a cell on stretch.
    - Stress relaxation and reorganization of cells on a microtubule level along the axis of stress to limit tension allow the skin to stretch along axis.
    - Results in loss of elastic recoil.
  - Biologic Creep.
    - Synthesis of new cells along the axis of stress to relieve tissue tension induced by expansion.
- Allows for tissue elongation and changes the nature of tissues during stretch:
  - Epidermis: thickens.
  - Dermis: thins.
  - Muscle and subcutaneous fat: thins.
  - Hypertrophy of vascularity.
- Given the need for elasticity in tissue to allow for accommodation, areas under more tension or that have been radiated are unable to be expanded properly.

A. Lopez (✉)
Division of Plastic Surgery, The University of Texas Medical Branch, Galveston, TX, USA
e-mail: annlopez@utmb.edu

Applications [10, 11]

- Tissue expanders are diverse and used in almost any body part, including the trunk, scalp, and extremities, for various oncologic, congenital, or traumatic reconstructive applications.
- After placement, the expansion process can begin after the incisional wound has healed. Time after expander placement to expansion can range from a week to 3 weeks, depending on the patient's healing ability.
- Expansion sessions are typically held weekly, with the amount of expansion relying upon the size of the expander, the amount of tissue needed, and patient pain tolerance.
- This amount injected (saline or air) is tailored to each patient.
- Typically, the amount of height of expanded tissue is equivalent to the amount of advancement.
- Specific uses:
    - Breast: remains the most common option for breast reconstruction. An expander is placed first and is used to shape a breast pocket and augment skin envelope for a later implant or free flap.
    - Scalp: Placed subgaleal, can expand 50% of the scalp to reconstruct without major thinning of hair.
    - Lower extremity: associated with large rate of complication, especially in children, mainly neuropraxia.
    - Abdomen: placed interoblique.
- Types of tissue expanders:
    - Can be internal or external (DermaClose).
    - Ports can be integrated or connected/external:
        - External ports often better for children (Fig. 4.1).

Contraindications and Complications [12, 13]

Contraindications of tissue expansion include the presence of or planned radiated tissue, obesity, expansion of skin grafts, and expansion in active areas of soft tissue infections. These tissues do not expand well and thin, leading to expander extrusion.

Complications include infection (prosthetic device), pain from expansion, skin necrosis from excess pressure from expansion, expander extrusion from wound dehiscence, seroma, and hematoma.

Fig. 4.1 Top: tissue expander ex vivo. Bottom: in vivo placement with expansion of the lateral cheek

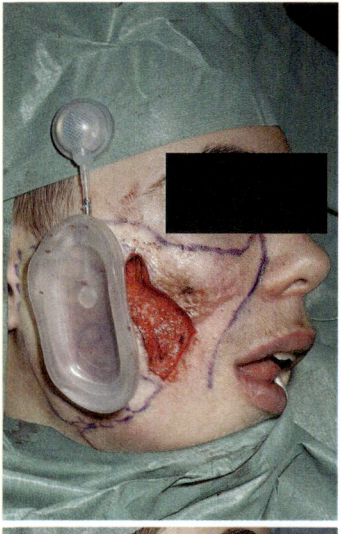
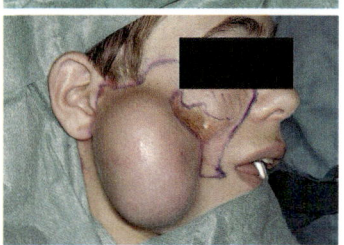

References

1. Codivilla A. On the means of lengthening, in the lower limbs, the muscles and tissues which are shortened through deformity. JBJS. 1905;2(4):353–69.
2. Putti V, Peltier LF. The operative lengthening of the femur. Clin Orthop Relat Res. 1990;250:4–7.
3. Radovan C. Tissue expansion in soft-tissue reconstruction. Plast Reconstr Surg. 1984;74(4):482–92.
4. Yousef H, Alhajj M, Sharma S. Anatomy, skin (integument), epidermis. In: StatPearls [Internet]. Treasure Island: StatPearls Publishing; 2025.
5. Kolarsick PA, Kolarsick MA, Goodwin C. Anatomy and physiology of the skin. J Dermatol Nurses Assoc. 2011;3(4):203–13.
6. Takei T, Mills I, Arai K, Sumpio BE. Molecular basis for tissue expansion: clinical implications for the surgeon. Plast Reconstr Surg. 1998;102(1):247–58.
7. De Filippo RE, Atala A. Stretch and growth: the molecular and physiologic influences of tissue expansion. Plast Reconstr Surg. 2002;109(7):2450–62.
8. Siegert R, Weerda H, Hoffmann S, Mohadjer C. Clinical and experimental evaluation of intermittent intraoperative short-term expansion. Plast Reconstr Surg. 1993;92(2):248–54.
9. Kane WJ, McCaffrey TV, Wang TD, Koval TM. The effect of tissue expansion on previously irradiated skin. Arch Otolaryngol Head Neck Surg. 1992;118(4):419–26.
10. Bertozzi N, Pesce M, Santi P, Raposio E. Tissue expansion for breast reconstruction: methods and techniques. Ann Med Surg. 2017;21:34–44.

11. Agrawal K, Agrawal S. Tissue regeneration during tissue expansion and choosing an expander. Indian J Plast Surg. 2012;45(1):7.
12. Malata CM, Williams NW, Sharpe DT. Tissue expansion: clinical applications. J Wound Care. 1995;4(2):88–94.
13. Manders EK, Schenden MJ, Furrey JA, Hetzler PT, Davis TS, Graham WP 3rd. Soft-tissue expansion: concepts and complications. Plast Reconstr Surg. 1984;74(4):493–507.

Chapter 5
Microsurgery

Edward H. Nahabet

Introduction

- Microsurgery encompasses microvascular coaptation of vessels usually less than 3 mm in diameter, microneural repair or reconstruction, and microlymphatic anastomoses under microscopic magnification.
- Within the field of plastic surgery, microsurgery is synonymous with reconstructive microsurgery.
- Historically, microsurgery was first used for digital replantations and revascularizations.
- The field has since expanded significantly to include nerve repair, reconstruction, or transfers, breast, head and neck, and extremity reconstruction.
- In more recent years, the field has grown to include perforator flap surgery, supermicrosurgery, and lymphatic surgery [1].
- Microsurgery does have a steep learning curve and longer operative durations and needs for special equipment and technical expertise.

Evaluation

- Whereas previously free tissue transfer was considered the final step on the reconstructive ladder, advancements in technique and instrumentation have made free flap reconstruction a first-line option, especially in the reconstruction of complex defects, providing superior outcomes while maximizing function and aesthetics [2, 3]:

E. H. Nahabet (✉)
Division of Plastic Surgery, Department of Surgery, UCLA, Los Angeles, CA, USA
e-mail: edwardnahabet@mednet.ucla.edu

- This is known as the "reconstructive elevator."
- Discussion with patients includes surgical goals, risks, and a complete discussion of donor site morbidity with regard to the flaps that are being considered.

Contraindications

- While there are no absolute contraindications to microsurgical reconstruction, patients should undergo complete evaluation and medical optimization of comorbidities including good hypertensive and diabetic control.
- Relative contraindications include poorly controlled systemic disease, hypercoagulable disorders, and smoking [4].
- Age alone is not a contraindication, and outcomes of microsurgical reconstruction in the elderly are comparable to the general population [5, 6].

Equipment

- Surgical loupes provide 2.5–8× magnification and are used for dissection during flap harvest.
- Surgical microscopes provide magnification up to 40×, but most surgeons use magnification in the 10–15× range for vessel preparation and anastomosis [7].
- Most microscopes are dual viewing and contain video output to a monitor for observation during a case.
- Microsurgical instruments include specialized forceps, microscissors, vessel dilators, needle holders, and vascular clamps.
- Suture is typically monofilament nylon or polypropylene and can range from 8–0 to 11–0 [4].

Planning

- Free tissue transfer requires meticulous planning that includes appropriate flap and recipient vessel selection.
- The operative plan should be discussed with the anesthesiologist including fluid intake, blood pressure goals, and muscle paralysis that may be crucial during perforator dissections.

- Perioperative vasopressor administration has not demonstrated any detrimental impact on free flap survival and is acceptable as hemodynamic stability can be crucial to flap perfusion [8].
- It is important to avoid intravenous lines, arterial lines, or blood pressure cuffs at flap harvest sites [4].
- Patient positioning is meant to optimize both flap harvest and recipient vessel preparation and should take into account the possible need for skin graft.
- Posture and position are critical to minimize strain and optimize technique.
- Surgeons should be either seated or standing, feet flat, elbows at approximately 90 degrees and forearms at approximately the level of the anastomosis.
- If operating on an uneven surface, make use of folded towels to support your wrists as necessary.

Operative Steps

- Prior to harvesting the flap, prepare the recipient vessels to minimize your ischemia time.
- Recipient vessels should demonstrate adequate inflow and outflow.
- The flap should be secured either temporarily or with suture to the site of inset prior to beginning the anastomosis to correctly identify the length of pedicle needed and to avoid placing undue tension on the anastomosis.

Vessel Preparation

- Vessels are kept moist to prevent desiccation.
- Arteries and veins both consist of the tunica intima, media, and adventitia (Fig. 5.1).
- Consider grasping power when grabbing vessels to avoid trauma and grasp adventitia only when possible.
- After ensuring adequate recipient vessel and pedicle length, trim vessels back to healthy tissue, and trim a few mm of the adventitia (Fig. 5.2).
- Vascular clamps are placed proximally on both recipient artery and vein to allow for anastomosis in a bloodless field.
- Flush both artery and vein with heparinized saline.
- If inadequate length of pedicle and recipient vessel resulting in undue tension, you may consider an interpositional vein graft.

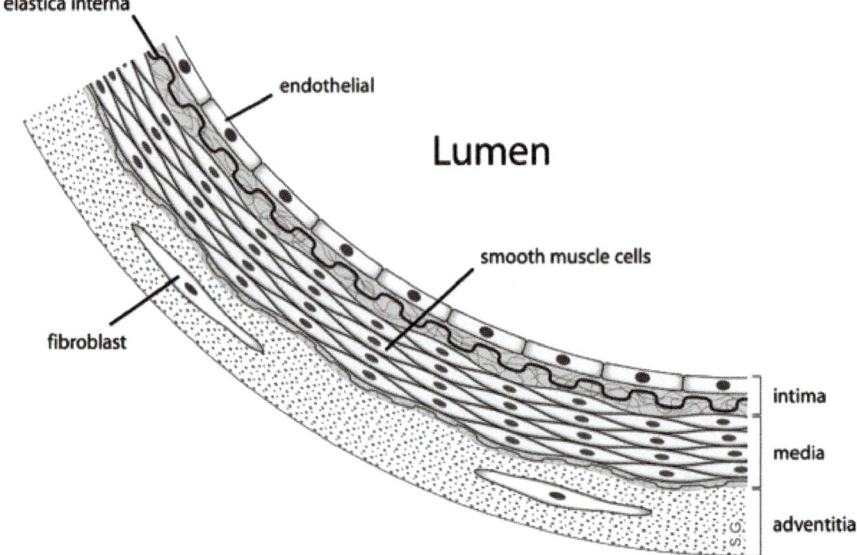

Fig. 5.1 Cross-sectional view of the artery

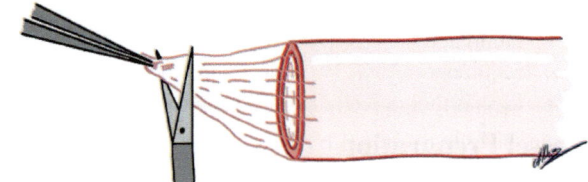

Fig. 5.2 Sharp trimming of adventitia

Anastomosis

Venous

- Venous anastomosis can be performed using either suture or a coupling device.
- Venous couplers are an anastomotic device that obviate the need for suturing:
    - Poiseuille's Law: Radius of coupler increases flow by a factor of r^4.
- They consist of two coupled rings with interlocking pins that come in range of sizes from 1 to 4 mm (Fig. 5.3).
- Some couplers come with an implantable Doppler allowing for internal monitoring of anastomosis.
- Venous couplers have demonstrated excellent patency rates while significantly decreasing the operative time needed to complete a venous anastomosis [9, 10].

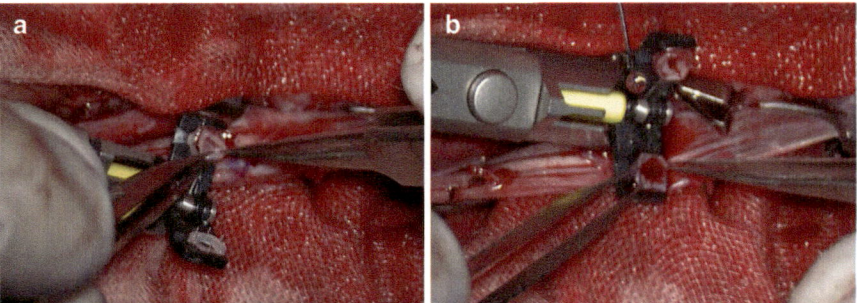

Fig. 5.3 (**a**) Ends of the veins are pulled through the opposing rings and spiked onto the pins. (**b**) Donor and recipient veins set on opposing rings. Coupler knob rotated to bring together the opposing rings and vein

Arterial

- While arterial anastomoses have been performed with coupler devices with acceptable results, it is not common practice as arterial walls are thicker and less malleable making them difficult to fold over the pins in the device [11].
- A double-approximating vascular clamp can be quite useful in stabilizing the vessels prior to beginning your anastomosis.
- There are several published techniques for hand-sewing vessels [12].
- Most commonly, two initial sutures are placed at 180 degrees from one another—these are often called the stay sutures.
- Interrupted, running continuous, running locking, or running mattress sutures can be used to suture the anterior wall, followed by flipping the vessels and suturing the back wall (Fig. 5.4).
- Needles should enter the vessel at 90 degrees, purchase all layers of the vessel including media and intima, and follow the curve of the needle.
- Care should be taken not to purchase the back wall while suturing the anterior vessel edges as this would result in an anastomotic occlusion.
- All knots should be tied square with minimal upward tension while tightening.

End to Side

- The end-to-side technique can be used in situations where there is significant size discrepancy between vessels, or as often encountered in extremity reconstruction, to maintain flow and distal perfusion.
- End-to-side anastomosis has demonstrated no differences in flap outcomes when compared to end-to-end [13, 14].
- End-to-side anastomosis involves making an arteriotomy/venotomy, or punch hole to anastomose the flap vessels to.

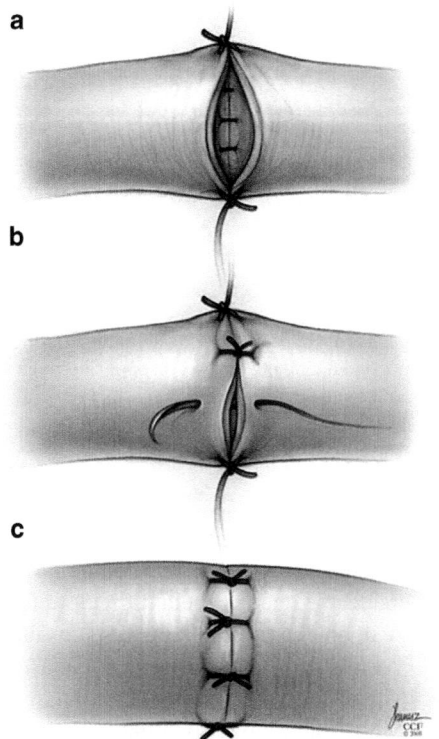

Fig. 5.4 Schematic illustration of the simple interrupted technique. The vessel ends are bisected with two stay sutures places at 180° (the posterior wall has already been sutured) (**a**). The suture is passed full thickness from the outside-in direction of one vessel end into the lumen and then from the inside-out through the other vessel end (**b**). The knots are tied along the anterior wall completing the entire anastomosis (**c**)

Monitoring

- There are various ways of monitoring flap inflow and outflow.
- Once the anastomosis is complete and the vascular clamps have been removed, one can observe as flap turgor increases the flap demonstrates bleeding from the edges and if a skin paddle is present demonstrates appropriate capillary refill:
  - Capillary refill should be around 2–3 s:
    - Slower capillary refill suggests arterial compromise.
    - Quick refill suggests venous compromise.
- Additional methods of monitoring flow include the implantable Cook-Swartz Doppler probe which incorporates an ultrasound Doppler within the venous coupler that can allow for intraoperative and postoperative monitoring.
- Implantable Dopplers can be particularly useful when performing a flap that does not contain a skin paddle for monitoring.
- Laser angiography using the SPY system and indocyanine green (ICG) is an additional method for assessing flap perfusion intraoperatively.

Postoperative Monitoring

- Clinical evaluation including assessing color, capillary refill, turgor, temperature, and handheld Doppler signals are the most common forms of postoperative monitoring.
- Well-perfused flaps are pink, warm, demonstrate a capillary refill time of about 2 s, and are within range of the patient's body temperature.
- A flap that is pale, flaccid, cold, and demonstrates no capillary refill is demonstrating signs of arterial insufficiency.
- A flap that appears blue or purple, is swollen, and has a brisk capillary refill is demonstrating signs of venous congestion.
- Transcutaneous near-infrared tissue oximetry is a form of infrared spectroscopy that measures tissue oxygenation saturation rather than flow and can identify flap compromise before clinical signs of arterial or venous thrombosis and demonstrates an increased flap salvage rate [15].

Flap Compromise

- Risk for flap failure is variable based on flap and indication, but is usually less than 5%.
- In the event of arterial or venous insufficiency, timely re-exploration in the operating room greatly increases chance of flap salvage.
- Flap failure is typically venous in nature, often due to kinking or thrombosis, and is most evident in the first 24 h after surgery.

Systemic Anticoagulation

- No systemic medications have been demonstrated to improve anastomosis patency; however, several are commonly used in the postoperative period including heparin and aspirin.

Nerve Repair

- Microneural repair requires healthy nerve tissue—any crushed, scarred, or damaged nerve should be cut back until healthy fascicles are identified.
- Repair should be performed without undue tension.
- If mobilization of cut nerve ends does not close the nerve gap, interpositional nerve grafts or conduits can be used.

- Vein grafts or conduits can be used for nerve defects of up to 3 cm [16].
- Processed human allografts demonstrate similar recovery in nerve defects of up to 7 cm [17].
- For larger defects, autografts such as the sural nerve and lateral or medial antebrachial cutaneous nerves remain the gold standard; however, it will result in donor site anesthesia.
- Types of microneural repair include epineural, fascicular, or grouped fascicular repairs.
- Epineurial repair involves suturing the epineurium alone.
- Fascicular repair involves repairing the individual fascicles, is technically more difficult, and demonstrates similar outcomes.
- Grouped fascicular repair is a technique employed for larger more proximal nerves within which the terminal branches can be identified [4].

Lymphatics

- Lymphatic surgery attempts to restore physiological lymphatic drainage by methods such as lymphaticovenous bypass or vascularized lymph node transfers.
- Lymphaticovenous anastomosis is a bypass operation that redirects excess lymphatic fluid into the venous circulation by anastomosing lymphatic vessels to nearby venules.
- When native lymph node basins are dysfunctional either after lymphadenectomy or radiation therapy, a vascularized lymph node transfer can transfer functional lymph nodes to promote lymphatic drainage.
- The most common donor nodes are the supraclavicular and superficial inguinal basins—these node basins are transferred with their accompanying vessels which are anastomosed to recipient vessels within the indicated extremity [18].

Supermicrosurgery

- Supermicrosurgery involves the anastomosis of vessels less than 0.8 mm and/or single nerve fascicles [19].
- It is used for lymphaticovenous anastomoses, distal fingertip or toe replantations and transfers, and more.

References

1. Park JE, Chang DW. Advances and innovations in microsurgery. Plast Reconstr Surg. 2016;138(5):915e–24e.

2. Gottlieb LJ, Krieger LM. From the reconstructive ladder to the reconstructive elevator. Plast Reconstr Surg. 1994;93(7):1503.
3. Bennett N, Choudhary S. Why climb a ladder when you can take the elevator? Plast Reconstr Surg. 2000;105(6):2266.
4. Janis J, editor. Chapter 8. Basics of microsurgery. In: Essentials of plastic surgery. Quality Medical Publishing; 2014.
5. Serletti JM, Higgins JP, Moran S, et al. Factors affecting outcome in free–tissue transfer in the elderly. Plast Reconstr Surg. 2000;106:66–70.
6. Coskunfirat OK, Chen HC, Spanio S, et al. The safety of microvascular free tissue transfer in the elderly population. Plast Reconstr Surg. 2005;115:771–5.
7. Neligan P. Chapter 26. Principles and techniques of microvascular surgery. In: Plastic surgery, vol. 1. Elsevier; 2018.
8. Goh CSL, Ng MJM, Song DH, et al. Perioperative vasopressor use in free flap surgery: a systematic review and meta-analysis. J Reconstr Microsurg. 2019;35(7):529–40.
9. Jandali S, Wu LC, Vega SJ, Kovach SJ, Serletti JM. 1000 consecutive venous anastomoses using the microvascular anastomotic coupler in breast reconstruction. Plast Reconstr Surg. 2010;125(3):792–8.
10. DeLacure MD, Wong RS, Markowitz BL, Kobayashi MR, Ahn CY, Shedd DP, Spies AL, Loree TR, Shaw WW. Clinical experience with a microvascular anastomotic device in head and neck reconstruction. Am J Surg. 1995;170(5):521–3.
11. Pafitanis G, Nicolaides M, O'Connor EF, Raveendran M, Ermogenous P, Psaras G, Rose V, Myers S. Microvascular anastomotic arterial coupling: a systematic review. J Plast Reconstr Aesthet Surg. 2021;74(6):1286–302.
12. Alghoul MS, Gordon CR, Yetman R, Buncke GM, Siemionow M, Afifi AM, Moon WK. From simple interrupted to complex spiral: a systematic review of various suture techniques for microvascular anastomoses. Microsurgery. 2011;31(1):72–80.
13. Cho EH, Garcia RM, Blau J, Levinson H, Erdmann D, Levin LS, Hollenbeck ST. Microvascular anastomoses using end-to-end versus end-to-side technique in lower extremity free tissue transfer. J Reconstr Microsurg. 2016;32(2):114–20.
14. Black C, Fan KL, Defazio MV, Luvisa K, Reynolds K, Kotha VS, Attinger CE, Evans KK. Limb salvage rates and functional outcomes using a longitudinal slit arteriotomy end-to-side anastomosis for limb-threatening defects in a high-risk patient population. Plast Reconstr Surg. 2020;145(5):1302–12.
15. Lin SJ, Nguyen MD, Chen C, et al. Tissue oximetry monitoring in microsurgical breast reconstruction decreases flap loss and improves rate of flap salvage. Plast Reconstr Surg. 2011;127(3):1080–5.
16. Chiu DTW, Strauch B. A prospective clinical evaluation of autogenous vein grafts used as a nerve conduit for distal sensory nerve defects of 3 cm or less. Plast Reconstr Surg. 1990;86(5):928–34.
17. Safa B, Jain S, Desai MJ, Greenberg JA, Niacaris TR, Nydick JA, Leversedge FJ, Megee DM, Zoldos J, Rinker BD, McKee DM, MacKay BJ, Ingari JV, Nesti LJ, Cho M, Valerio IL, Kao DS, El-Sheikh Y, Weber RV, et al. Peripheral nerve repair throughout the body with processed nerve allografts: results from a large multicenter study. Microsurgery. 2020;40(5):527–37. https://doi.org/10.1002/micr.30574.
18. Kung TA, Champaneria MC, Maki JH, Neligan PC. Current concepts in the surgical management of lymphedema. Plast Reconstr Surg. 2017;139(4):1003e–13e.
19. Koshima I, Yamamoto T, Narushima M, Mihara M, Iida T. Perforator flaps and supermicrosurgery. Clin Plast Surg. 2010;37(683689):vii.

Chapter 6
Transplantation Biology and Vascularized Composite Allotransplantation

Jasmine Lee, Kshipra Hemal, and Allyson R. Alfonso

Overview

- Vascularized composite allotransplantation (VCA) is the transplantation of tissues such as skin, muscle, nerves, and blood vessels from an immunologically compatible donor to recipient. Examples include abdominal wall, penis, and larynx transplantation. Discussed here are facial transplantation (FT) and hand transplantation (HT), the two most common examples of VCA.

Historical Perspective

- The first hand transplant was performed in 1964 in Ecuador, which resulted in rejection and reamputation. In 1998, a successful hand transplant was performed in France. Although the graft was lost at 2.5 years, the procedure demonstrated the feasibility of the surgical technique alongside immunosuppression. By 2020, nearly 150 hand transplants have been reportedly performed worldwide [1].
- The first face transplant was performed in 2005 in France for a 38-year-old woman who suffered a severe dog bite injury. The transplant was a success though the patient passed from cancer 11 years after the operation. By 2020, nearly 50 face transplants have been performed in 46 patients [2].

Demographics, Incidence, and Epidemiology

- The annual incidence of severe nonfatal craniofacial injuries in adults aged 20–64 years the United States lies between 32 and 58 per 100,000 [3].
- Upper extremity amputation proximal to the wrist accounts for 8% of the amputations affecting the 1.5 million individuals living with limb loss. Trauma is the most common cause of upper extremity amputation [4].

Anatomy

- Vascularized composite allografts are intact anatomical/structural units containing multiple tissue types and require blood flow through surgical connection of blood vessels [5].
- Facial allografts are individualized to recipients with variable vascular pedicles and inclusion of soft tissue, bone, and skin.
- Depending on level of amputation, commonly repaired nerves during upper extremity transplantation include the median, ulnar, and radial. Most commonly repaired arteries are the radial and ulnar arteries, while unspecified/unnamed veins are often repaired for venous drainage [1].

Immunology

- Lifelong immunosuppression is required after VCA. Current standard protocols include induction and maintenance immunotherapy.
- Induction immunosuppression agents vary and include tacrolimus, mycophenolate mofetil (MMF), alemtuzumab, rapamycin, antithymocyte globulin (ATG), humanized IL-2 antibody, and steroids [1, 6].
- Maintenance immunosuppression is most often comprised of triple therapy: tacrolimus, mycophenolate mofetil (MMF), and steroid taper [6, 7].

Patient Selection

- Indications
    - There are no universal guidelines regarding indications/contraindications for VCA and each patient must be evaluated individually.
    - In general, VCA is only indicated in patients with functional deficits that have failed conventional tissue reconstruction and/or prosthetic use.

- Contraindications
    - Common contraindications include active malignancy, history of malignancy, poor medication adherence, or lack of social support as patients must remain on lifelong immunosuppression for graft survival.
    - Given the unique psychological impact of certain VCAs, such as FT, many institutions require psychiatric evaluation to demonstrate psychological stability prior to transplantation.

Surgical Technique

- Procurement
    - In the USA, VCA falls under the scope of organ transplantation. As a general rule, face or limb recovery should not compromise any multi-organ procurement.
    - Procurement of VCA requires coordination of multiple organ transplantation teams. A planned sequence for limb, face, and organ recovery must be established preoperatively to reduce ischemia time.
- Recipient Preparation and Transplantation
    - HT is performed under tourniquet control. Although sequence of repair may vary depending on surgical team, generally bone osteosynthesis is followed by tendon/muscle repair, definitive vessel repair, and neural repair [8].
    - In FT, all scar tissue is debrided and recipient muscle is preserved. Rigid fixation is performed first, followed by vascular anastomoses and neural repair [8] (Fig. 6.1).

Postoperative Care

- Infection Prevention and Treatment
    - Infection is an important factor to control in immunocompromised patients, particularly in the early postoperative period, as this is when the highest incidence of infections has occurred [9, 10].
    - Important pathogens to keep in mind include cytomegalovirus (CMV), Epstein-Barr virus (EBV), and *Pneumocystis carinii* (PCP). Preventative treatment includes performing CM-compatible transplant or providing prophylaxis of valganciclovir for 6 months. PCP prophylaxis includes trimethoprim-sulfamethoxazole for 6 months.

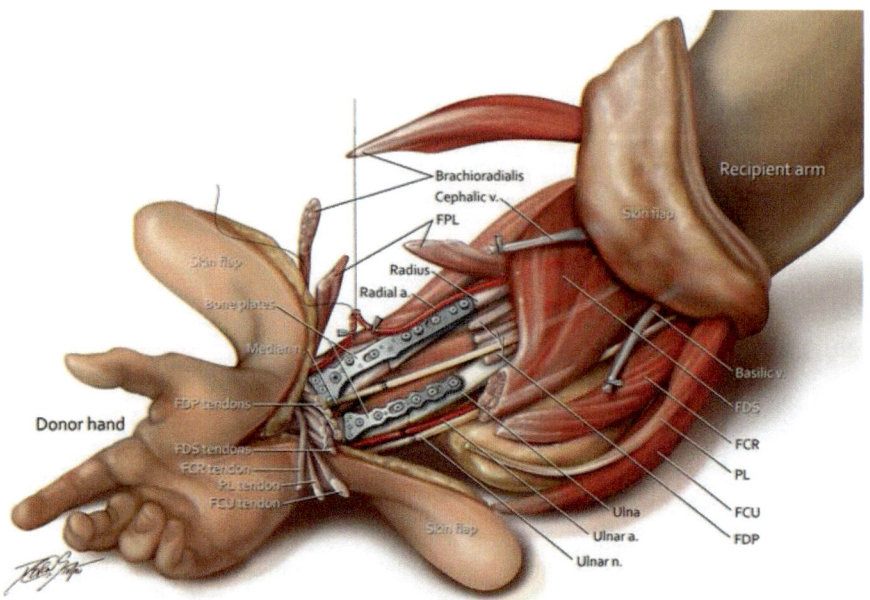

Fig. 6.1 Demonstration of anastomoses and fixation for a hand transplant

- Immunotherapy and Risk of Rejection
  - VCA rejection is monitored using the Banff classification, which utilizes histologic assessment of skin biopsies. Less invasive and locally traumatic methods are currently being developed [11, 12].
  - Acute rejection is common among both HT and FT recipients. Episodes are treated with pulse steroids [8].
  - Chronic rejection has recently been described as a threat to graft loss [13].

Ethical Considerations

- As VCAs are not life-saving procedures, but require lifelong immunosuppression, which increases the risk of opportunistic infections and malignancy, individualized risk benefit analyses must be performed for each VCA candidate.

Future Directions

- The future lies in developing an understanding of long-term outcomes, implications of lifelong immunosuppression, and educating the general public to expand the donor pool.

References

1. Wells MW, Rampazzo A, Papay F, Gharb BB. Two decades of hand transplantation: a systematic review of outcomes. Ann Plast Surg. 2022;88(3):335–44. https://doi.org/10.1097/sap.0000000000003056.
2. Kantar RS, et al. Facial transplantation: principles and evolving concepts. Plast Reconstr Surg. 2021;147(6):1022e–38e.
3. Kantar RS, et al. Incidence of preventable nonfatal craniofacial injuries and implications for facial transplantation. J Craniofac Surg. 2019;30(7):2023–5.
4. Ziegler-Graham K, MacKenzie EJ, Ephraim PL, Travison TG, Brookmeyer R. Estimating the prevalence of limb loss in the United States: 2005 to 2050. Arch Phys Med Rehabil. 2008;89(3):422–9. https://doi.org/10.1016/j.apmr.2007.11.005.
5. Thuong M, et al. Vascularized composite allotransplantation – a Council of Europe position paper. Transpl Int. 2019;32(3):233–40. https://doi.org/10.1111/tri.13370.
6. Rifkin WJ, et al. Achievements and challenges in facial transplantation. Ann Surg. 2018;268(2):260–70. https://doi.org/10.1097/sla.0000000000002723.
7. Giannis D, Moris D, Cendales LC. Costimulation blockade in vascularized composite allotransplantation. Front Immunol. 2020;11:544186. https://doi.org/10.3389/fimmu.2020.544186.
8. Pomahac B, Gobble RM, Schneeberger S. Facial and hand allotransplantation. Cold Spring Harb Perspect Med. 2014;4(3) https://doi.org/10.1101/cshperspect.a015651.
9. Knoll BM, et al. Infections following facial composite tissue allotransplantation–single center experience and review of the literature. Am J Transplant Off J Am Soc Transplant Am Soc Transplant Surg. 2013;13(3):770–9. https://doi.org/10.1111/ajt.12013.
10. Gordon CR, Avery RK, Abouhassan W, Siemionow M. Cytomegalovirus and other infectious issues related to face transplantation: specific considerations, lessons learned, and future recommendations. Plast Reconstr Surg. 2011;127(4):1515–23. https://doi.org/10.1097/PRS.0b013e318208d03c.
11. Cendales LC, et al. The Banff 2007 working classification of skin-containing composite tissue allograft pathology. Am J Transplant Off J Am Soc Transplant Am Soc Transplant Surg. 2008;8(7):1396–400. https://doi.org/10.1111/j.1600-6143.2008.02243.x.
12. Rabbani PS, Kadle RL, Rao N, Park C, Ceradini D. Optimization of a differential cytokine profile-based non-invasive diagnostic and predictive tool for reliable diagnosis of acute rejection in VCA. VCA. 2016;3:24.
13. Krezdorn N, et al. Chronic rejection of human face allografts. Am J Transplant. 2019;19(4):1168–77. [Online]. Available: http://proxy.library.nyu.edu/login?url=http://ovidsp.ovid.com/ovidweb.cgi?T=JS&CSC=Y&NEWS=N&PAGE=fulltext&D=emexb&AN=624871973, http://sfx.med.nyu.edu/sfxlcl3?sid=OVID:embase&id=pmid:30312535&id=doi:10.1111%2Fajt.15143&issn=1600-6135&isbn=&volume=19&issue=4&spage=1168&pages=1168-1177&date=2019&title=American+Journal+of+Transplantation&atitle=Chronic+rejection+of+human+face+allografts&aulast=Krezdorn&pid=%3Cauthor%3EKrezdorn+N.%3BLian+C.G.%3BWells+M.%3BWo+L.%3BTasigiorgos+S.%3BXu+S.%3BBorges+T.J.%3BFrierson+R.M.%3BStanek+E.%3BRiella+L.V.%3BPomahac+B.%3BMurphy+G.F.%3C%2Fauthor%3E&%3CAN%3E624871973%3C%2FAN%3E&%3CDT%3EArticle%3C%2FDT%3E.

Chapter 7
Local Anesthesia

Jacquelynn P. Tran and Yara Samman

Types and Mechanism of Action [1, 2]

- *Mechanism of action*: Local anesthetics (LA) block conduction in peripheral nerves by preventing depolarization:
    - Reversibly binds to sodium channels and inhibits sodium ion influx.
    - The rate of onset is determined by the pKa:
        - pKa is the acid dissociation constant; the lower the pKa, the stronger the acid.
        - The closer the pKa is to physiologic pH (7.4), the higher the nonionized concentration of local anesthetic → faster onset.
        - The nonionized form that crosses cell membrane then is converted to ionized state → ionized form binds to sodium channel and inhibits sodium ion influx.
    - The length of effect is due to protein binding (the more binding, the longer onset).
- *Ester-linked*: [3]
    - Metabolized by plasma pseudocholinesterase → shorter half-lives.
    - Risk of true allergy due to metabolism to para-aminobenzoic acid.
- *Amide-linked* [3]
    - Liver metabolism.
    - Chemically stable.

J. P. Tran (✉) · Y. Samman
University of Texas, Medical Branch Plastic Surgery, Austin, TX, USA
e-mail: jptran@utmb.edu; ybsamman@utmb.edu

- Lower risk of allergic reactions.
- Nomenclature: *i* before *-aine*.
  - Examples: bupivacaine, lidocaine, mepivacaine, prilocaine, ropivacaine.

Uses and Timing [4]

- Local anesthetic blockage inversely related to nerve fiber diameter. [5, 6]
- Smaller fibers are blocked quicker.
- Local anesthetics are less effective in infected fields; infected tissues are acidic leading to decreased concentration of nonionized form.
- *Block Onset: Sequence of Effect on Nerve Fibers* [4, 6]
  - Block recovery follows the same sequence:

  ↓ Last

  B (myelinated): vasodilation
  C, A-delta: loss of pain and temperature
  A (myelinated)

  Gamma—loss of proprioception
  Beta—loss of pressure sensation
  Alpha—loss of motor function

Additives

- *Epinephrine*
  - Vasoconstricts the infiltrated region, assists with hemostasis upon skin incision, less vascular absorption allowing for slight increase in maximum dose.
  - Optimal time delay after epinephrine injection to minimize bleeding is 25 min, but often surgeons do not wait this long.
  - Increases duration of anesthesia, shortens time to onset.
  - Use with caution in digits of patients with vascular disease, diabetes, Raynaud's:
    - Epinephrine is *not* contraindicated in the hand of neonates or adults without underlying vascular disease.

- Additionally, use with caution in the nasal tip.
- Absolute contraindication: penile shaft.
- Common concentrations: 1:100,000 (1 mg/100 ml or 10 μg/ml), 1:200,000 (1 mg/200 ml or 5 μg/ml), 1:400,000 (1 mg/400 mL or 2.5 μg/mL).
- Epinephrine comes in a 1-mg/mL vial commonly known as "1 amp of epinephrine"; the concentration is 1:1000. To prepare a 1:100,000 local anesthetic solution from plain epinephrine (1 mg/mL), add 0.1 mL to 10 mL of local anesthetic solution.
- Often used with lidocaine in a tumescent solution:
    - 1 L normal saline, 30 cc 1% lidocaine, 1 amp of epinephrine
    - Diluting lidocaine with epinephrine allows for slow absorption of local anesthetic, resulting in the ability to give higher doses and longer-lasting effect (35–55 mg/kg).

- *Sodium Bicarbonate*
    - Buffers the pH, reduces acidity of local anesthetic, increases the ratio of non-ionized fraction resulting in less burning sensation upon injection, and reduces time to blockage onset.
    - Common dose: 8.4% NaHCO3, 1 mL of sodium bicarbonate with 9 mL of lidocaine.

Topical Anesthesia

- *EMLA (Eutectic Mixture of Anesthetics)*
    - Mixture of 2.5% lidocaine and 2.5% prilocaine oil-in-water emulsion.
    - Use for superficial procedures.
    - Takes 45–60 min to achieve dermal analgesia.
    - Toxicity: methemoglobinemia (due to prilocaine component) potentially life-threatening in infants.
- *Cocaine* [7]
    - Topical solution strengths 4% and 10%.
    - Use mainly for vasoconstriction effects of mucosal membranes: nose, oral cavity.
    - Takes 4–10 min to achieve effect.

Maximum Safety Dose [8]

- Calculating maximum volume allowed = patient weight (kg) × [local anesthetic] × maximum safety dose.

Table 7.1 Local anesthetic characteristics and dosages

Class	Drug	pK$_a$	Onset	Duration (hrs) Plain	w/epi	Maximum dose (mg/kg) Plain	w/epi
Amide	Bupivacaine 0.25–0.75%	8.1	Slow	4	8	2.5	3
	Lidocaine 1–5%	7.9	Rapid	2	4	5	7
	Prilocaine 4%	7.9	Medium	1.5	6	5	7.5
	Ropivacaine 0.5%	8.1	Medium	3	6	2	3
Ester	Chloroprocaine 2–3%	8.7	Rapid	0.5	1.5	10	15
	Procaine 0.5–1%	8.9	Rapid	0.75	1.5	8	10
	Tetracaine 0.1–0.5%	8.5	Slow	3	10	1.5	2.5

- Example: 1% lidocaine plain in a 70-kg man.
  - 70 kg × 1 mL/10 mg × 5 mg/kg = 35 mL
- Example: 0.25% bupivacaine with epinephrine in a 5-kg child.
  - 5 kg × 1 ml/2.5 mg × 3 mg/kg = 6 mL.
  - Easy way to remember for bupivacaine is that maximum dose is roughly equivalent to concentration, so a 5-kg child can receive 5 mL (Table 7.1).

Local Anesthetic Toxicity

- Symptoms in order of increasing plasma concentration:

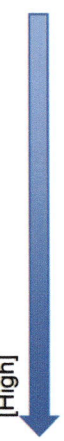

Metallic taste
Perioral paresthesia, tongue numbness
Disorientation, lightheadedness
Audiovisual disturbances
Muscle spasms, twitching

Agitation, reduced level of consciousness
Seizures
Hypotension, cardiac arrhythmias (drives resting membrane potential more negative → prolong QT interval
Respiratory arrest
Cardiac arrest

Toxicity Treatment

- Discontinue agent.
- Supportive care:
    - "ABCs": manage airway, breathing, circulation
        - Airway management: Have secure airway if patient is unconscious.
        - Breathing: Give 100% supplemental oxygen; hyperventilate to prevent hypoxia, hypercarbia, and acidosis.
        - Circulation.
    - 20% intravenous lipid emulsion (Intralipid® 20%) as binding agent for local anesthetic in plasma (shuttles LA from high-flow organs (brain, heart) to storage or detoxification (liver, muscle))
    - An initial bolus of 100 mL should be administered over 2–3 min (or 1.5 mL/kg if the lean body weight <70 kg).
    - Followed by a 20% lipid emulsion infusion of 200–250 mL over 15–20 min (or 0.25 ml/kg/min if the lean body weight is <70 kg).
    - Note: Although Propofol is a lipid containing emulsion, it is *not* equivalent to 20% IV lipid emulsion, and large doses can further depress cardiac function [9].
    - Fluid resuscitation, antiarrhythmic therapy, vasopressor support.
    - Suppress seizures with benzodiazepines—first line.

References

1. Covino BG, Giddon DB. Pharmacology of local anesthetic agents. J Dent Res. 1981;60:198108.
2. Strichartz GR. Current concepts of the mechanism of action of local anesthetics. J Dent Res. 1981;60:1460–7.
3. Shah J, Votta-Velis EG, Borgeat A. New local anesthetics. In: Best practice and research: clinical anaesthesiology, vol. 32. Bailliere Tindall Ltd; 2018. p. 179–85.
4. Lirk P, Picardi S, Hollmann MW. Local anaesthetics: 10 essentials. Eur J Anaesthesiol. Lippincott Williams and Wilkins. 2014;31:575–85.
5. Day TK, Skarda RT. Standing surgery the pharmacology of local anesthetics. Vet Clin North Am Equine Pract. 1991;7:489–500.

6. Huang JH, Thalhammer JG, Raymond SA, Strichartz GR. Susceptibility to lidocaine of impulses in different somatosensory afferent fibers of rat sciatic nerve. J Pharmacol Exp Ther. 1997;282:802–11.
7. Pearman K. Cocaine: a review. J Laryngol Otol. 1979;93(12):1191–9.
8. Williams DJ, Walker JD. A nomogram for calculating the maximum dose of local anaesthetic. Anaesthesia. 2014;69(8):847–53.
9. El-Boghdadly K, Pawa A, Chin KJ. Local anesthetic systemic toxicity: current perspectives. In: Local and regional anesthesia, vol. 11. Dove Medical Press Ltd; 2018. p. 35–44.

Chapter 8
Lasers in Plastic Surgery

Andi J. Cummins

Overview

Laser is an acronym for *l*ight *a*mplification by *s*timulated *e*mission of *r*adiation, which becomes a self-explanatory moniker for a laser's function. Lasers can be powerful tools for the plastic surgeon in the treatment of cutaneous lesions that may be congenital, acquired, or due to the normal effects of aging. Lasers are most well-known for use in hair removal, tattoo removal, treatment of scars, vascular lesions, and facial resurfacing for facial aging. In this chapter, we will discuss laser basics, common types of lasers in practice, and treatment of different cutaneous pathologies with different lasers.

How Does a Laser Work?

- Parts of a Laser (Fig. 8.1).
- Basic Steps to Producing Laser Light.
    - Energy is pumped into the lasing medium:
        - Energy is usually light or electricity.
        - Excites atoms of the medium from ground or resting state into excited state:
            - Medium, may be solid, liquid, or gas.
            - Laser derives name from medium.

A. J. Cummins (✉)
University of Texas Medical Branch, Department of Surgery, Division of Plastic Surgery, Galveston, TX, USA
e-mail: andcummi@utmb.edu

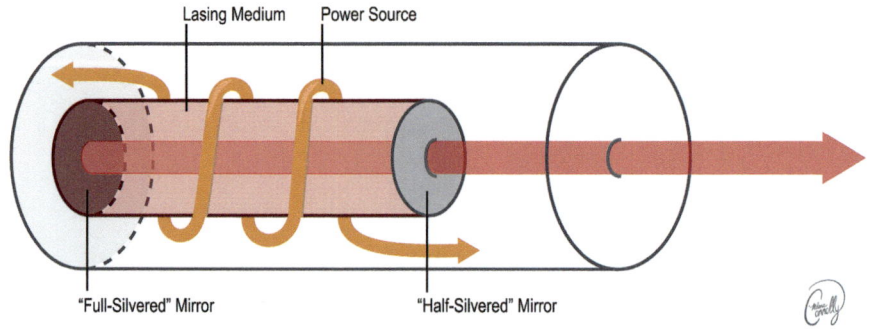

Fig. 8.1 Diagram of a basic ruby laser (first laser developed) and its parts

- Excited atoms release their energy to get back to ground state:
  - Energy, or photons, released is light of a specific wavelength.
  - Stimulated emission cascade begins—one photon will excite other excited electrons to release photons in the same phase.
- Photons are reflected off mirrors within the laser apparatus:
  - Bouncing back and forth creates positive feedback and even more opportunities for stimulated emission.
- "Half-silvered" mirrors reflect the light through opening to the outside world, generating a beam of light.

- The Three "Cs" of Laser Properties [1].
  - *C*ollimated: All light is emitted in one direction or a solid beam.
  - *C*oherent: All light is in the same phase, aka the peaks and troughs of the light wave line up, increasing the focus.
  - Mono*c*hromatic: Light is emitted in only one wavelength and is therefore all the same color.

- Laser Interaction with Tissues [2]: Selective Photothermolysis.
  - Light can be:
    - Absorbed.
    - Transmitted (passes through).
    - Reflected (bounces back).
    - Scattered (diffuses within target).
  - Treatment with lasers focus on tissues that *absorb* the light:
    - Remember from physics—the colors that are *reflected*, not absorbed, generate the appearance to the human eye. For example, chlorophyll appears green because it absorbs all wavelengths except green.

- The corresponding laser to a given chromophore is likely a complimentary color, for example, most lasers targeting the red pigment hemoglobin are not in the red spectrum, because red is reflected.
  - Chromophore [3]—a component of tissue or pigment that absorbs a certain wavelength of light such as:
    - Hemoglobin (oxy, deoxy, methmo, etc.)
    - Melanin.
    - Water.
    - Tattoo ink.
  - Because all light produced by a laser is of the same wavelength, the surgeon may effectively choose their wavelength to specifically target the chromophore while minimizing damage to the surrounding tissue:
    - The non-chromophore tissue will harmlessly transmit or scatter the light within the matrix.
  - Lasers essentially damage the chromophore using thermal energy or heat:
    - For example, heat coagulates a small blood vessel to treat spider veins in the leg.
- Laser Parameters [4].
  - Energy/power—amount of heat energy delivered:
    - Measured in Joules.
  - Spot size—area over which treatment is delivered:
    - Measured in millimeters.
  - Energy + spot size = "fluency" or "power density":
    - Inverse relationship in how much energy is required as spot size becomes larger, aka less energy is required for larger spot size.
  - Pulse width—the amount of time a target is exposed to laser, based on thermal relaxation time of each target:
    - Larger targets, like a hair follicle, require longer pulse widths.
  - Cooling—selective cooling of superficial skin to prevent collateral damage, done through contact methods.
- Q-Switching.
  - Technique of alternating laser resonance capacity to produce short, very powerful pulses.
  - Useful for generating enough energy to target the deep dermis while minimizing damage to the overlying and surrounding tissues.
  - Excellent for tattoo removal (pigments within dermis) and deep pigmented lesions like nevi.

Patient Selection Criteria

- Fitzpatrick (FP) skin type [5] and laser selection:
    - Scale that defines skin types and features based on the propensity to sunburn, surrogate for melanin content.
    - Melanin is a common chromophore, so this can make selective photothermolysis more challenging with FP types 4–6, essentially making the target and background tissue similar.
    - Additionally, higher risk of complication of post-inflammatory hyperpigmentation.
- FP types IV–VI is not a contraindication for laser but important that patients understand the risk (Fig. 8.2).
- Previous scar history:
    - Patients with prior hypopigmentation or keloids may need adjunctive treatment for prevention with laser therapy:
        - Especially ablative lasers like CO2.
- Patients actively using isotretinoin or other retinoids may have an unfavorable reaction.
- Psychological considerations:
    - Does the patient have reasonable expectations?
    - Can the patient provide themselves with the extremely important postoperative maintenance regimen?
    - Does the patient have body dysmorphic disorder?
    - Can the patient sit still to tolerate the procedure (may require general anesthesia vs in-office procedure or moderate sedation)?

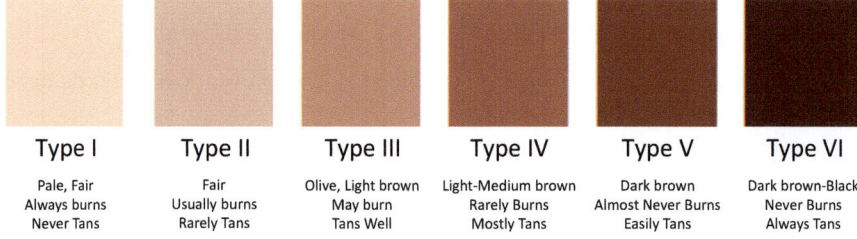

Fig. 8.2 Approximated color scale of Fitzpatrick skin types [5] I–VI

Laser Safety

- Laser safety [2] in the OR:
  - All lasers can cause damage to the patient, operative area, or operators involved and must be handled with caution.
- Important to designate areas where the laser is being used with signage and notifications to avoid inadvertent harm to untrained personnel.
- Eye protection:
  - All lasers targeting melanin or hemoglobin have the potential for retinal damage.
  - Important to utilize protective eyewear that has the following:
    - Compatible wavelength filter to block the specific wavelength of your device.
    - Recommended optical density (OD) protection.
  - All ablative and fractional lasers that target water have potential to damage the cornea:
    - In this case, the eyewear plastic is creating a physical barrier but just as important for vision!
- Laser plume and ventilation:
  - Vaporized cells and proteins from patients can contain aerosolized bacteria, viruses, and other biohazardous materials.
  - It is important to utilize smoke evacuation to prevent inhalation by OR personnel.
- Heat and flame protection:
  - All lasers have the potential to cause thermal damage and hence are flame risks.
  - Minimizing field fuel in case of ignition—surrounding area with wet towels or ultrasound gel.
  - Ensuring contact cooling mechanism is functioning to avoid unwarranted thermal damage to the patient.
  - Standard fire safety to be practiced in all operating rooms.

Common Chromophores and Treatment Options (Fig. 8.3)

- Vascular lesions [2, 3]:
  - Target chromophore is hemoglobin, either oxyhemoglobin (arterial or capillary) or deoxyhemoglobin (venous).
  - Examples of treatable vascular lesions:

Fig. 8.3 Pretreatment and posttreatment effect of laser resurfacing

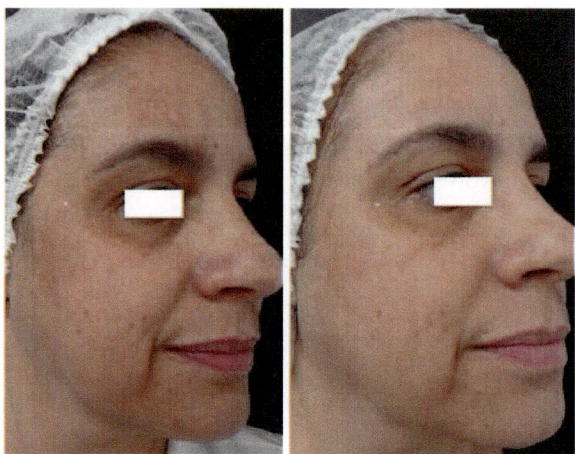

- Hemangioma.
- Telangiectasia.
- Small arteriovenous (AV) malformations.
- Capillary malformation (formerly port-wine stain).
- Spider veins/small varicosities.

- Peak wavelength: 420–800 nm for both oxyhemoglobin and deoxyhemoglobin:
  - Difference between oxy and deoxy at 630 nm.
- Useful laser modalities [2–4]:
  - KTP (potassium titanyl phosphate).
    - 532 nm
    - High affinity for Hgb, low for H20.
  - Pulse dye laser (PDL).
    - 585–595 nm
  - Intense pulsed light (IPL):
    - 510–1400 nm
    - Not a laser, instead emits polychromatic light that can be filtered to omit certain wavelengths.
    - Useful for diffuse red pigments like telangiectasias, capillary malformations, rosacea.
- Tips and tricks:
  - Many wavelengths with high affinity for hemoglobin also have a high affinity for melanin:
    - Careful targeting with small spot size.
    - Constant cooling.

- Do not compress vessels as hemoglobin will not fill in, no target:
  - Avoid vasodilators or constrictors (local anesthetics with epinephrine).
- Modalities may cause bruising or discomfort, well-tolerated awake.

- Pigmented lesions:
  - Target chromophore is melanin, which is actually brown (a mix of wavelengths) but has peaks at blue and violet wavelengths (400–600).
  - Lesions are often located deep in the dermis, so Q-switched modalities are often useful in penetrating deep while minimizing superficial damage.
  - Lesion examples:
    - Melanocytic lesions (nevi, lentigines, photoaging).
    - Tattoo pigments:
      - Pigments are fractured into microscopic pigments which are then phagocytosed by macrophages.
    - Hair follicles:
      - Target is the base of hair follicle, which heats and destroys its own blood supply and epidermis as it reaches thermal relaxation.
  - Useful laser modalities:
    - IPL—older method, primarily for hair removal and photoaging/freckles.
    - Q-switched ruby:
      - 694 nm
      - High affinity for dark pigments, violet + blue tattoo ink.
    - Alexandrite:
      - 755 nm
      - Excellent hair removal.
      - Superior for green and light blue tattoo ink.
    - Nd:YAG (neodymium-doped yttrium aluminum garnet):
      - 1064 nm (+ Q switched 532 nm)
      - Best for hair removal (penetrates deepest).
      - Also has some activity with vascular lesions.
      - Excellent red tattoo ink removal.
  - Tips and tricks:
    - Compressing the skin can avoid targeting blood vessels.
    - Hair should be shaved 1 day before treatment to ensure a uniform short "fuse" and avoid burning epidermis.
    - For skin types with low differentiation between hair and skin color (blonde on pale or dark on dark), selectivity is less useful. May need electrolysis (non-laser hair removal).

- Textural changes/skin resurfacing [2]:
  - The principal chromophore is water (H2O), which is ubiquitous in all skin layers.
  - The goal is to create controlled damage to the epidermis and papillary dermis in order to stimulate new collagen growth, remodeling and skin tightening:
    - Useful for normal aging and hypertrophic scarring (acne, burns, surgical scar).
  - Ablative lasers—causes vaporization of the entire epidermis and papillary dermis.
  - Useful modalities:
    - CO2 laser:
      - 10,600 nm
      - Earlier model.
      - Heat coagulation of the epidermis and dermis.
    - Er:YAG (erbium yttrium aluminum garnet):
      - 2940 nm
      - Greater affinity for water than CO2.
      - Can be used as heat coagulation or cool coagulation.
    - Fractionated ablative lasers:
      - CO2 and Er:YAG.
      - Delivers selected pulses of energy to drill microscopic holes through the dermis.
      - Preserving dermal appendages allows collagen contraction with shorter healing time.
    - Non-ablative:
      - Nd:YAG, PDL, and KTP can be used for dermal-only tightening, not as well studied as ablative (Table 8.1).

Postoperative Laser Care

- Skin resurfacing:
  - Important to keep area moisturized to avoid crusting/flaking (can be uncomfortable).
  - Frequent cleansing to avoid infection:
    - Antibacterial soaps, no need for systemic antibiotics.
    - Treatment on the face requires prophylactic antiviral medications to prevent herpes reactivation.

8 Lasers in Plastic Surgery

Table 8.1 Summary of the most commonly used lasers in plastic surgery

Laser type/medium	Wavelength (nm)	Target chromophore	Conditions treated
KTP	532	Hemoglobin	Vascular lesions
PDL	595	Hemoglobin	Capillary malformation, vascular lesions
Ruby (Q-switch)	694	Deoxyhemoglobin, melanin, dark blue/violet pigments	Venous lesions, tattoo removal (violet, indigo, blue)
Alexandrite	755	Melanin + green/blue pigment	Hair removal, tattoo removal (green, black)
Nd:YAG	1064	Melanin + red/orange pigments	Vascular lesions, pigmented lesions, hair removal, tattoo removal (red, orange)
IPL	512–1200	N/A (not a laser)	Diffuse redness (rosacea, capillary malformation, telangiectasia), hair removal
Er:YAG	2940	Water	Skin resurfacing, scar remodeling
CO2	10,600	Water	Skin resurfacing, scar remodeling

- Postoperative dressings:
  - Open dressings (bacitracin, no bandages, etc.):
    - Typically easier to manage on the face.
    - May cause patient discomfort if not adequately moisturized.
  - Occlusive dressings:
    - Evidence for decreased reepithelialization time.
- Complications:
  - Pain—usually Tylenol is sufficient.
  - Infection:
    - Viral reactivation—Herpes simplex, especially in the face, requires prophylaxis with acyclovir with history of any herpetic lesions in the past.
    - Bacterial infection—very uncommon if patient washing regularly, however can develop impetigo or cellulitis to open areas.
  - Need for multiple treatments—important to set expectations early on.
  - Erythema can persist for 6–12 months following skin resurfacing.
  - Intensive sun care including sunblock after reepithelialization, high coverage clothing, and wide brimmed hats are critical.
  - Post-inflammatory hyperpigmentation:
    - Fitzpatrick type ≥3 are more prone to post-inflammatory hyperpigmentation.
    - Often see hyperpigmentation in the short term and hypopigmentation in the long term.

– Option for lightening of hyperpigmented areas after laser:
    - Azelaic acid.
    - Tretinoin or topical retinoids only for post-laser care.
 – Option for darkening of hypopigmented scar:
    - Bimatoprost.

Acknowledgments William B. Norbury, MD: for many of the laser aphorisms utilized in this chapter.
Melanie Connolly, MS: for generation and editing of the figures and diagrams in this chapter.

References

1. Meamber M, Jett J. NIF's guide to how lasers work. Available at: https://lasers.llnl.gov/education/how-lasers-work. Accessed 28 June 2022.
2. Basci D, Kenke J. Nonsurgical facial rejuvenation and skin resurfacing. In: Chung K, editor. Grabb and smith's plastic surgery. 8th ed. Philadelphia: Wolters Kluwer; 2020. p. 458–71.
3. Silva AK, Teven CM, Hoopman JE. Lasers in plastic surgery. In: Janis J, editor. Essentials of plastic surgery. 2nd ed. Boca Raton: Taylor&Francis; 2014. p. 115–24.
4. Schierle C. Injectables, skin resurfacing, lasers, and hair restoration. In: Buck D, editor. Review of plastic surgery. 1st ed. Toronto: Elsevier; 2019. p. 299–307.
5. Wanner M, Sakamoto FH, Avram MM, Anderson RR. Immediate skin responses to laser and light treatments: warning endpoints: how to avoid side effects. J Am Acad Dermatol. 2015;74(5):807–19.

Chapter 9
Skin Lesions: Benign and Malignant

Evelyn Reed

Evaluation [1]

- The history and physical exam findings should allow for the generation of a differential diagnosis.
- History: There are several key questions to ask about all skin lesions and masses.
  - How long has the lesion been present?
  - Is it growing or changing?
  - Does it have symptoms such as pain or bleeding?
  - Does the patient have relevant risk factors?
- Physical Exam: There are several key signs to note about every lesion.
  - Morphology and color of the lesion.
  - Location and distribution of lesion(s).
  - Palpation of the lesion can identify if it is tender, its consistency, its depth, and any fixation.
- Signs that can be red flags for malignancy include bleeding, ulceration, rapid growth, and size >6 mm.

E. Reed (✉)
Division of Plastic Surgery, University of Utah Health, Salt Lake City, UT, USA
e-mail: evelyn.reed@hsc.utah.edu

Benign Skin Lesions

Acrochordon or "Skin Tag" [2]

- Common, benign, pedunculated lesions often associated with obesity and increased age.
- Findings:
  - Often found in the neck, axilla, and groin areas
  - Skin-colored or hyperpigmented
  - If symptomatic, often pruritic or irritated due to friction
- Treatment options for irritated lesions include sharp excision, cryotherapy, or electrodessication.

Seborrheic Keratosis [3]

- Benign skin lesions resulting from proliferations of immature keratinocytes
- Common in patients middle-aged and older
- Findings:
  - "Stuck-on" appearance with a dull, waxy surface
  - Well-demarcated and slow-growing
  - Variable color and location on the body
- Leser-Trélat sign: Sudden emergence and growth of multiple seborrheic keratoses can signal an underlying malignancy.
- Treatment options for irritated lesions include shave excision, cryotherapy, or electrodessication (Fig. 9.1).

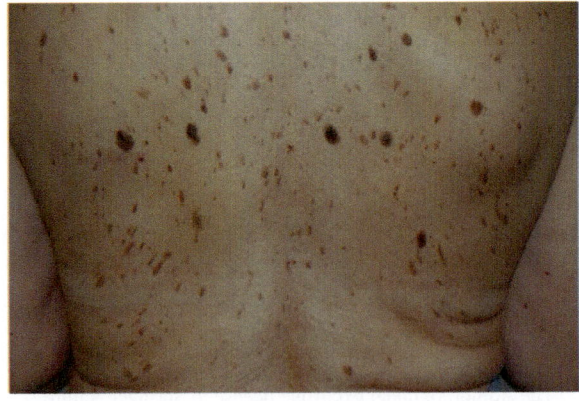

Fig. 9.1 Seborrheic keratoses on an elderly man's back [4]

Cherry Angioma [5]

- Benign vascular proliferations that increase in frequency with age.
- Findings:
  - Round, well-demarcated, red papules with a surrounding paler halo
  - Usually several mm in size
- Treatment for lesions that are irritated or bleed with trauma is excision (Fig. 9.2).

Nevus of Ota and Ito [7]

- Both conditions are benign dermal melanoses that arise in specific nerve distributions.
- Most commonly seen in Asian females, often present at birth but can develop during puberty.
- Findings:
  - Unilateral with a characteristic blue-gray color
  - Nevus of Ota: Present in the trigeminal ophthalmic (V1) and maxillary (V2) distributions, often includes hyperpigmentation of the eye
  - Nevus of Ito: Present in the distribution of the posterior supraclavicular and lateral cutaneous brachial nerves of the shoulder
- Treatment options depend on the goal.
  - Cosmetic improvement can be achieved with laser therapy.
  - Mohs micrographic surgery is recommended for areas suspicious for malignancy or delicate areas that would benefit from excision (Fig. 9.3).

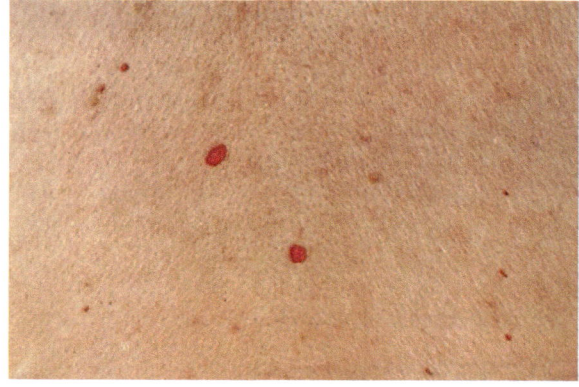

Fig. 9.2 Cherry angioma [6]

Fig. 9.3 Nevus of Ota [8]

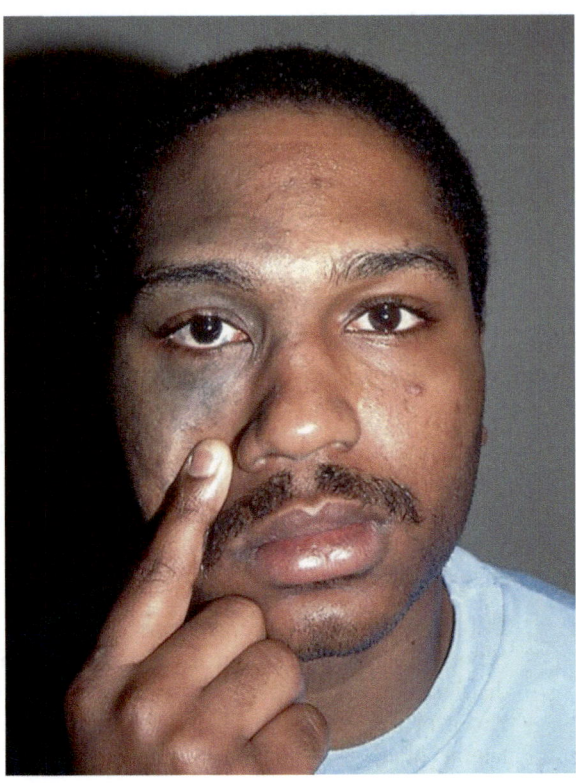

Melanocytic Nevus [9]

- Benign nevi should be ≤6 mm in diameter, homogeneously colored, with well-demarcated borders.
- Patients with many benign nevi may be at increased risk of melanoma and should be followed by a dermatologist.
- Different types of benign nevi include:
  - Congenital: Nevi can be present at birth, but most appear after the first 6 months of age.
  - Intradermal: The cells of these nevi live in the dermis, where they can lose their ability to produce melanin and present as flesh-colored papules. They are often soft and rubbery.
  - Junctional: These nevi consist of cells at the dermal-epidermal junction. They are usually flat or minimally raised, with darker pigmentation than surrounding skin.
  - Compound: These nevi involve cells both in the dermis and at the dermal-epidermal junction. They can be nearly flat or raised papules and often contain more pigment than the surrounding skin.

- Blue: These nevi contain dermal melanocytes that are actively producing melanin. The color is due to the "Tyndall effect," which is the scattering of shorter light wavelengths by the melanin itself.

Spitz Nevus or "Benign Juvenile Melanoma" [10]

- Acquired proliferations of melanocytes that appear in childhood and adolescence.
- Findings:
  - Pink or tan dome-shaped nodules.
  - Surface can be smooth or verrucous.
  - Often appear on the face.
  - Can exhibit rapid growth and "atypical" features suspicious for melanoma.
- Treatment options include monitoring (for truly benign-appearing spitz nevi) or excision:
  - Nevi with suspicious features should be excised with margin clearance appropriate for degree of melanoma suspicion (3–5 mm vs. up to 1 cm) (Fig. 9.4).

Nevus Sebaceous of Jadassohn [11]

- Congenital hamartomas of the pilosebaceous follicular unit.
- Present in about 0.3% of people, often on the scalp.
- Findings:
  - Initially appear yellow, waxy, and smooth
  - Grow and transition to more prominent, verrucous lesions during puberty

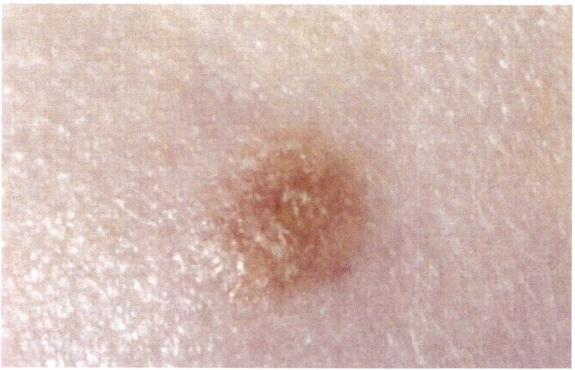

Fig. 9.4 Spitz nevus

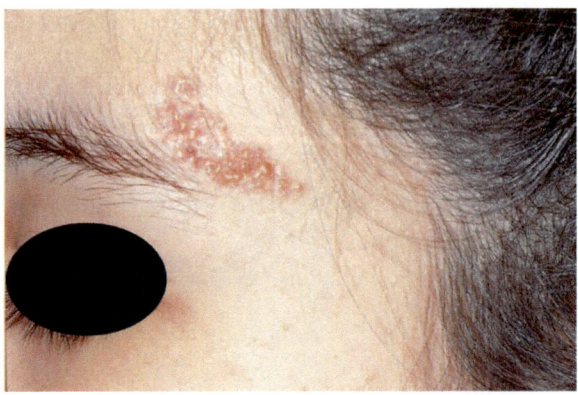

Fig. 9.5 Nevus sebaceous [12]

- Treatment is excision in late childhood due to the risk of malignant transformation to basal cell carcinoma, trichoblastoma, or other sebaceous tumors later in life (Fig. 9.5).

Dermatofibroma or "Fibrous Histiocytoma" [13]

- Benign, subcutaneous lesions made up of fibrous cells.
- Often develop after a traumatic event.
- More common in females (2:1) in ages 20–40
- Findings:
  - Firm, smooth, nontender nodules
  - Brown or reddish coloration
  - Usually <1 cm
- Treatment recommendation is for excisional biopsy to confirm diagnosis—recurrence afterward is very rare (Fig. 9.6).

Pilomatricoma or "Calcifying Epithelioma" [15]

- Benign, subcutaneous lesions originating from hair follicles.
- Often present in the head and neck region.
- Findings:
  - Characteristic feature is microcalcifications, which can be palpable and give an irregular appearance
- Treatment is excision with 1 cm margins to eliminate the risk of recurrence:

Fig. 9.6 Dermatofibroma [14]

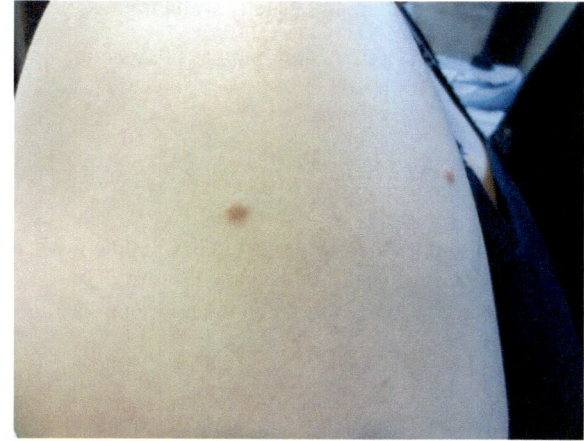

- In very rare case reports, pilomatricomas have undergone malignant transformation into pilomatrix carcinoma.

Epidermal Inclusion Cyst [16]

- Very common cysts from epidermal contents becoming trapped in the dermis, often related to a plugged hair follicle.
- Epithelialized cyst wall containing keratinous debris.
- Findings:
  - Mobile masses directly under the skin.
  - Often have a central punctum that can drain "cheesy" white material, causing size fluctuations.
  - Cysts can become inflamed and infected, which can lead to rupture.
- Treatment is excision of the cyst with its walls intact:
  - Easier to do when the cyst is not actively inflamed.

Lipoma [17]

- Very common benign, subcutaneous tumors of adipocytes.
- Can be found anywhere on the body.
- Findings:
  - Can be found in subcutaneous plane, where they are usually highly mobile, or deeper planes where they may be firmer

Dermoid Cyst [18]

- Benign tumors that occur during development when ectodermal components get trapped along sites of embryonic closure.
- Congenital, usually identified in children under age 5
- Findings:
  - Nontender, slow-growing, firm
  - Adherent deep to the subcutaneous tissue
  - Most often seen in the lateral third of the eyebrow
- Treatment is early excision, as the lesions are easier to remove before they continue to grow:
  - Midline or nasal dermoid cysts can be associated with intracranial extension, and MRI or CT can be used to evaluate this prior to excision (Fig. 9.7).

Pyogenic Granuloma or "Lobular Capillary Hemangioma" [20]

- Acquired vascular tumor of skin and mucous membranes.
- Likely reactive to trauma, hormonal changes, infection.
- Findings:
  - Reddish, pedunculated papule.
  - Friable, often ulcerated.
  - Rapid growth, then stabilizes.
- Treatment is complete excision to reduce recurrence (Fig. 9.8).

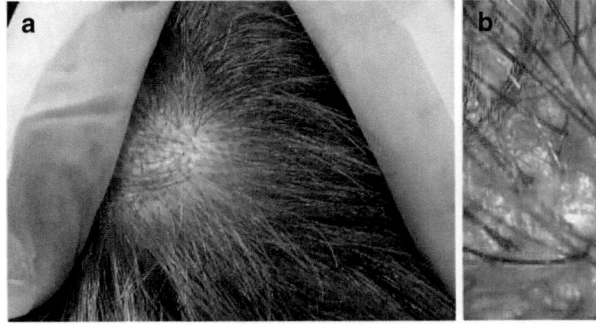
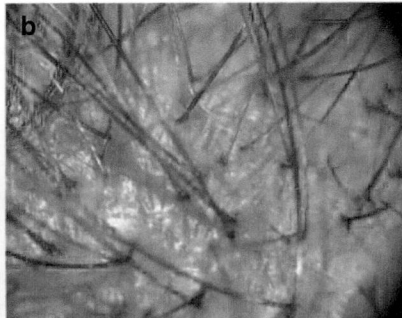

Fig. 9.7 A dermoid cyst under the scalp [19]

Fig. 9.8 Pyogenic granuloma

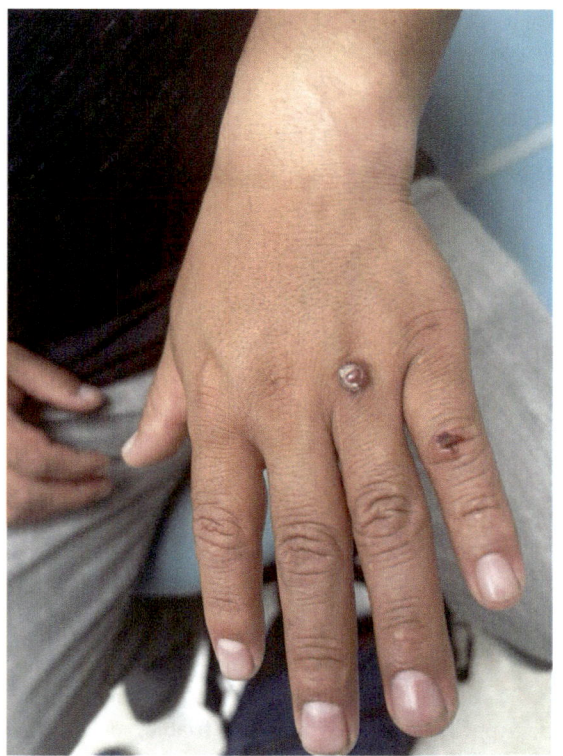

Malignant Skin Lesions

Basal Cell Carcinoma (BCC) [21, 22]

- Etiology: Most common malignancy. Locally aggressive, but unlikely to metastasize.
- Risk factors: UV exposure, lighter skin, and immunosuppression.
- Appearance: Usually flesh-colored or pink, often with a "pearly" appearance. Can have telangiectatic vessels or ulceration. Often sun-exposed areas.
- Diagnosis: Biopsy suspicious lesions.
- Treatments:
  - Surgical: If cosmetically or anatomically sensitive areas, Mohs micrographic surgery is recommended. For other areas, surgical excision with 4 mm margins.

Table 9.1 Common indications for Mohs surgery

Common indications for Mohs surgery
Indistinct margins
Cosmetically/functionally sensitive areas (face, ear, hands)
Recurrent disease in scar or radiated fields
Aggressive patterns (morpheaform)
Immunosuppressed patients

- Nonsurgical: Cryosurgery or curettage and electrodessication (EDC) can be used for superficial, low-risk tumors or for patients who are poor surgical candidates. Phototherapy, radiation, or topical imiquimod are other options. Systemic therapies only for very locally advanced or metastatic disease (Table 9.1).

Squamous Cell Carcinoma (SCC) [23, 24]

- Etiology: Second most common skin cancer. From keratinocytes and adnexal cells.
- Risk factors: UV exposure, lighter skin, immunosuppression, and HPV+ status.
- Appearance: Often appear as friable, scaly patches, can have ulceration. Variable depending on additional subtypes:
    - Keratoacanthoma: Benign or low-grade rapidly growing, protruding dome-shaped lesion with a central keratin plug that often stabilizes and can even involute.
    - Actinic Keratosis: Premalignant precursor. Scaly, flesh-colored plaque, often on the head and neck.
    - Bowen's Disease: SCC in situ. Erythematous, scaly plaque that is well-demarcated.
    - Marjolin's Ulcer: Aggressive, invasive SCC that originates from a chronic wound, typically a burn. Often seen as a persistent, ulcerated area.
- Diagnosis: Biopsy suspicious lesions. High-risk features such as increased depth, poor differentiation, and perineural or lymphovascular invasion will be identified.
- Treatments:
    - Surgical: If cosmetically or anatomically sensitive areas, Mohs micrographic surgery is recommended. For other areas, surgical excision with 4–6-mm margins.
    - Nonsurgical: Precursor or low-risk lesions can be treated with cryosurgery, phototherapy, or EDC. Radiation or systemic therapies reserved for very locally advanced or metastatic disease (Fig. 9.9).

Fig. 9.9 Squamous cell carcinoma

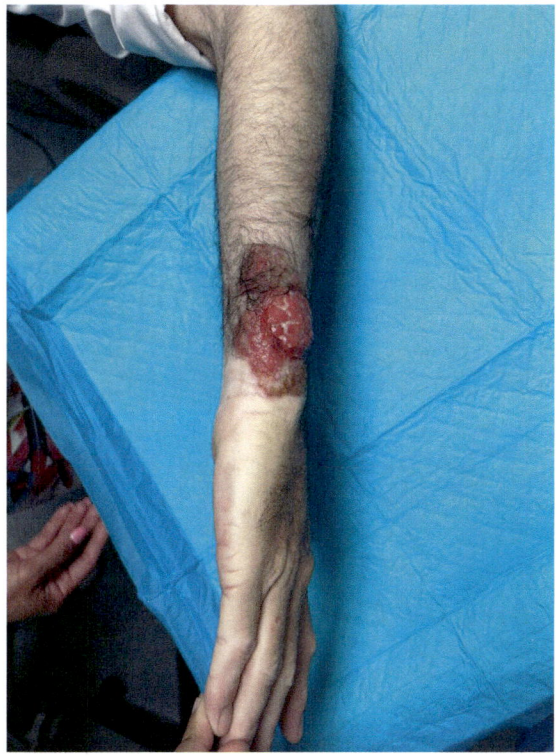

Melanoma [25–27]

- Etiology: Mutation in neural crest-derived melanocytes.
- Risk factors: UV exposure, lighter skin, number of melanocytic nevi, family history.
- Appearance—Think of the ABCDEs:
    - *A*symmetry
    - Irregular *b*order
    - *C*olor variation
    - *D*iameter >6 mm
    - *E*volving
- Diagnosis: Perform excisional biopsy to allow assessment of depth.
    - Staging criteria include depth, ulceration, lymph node status, and presence of metastatic disease.
- Treatments:
    - Surgical: Wide local excision with 1–2 cm margins. SNLB for stage 1B or higher (<0.75 cm diameter with ulceration or >0.75 cm in diameter).

Fig. 9.10 Melanoma

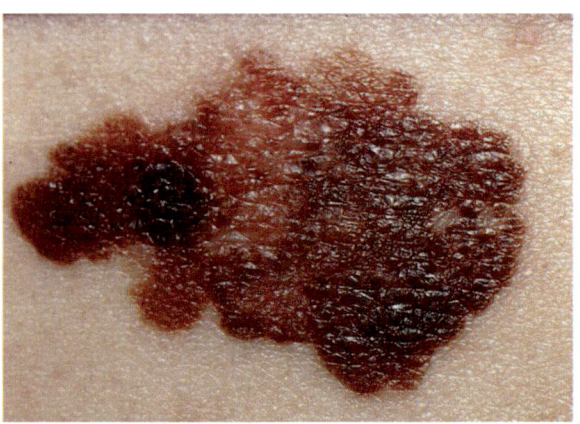

- Nonsurgical: Immunotherapy preferred for systemic disease. Consider radiation for positive nodes (Fig. 9.10).

Merkel Cell Carcinoma [28, 29]

- Etiology: Rare, aggressive cutaneous neuroendocrine tumor.
- Risk factors: Elderly white males, immunosuppression, UV exposure.
- Appearance: Rapidly growing, tender, erythematous nodule in sun-exposed skin.
- Diagnosis: Biopsy suspicious lesions.
- Treatments:
  - Surgical: Wide local excision with 1–2 cm margins, including SLNB.
  - Nonsurgical: Adjuvant chemotherapy, immunotherapy, or radiation recommended for nonlocal disease (Fig. 9.11).

Dermatofibrosarcoma Protuberans [31]

- Etiology: Dermal fibrohistiocytic neoplasm caused by a t(17:22) chromosomal translocation. Low rate of metastasis.
- Risk factors: African ethnicity.
- Appearance: Indolent, nontender, pink or violet plaque. Often on the trunk or upper extremities.
- Diagnosis: Biopsy suspicious lesions.
- Treatments:
  - Surgical: Wide local excision with 2–3 cm margins.
  - Nonsurgical: Radiation can be considered; use of systemic therapy is rare.

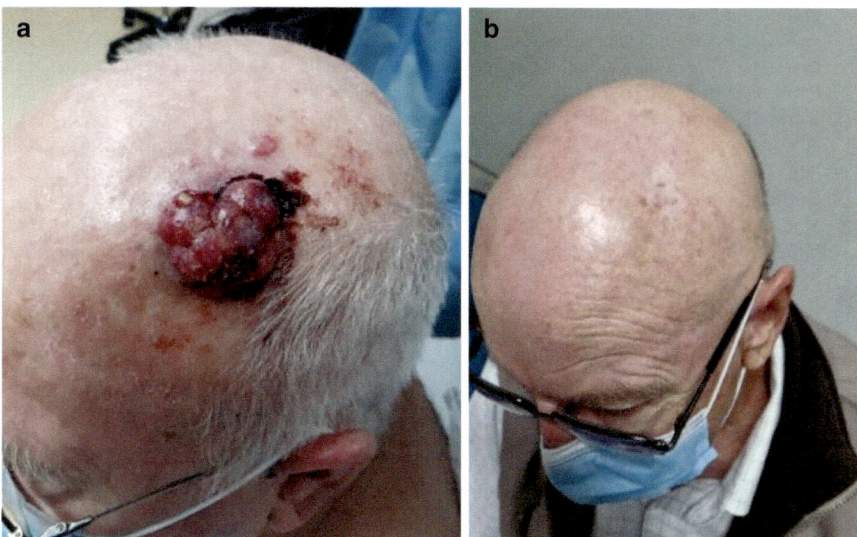

Fig. 9.11 Merkel cell cancer [30]

References

1. Armstrong C. Approach to the clinical dermatologic diagnosis. In: Corona R, editor. UpToDate [Internet]; 2021. http://www.uptodate.com/contents/approach-to-the-clinical-dermatologic-diagnosis.
2. Syed S, Lipoff J, Chatterjee K, LLC SP, editors. Acrochordon. StatPearls Publishing LLC; 2021.
3. Greco M, Bhutta B. Seborrheic keratosis. In: StatPearls [Internet]. StatPearls Publishing LLC; 2022.
4. Picoto A. Seborrhoeic keratosis. In: Katsambas AD, Lotti TM, Dessinioti C, D'Erme AM, editors. European handbook of dermatological treatments. Berlin, Heidelberg: Springer; 2015. https://doi.org/10.1007/978-3-662-45139-7_88.
5. Qadeer H, Singal A, Patel B. Cherry Hemangioma. In: StatPearls, editor. StatPearls [Internet]. StatPearls Publishing LLC; 2021.
6. Müller H. Vascular tumors. In: Plewig G, French L, Ruzicka T, Kaufmann R, Hertl M, editors. Braun-Falco´s dermatology. Berlin, Heidelberg: Springer; 2022. https://doi.org/10.1007/978-3-662-63709-8_107.
7. Agarwal P, Patel B. Nevus of Ota and Ito. In: StatPearls, editor. StatPearls [Internet]. StatPearls Publishing LLC; 2021.
8. Treadwell P. Nevus of Ota and Ito. In: Treadwell P, Smith ML, Prendiville J, editors. Atlas of adolescent dermatology. Cham: Springer; 2021. https://doi.org/10.1007/978-3-030-58634-8_23.
9. Hunt R, Schaffer J, Bolognia J. Acquired melanocytic nevi (moles). In: Corona R, editor. UpToDate; 2022. https://www.uptodate.com/contents/acquired-melanocytic-nevi-moles#H29.
10. Barnhill R, Kim J. Spitz nevus and atypical Spitz tumors. In: Corona R, editor. UpToDate [Internet]; 2020. https://www.uptodate.com/contents/spitz-nevus-and-atypical-spitz-tumors?sectionName=MANAGEMENT&topicRef=4846&anchor=H53356221&source=see_link#H53356221.
11. Baigrie D, Troxell T, Cook C. Nevus Sebaceus. In: StatPearls, editor. StatPearls [Internet]. StatPearls Publishing LLC; 2021.

12. Prendiville J. Nevus sebaceous. In: Treadwell P, Smith ML, Prendiville J, editors. Atlas of adolescent dermatology. Cham: Springer; 2021. https://doi.org/10.1007/978-3-030-58634-8_22.
13. Myers D, Fillman E. Dermatofibroma. In: StatPearls, editor. StatPearls [Internet]. StatPearls Publishing LLC; 2021.
14. Sanyal R, Terrano D, Singh R, Phelps R. Common soft tissue tumors. In: Smoller B, Bagherani N, editors. Atlas of dermatology, dermatopathology and venereology. Cham: Springer; 2022. https://doi.org/10.1007/978-3-319-53805-1_82.
15. DeRosa DC, Lin-Hurtubise K. Pilomatricoma: an unusual dermatologic neoplasm. Hawaii J Med Public Health. 2012;71(10):282–6.
16. Weir C, St. Hilaire N. Epidermal inclusion cyst. In: StatPearls, editor. StatPearls [Internet]. StatPearls Publishing LLC; 2021.
17. Kolb L, Yarrarapu S, Ameer M, Rosario-Collazo J. Lipoma. In: StatPearls, editor. StatPearls [Internet]. StatPearls Publishing LLC; 2021.
18. Shareef S, Ettefagh L. Dermoid cyst. In: StatPearls, editor. StatPearls [Internet]. StatPearls Publishing LLC; 2021.
19. Wortsman X, Pizarro K, Corredoira Y, Morales C, Carreño L. Ultrasound of congenital cutaneous conditions. In: Wortsman X, editor. Textbook of dermatologic ultrasound. Cham: Springer; 2022. https://doi.org/10.1007/978-3-031-08736-3_7.
20. Sarwal P, Lapumnuaypol K. Pyogenic granuloma. In: StatPearls, editor. StatPearls [Internet]. StatPearls Publishing LLC; 2021.
21. McDaniel B, Badri T, Steele R. Basal cell carcinoma. In: StatPearls, editor. StatPearls [Internet]. StatPearls Publishing LLC; 2021.
22. Kim D, Kus K, Ruiz E. Basal cell carcinoma review. Hematol Oncol Clin North Am. 2019;33(1):13–24. https://doi.org/10.1016/j.hoc.2018.09.004.
23. Kallini JR, Hamed N, Khachemoune A. Squamous cell carcinoma of the skin: epidemiology, classification, management, and novel trends. Int J Dermatol. 2015;54(2):130–40. https://doi.org/10.1111/ijd.12553.
24. Zito P, Scharf R. Keratoacanthoma. In: StatPearls, editor. StatPearls [Internet]. StatPearls Publishing LLC; 2021.
25. Network NCC. Melanoma: cutaneous (Version 3.2022). Accessed 27 May 2022. https://www.nccn.org/professionals/physician_gls/pdf/cutaneous_melanoma.pdf.
26. Heistein J, Acharya U. Malignant melanoma. In: StatPearls, editor. StatPearls [Internet]. StatPearls Publishing LLC; 2021.
27. Leonardi GC, Falzone L, Salemi R, et al. Cutaneous melanoma: from pathogenesis to therapy (Review). Int J Oncol. 2018;52(4):1071–80. https://doi.org/10.3892/ijo.2018.4287.
28. Emge DA, Cardones AR. Updates on merkel cell carcinoma. Dermatol Clin. 2019;37(4):489–503. https://doi.org/10.1016/j.det.2019.06.002.
29. Coggshall K, Tello TL, North JP, Yu SS. Merkel cell carcinoma: an update and review: pathogenesis, diagnosis, and staging. J Am Acad Dermatol. 032018. 78(3):433–42. https://doi.org/10.1016/j.jaad.2017.12.001.
30. Veness MJ. Merkel cell carcinoma. In: Joseph KJ, Veness MJ, Barnes E, Rembielak A, editors. Radiotherapy in skin cancer. Cham: Springer; 2023. https://doi.org/10.1007/978-3-031-44316-9_12.
31. Allen A, Ahn C, Sangüeza OP. Dermatofibrosarcoma Protuberans. Dermatol Clin. 2019;37(4):483–8. https://doi.org/10.1016/j.det.2019.05.006.

Chapter 10
Burn

Katherine J. Choi and Christopher H. Pham

Epidemiology

- Every year, there are approximately 200,000 burn-related hospital admissions in the United States [1]:
  - Over 67% of those burned had a total body surface area (TBSA) % less than 10%, with an associated mortality rate less than 1%.
- Major predictors of case fatality include burn size, age, and the presence of inhalation injury [2], which is also known as the revised Baux score (r-Baux):
  - R-Baux = TBSA % + age + [17 × R], R = 1 if patient has inhalational injury, R = 0 if not [3].
  - Traditionally, the Baux score, which does not account for inhalational injury, was used, and a score of 110 was associated with 50% mortality, and a score of 160 was associated with 100% mortality.

Pathophysiology

- After the epidermis and dermis are injured after burn, the skin is no longer able to serve as a barrier to moisture loss and microbes:
    - This necessitates appropriate fluid administration and judicious wound care.
    - Burns develop in three zones: zone of coagulation (dead tissue), zone of stasis (questionable tissue), and zone of hyperemia (alive tissue) (Fig. 10.1).
        - Inadequate resuscitation of injured tissue results in microvasculature thrombosis in the zone of stasis, which can cause tissue to die and convert to necrosis.
- Initial injury depends on the temperature of the energy source and duration of contact.
- In adults with burns >15% TBSA, a systemic response ensues as injured tissue secretes inflammatory mediators that result in systemic vasodilation:
    - This results in a hypermetabolic state driven by catecholamines, prostaglandins, and glucocorticoids that predictably requires enteral supplementation to provide adequate nutritional support (Curreri formula) [4, 5].
    - The counterregulatory anti-inflammatory reaction results in relative immune dysfunction and predisposes to infection.

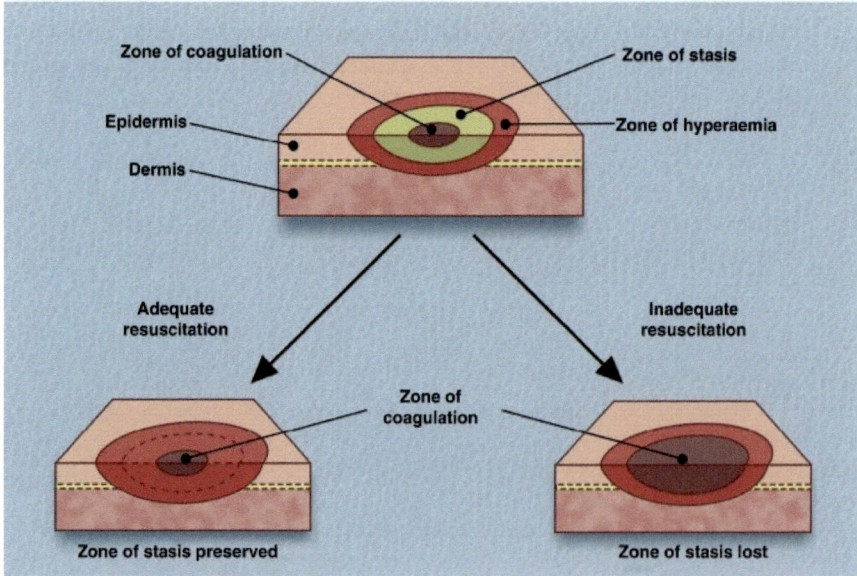

Fig. 10.1 Zones of burns with progression

Table 10.1 Degrees of burn with specific features of each type

First degree	Second degree	Third degree
Only the epidermis (i.e., sunburn, superficial scald burn) Pink, painful, and dry Heal with wound care alone	Dermal injury present (subdivided into superficial and deep) Pink, painful, and edematous Usually heal with local wound care	Full-thickness dermal injury Leather-like, painless, and dry Will not heal without surgery

Burn Depth and Histology [6] (Table 10.1)

Treatment of Acute Burns

- American Burn Association Burn Center Referral Criteria [7].
  - Partial-thickness burns greater than 10% of TBSA in patients younger than 10 years old or older than 50 years old:
    - Partial-thickness burns over more than 20% TBSA in other age groups.
  - Burns involving the face, hands, feet, genitalia, perineum, or major joints.
  - Third-degree burns.
  - Electrical burns (including lightning injury).
  - Chemical burns.
  - Inhalation injury.
  - Presence of preexisting medical conditions that could complicate management, prolong recover, or affect mortality.
  - Any concomitant trauma in which burn injury poses greatest risk of morbidity or death.
  - Children at hospitals without qualified personnel or equipment to care for children.
  - All patients who require special social, emotional, or long-term rehabilitative intervention.

Initial Assessment [6]

- The "rule of nines" is used to quickly estimate TBSA%, but the most consistent estimates are obtained with the Lund-Browder burn diagram [8] (Fig. 10.2).
- Inhalational Injury.
  - High index of suspicion with:
    - Enclosed space.

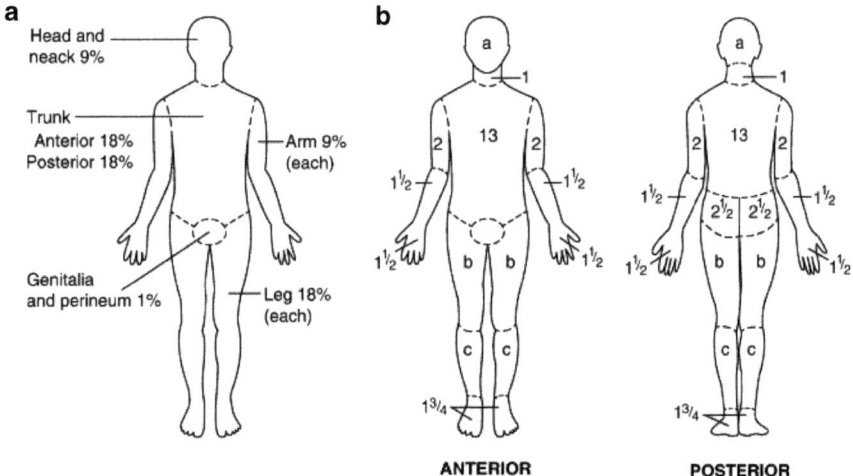

Fig. 10.2 Rule of nines in an adult

- Hoarse voice.
- Singed facial/nasal hairs*.
- Facial burns*.
- Soot in airway*.
- Carbonaceous sputum.
- *Has a low predictive value of inhalation injury when taken in isolation [9]

  – Carbon monoxide exposure (carboxyhemoglobin ≥10%) should be treated with 100% O_2.
  – Further workup with arterial blood gas analysis, chest radiograph (initially normal), direct laryngoscopy, or bronchoscopy.

- Compartment syndrome.
  – 5 Ps: Pain out of proportion or with passive extension, paresthesias, pallor, pulselessness, and paralysis
  – Higher risk with deep partial- or full-thickness circumferential burns (i.e., trunk burns can cause abdominal compartment syndrome; upper extremity burns can cause hand or arm compartment syndrome).

Treatments

- Initial resuscitation is followed by early excision of full-thickness burns and some deep partial thickness burns and appropriate daily wound care:
  - Excised wound beds can be immediately covered with a skin graft or temporized with dressings, dermal substitutes, or allograft.
  - Skin grafts can be split thickness (meshed or sheet) or full thickness, based on recipient site (e.g., sheet to the hands or face) and donor site availability.
- Prophylactic antibiotics are typically not indicated:
  - Most burns are colonized not infected.
  - Antibiotics without a clear infectious source lead to increased bacterial resistance.
- Fluid resuscitation by Parkland formula [10]:
  - Consider for >20% TBSA.
  - 4 mL × weight (kg) × %TBSA of second/third degree burned = total amount of lactated Ringer's to be given in 24 h:
    - First 8 h: Give half the total amount fluids.
    - Next 16 h: Give remaining half of fluids, adjusting rate with hourly urine output to avoid over-resuscitation and its complications.
    - Timing is set from burn onset, *not* arrival:
      - If patient gets to burn center 3 h after burn without any resuscitation, then give the 8-h component over 5 h.
    - Example:
      - 100-kg person, 60% TBSA second degree
      - 24 L to be given in first 24 h
      - 1.5 L/h for the first 8 h
      - 750 mL/h for the second 16
- Dressings (wound coverage)—The ideal dressing has effective antimicrobial coverage, minimizes pain to the patient, and minimizes wound care labor.
  - Silver sulfadiazine (Silvadene):
    - Broad-spectrum, gram-positive, and gram-negative coverage.
    - Side effects: transient leukopenia, poor eschar penetration.
  - Silver nitrate:
    - Staphylococcus and gram negatives.
    - Side effects: hyponatremia, hypokalemia.
  - Mafenide acetate (Sulfamylon):

- Gram-positive coverage.
- Side effects: metabolic acidosis (carbonic anhydrase inhibitor), compensatory hyperventilation.
  - Silver-impregnated dressings (e.g., Mepilex Ag, KerraContact Ag):
    - Staphylococcus and gram-negative coverage.
    - Can be changed every 3–7 days.
  - Enzymatic debridement (e.g., Santyl):
    - Collagenase (enzymatic debrider).
    - Does not have intrinsic antimicrobial activity.
  - Hypochlorous acid (Vashe):
    - Broad spectrum.
    - Less cytotoxic to fibroblasts than Dakin's.

Sequelae

- Complications.
  - Short term: pneumonia, sepsis, renal failure (from hypoperfusion).
  - Long term: hypertrophic scarring, keloid formation, joint stiffness due to scar contractures or heterotopic ossification (when near joints).

Delayed Burn Reconstruction

After acute phase, healed burns can result in contractures with functional limitations. The goal is typically to excise contracted scar with replacement with pliable tissue or Z-plasty to elongate the contracted tissue, depending on location and functional limitation.

References

1. Mosier MJ, et al. American Burn Association National Burn Repository 2017 report. https://ameriburn.site-ym.com/page/NBR. Accessed 10 Apr 2019.
2. Choi KJ, Pham CH, Collier ZJ, et al. The predictive capacity of American Society of Anesthesiologists Physical Status (ASA PS) score in burn patients. J Burn Care Res. 2020;41:803–8.
3. Dokter J, Meijs J, Oen IM, et al. External validation of the revised Baux score for the prediction of mortality in patients with acute burn injury. J Trauma Acute Care Surg. 2014;76:840–5.

4. Turner WW Jr, Ireton CS, Hunt JL, Baxter CR. Predicting energy expenditures in burned patients. J Trauma. 1985;25(1):11–6.
5. Pham CH, Fang M, Vrouwe SQ, et al. Evaluating the safety and efficacy of intraoperative enteral nutrition in critically ill burn patients. J Burn Care Res. 2020;41:841–8.
6. Grunwald TB, Garner WL. Acute burns. Plast Reconstr Surg. 2008;121:311e–9e.
7. Guidelines for the Operation of Burn Centers, Resources for Optimal Care of the Injured Patient. Committee on Trauma, American College of Surgeons; 2006.
8. Pham CH, Collier ZJ, Gillenwater TJ. Changing the way we think about burn size estimation. J Burn Care Res. 2019;40:1–11.
9. Ikonomidis C, Lang F, Radu A, et al. Standardizing the diagnosis of inhalation injury using a descriptive score based on mucosal injury criteria. Burns. 2012;38:513–9.
10. Baxter CR. Fluid volume and electrolyte changes of the early postburn period. Clin Plast Surg. 1974;1:693–703.

Chapter 11
Pressure Ulcers

Yara Samman and Jacquelynn T. Lee

Introduction

Pressure sores are defined as necrosis or ulceration in the skin and underlying tissue beds that result from prolonged pressure. They remain common, especially in acute, long-term, and home care settings.

- Prevalence [1]
  - Prevalence ranges between 5% and 15% in hospitalized patients:
    - 21.5% prevalence in intensive care units, with older patients at a higher risk of developing pressure ulcers
- Incidence [1]
  - 1–3 million per year in the United States.
  - 23% of patients in the neonatal and pediatric ICU may develop pressure ulcers:
    - Neonates who are hospitalized are at a higher risk of pressure ulcer than adults due to their decreased mobility, compromised perfusion, underdeveloped epidermal barrier, fluid retention, moisture, and medical devices [2, 3].
- Note name change designation to "pressure injury" by the National Pressure Ulcer Advisory Panel (NPAUP) in 2016:
  - The NPUAP changed their name to National Pressure Injury Advisory Panel (NPIAP) in 2019.

Y. Samman · J. T. Lee (✉)
University of Texas Medical Branch, Division of Plastic Surgery, Galveston, TX, USA
e-mail: ybsamman@utmb.edu

- Susceptible areas listed in order of occurrence
  - Device-related 50%:
    - Commonly associated with respiratory devices, tubes/drains, and compression wraps/splinters/braces [4].
    - 57% of patients in the ICU due to COVID-19 infection who are nursed in the prone position develop pressure ulcers [5].
  - Sacrum 27–48% [6].
  - Heels 19–40%
  - Ischial tuberosity 4–20%
  - Trochanter/hips 11–16%

Etiology

- Forces exerted on soft tissue leading to pressure necrosis—pressure, shear, and friction [7, 8]:
  - Pressure is the vertical force of body weight on a surface [9].
  - Shear is a horizontal force of pressure that contributes to pressure ulcer formation. It is the resistance force between the patient's skin surface and the plane in touch with that area such as chair or bed. This type of force will cause injury that is not seen on skin level but rather underneath it.
  - Friction is the force of rubbing two objects together such as the skin surface and clothing items. An example is when the skin is dragged across the hospital bed linens. This type of force causes visible injury on the skin, by injuring the epidermal layer of the skin and decreasing its integrity, thus increasing the chance of further damage in the layers underneath. This accounts for a minority of pressure ulcers.
- Tip of the iceberg phenomenon:
  - The skin can mask a much deeper and wider pressure injury, where underneath there may be damage to fat, muscle, and possibly bone. This is explained by the fact that muscle is more susceptible to ischemia than the skin and fat has much lower tensile strength and thus would be more at risk of an extrinsic tissue injury than the skin.
- Pressure sores can happen in a variety of clinical settings, the most common is related to immobility.

Diagnosis

- Imaging: MRI is typically used to assess for the presence of osteomyelitis; bone biopsy is gold standard for diagnosis of osteomyelitis.
- Labs: Nutrition labs (liver function, total protein, prealbumin, albumin) assess for anemia and inflammatory markers CRP and ESR if concerned for deep infection.

Presentation

- Stages defined by the National Pressure Injury Advisory Panel (Fig. 11.1):
    - Stage 1: nonblanchable erythema of intact skin
    - Stage 2: partial-thickness skin loss with exposed dermis
    - Stage 3: Full-thickness skin loss
        - Subcutaneous tissue is visible.
    - Stage 4: Full-thickness loss of the skin and tissue
        - Exposed or directly palpable fascia, muscle, tendon, ligament, or bone
    - Unstageable: obscure full-thickness skin and tissue loss
        - The extent of tissue damage within ulcer cannot be confirmed due to eschar or slough.
- Acute Skin Failure vs Pressure Injury
    - Pressure injury is a localized injury due to pressure, shear, or friction forces.
    - Acute skin failure is the death of the skin and underlying tissue due to hypoperfusion. It is often concurrent with severe failure or dysfunction of other organs [10].

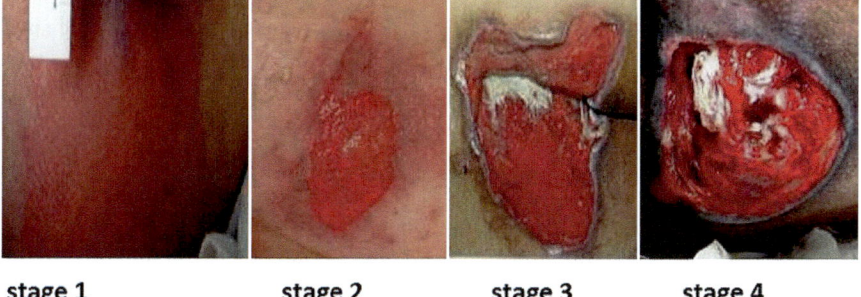

stage 1   stage 2   stage 3   stage 4

Fig. 11.1 Stages of pressure ulcers

- Distinguishing the two may be difficult since there is no clear diagnostic criteria for skin failure. Pressure ulcers can happen in both critically ill patients and healthy patients. However, skin failure will "mirror" the health of the individual and will often be associated with other organ failures [8].

Prevention and Treatment

Stages I and II

- Nonoperative
- Relieve pressure via turning schedule every 2–4 h, control external factors: shear, moisture, friction.
- Dressing changes: wet to dry and wet to moist.
  - Wet to dry or wet to moist is used to remove dead tissue from the wound. Wet gauze is placed on the wound and allowed to dry. Once gauze is dried, the removal of the gauze will mechanically debride the top layer of unhealthy tissue adherent to it. Frequency of dressing changes ranges widely from daily to every 4–6 h.
- Dakin's solution:
  - 0.5% buffered sodium hypochlorite solution, also known as household bleach.
  - General disinfectant; denatures proteins in bacterial biofilm and within the cell, thus irreversibly killing them. It is especially effective against *Staphylococcus aureus* biofilms and *Pseudomonas aeruginosa* [11].
- Collagenase topical agent:
  - Metallo-endoproteinase typically produced by keratinocytes, fibroblasts, macrophages, and neutrophils. It is isolated from fermented *Clostridium histolyticum*. [12]
  - An enzymatic debriding ointment that degrades collagen, especially in necrotic tissue.

Stages III and IV

- May require surgical intervention
  - Debridement is considered a component of wound management to decrease bioburden, remove slough and necrotic tissue, and prepare wound bed for soft tissue coverage [13].
- Wound coverage options based on anatomic site

- Ischial
  - Posterior thigh fasciocutaneous or myocutaneous V-Y advancement flap
  - Tensor fascia lata flap
- Trochanteric
  - Tensor fascia lata flap often used
- Sacral
  - Unilateral vs bilateral gluteal fasciocutaneous flap or myocutaneous rotation flap.
  - Unilateral vs bilateral gluteal fasciocutaneous flap or myocutaneous advancement flap.
  - Avoid taking muscle in ambulatory patients.
  - These flaps can be re-rotated or readvanced.

- Goals of reconstruction
  - Provide wound coverage over vital structures such as the bone, muscle, and fascia.
  - Prevent complications related to infection and sepsis.
- Postoperative management following soft tissue reconstruction
  - Strict pressure offloading
  - Medical optimization
  - Antibiotics for underlying osteomyelitis
  - Bowel regimen
  - Nutrition optimization
  - Sitting protocol
- Surgical complications
  - Recurrence of pressure injury following reconstruction 80% [13].
  - Wound dehiscence
  - New or unresolved infection
  - Hematoma
  - Seroma
- Risk factors for recurrence
  - HbA1C >6% [14].
  - Albumin levels <3.5 g/kg/day [15].
  - Smoking [13, 15].
  - Spinal cord injury population (paraplegia, quadriplegia) [13, 15, 16].
  - Obesity [17].

Prevention [18]

- Proper skin care to minimize excess moisture and skin maceration:
  - Use multilayer foam dressing on bony prominences.
  - Apply heel protectors.
  - Use skin moisturizer on dry skin, and use absorbent pads to avoid excess moisture.
- Use support surfaces to disperse pressure:
  - Use a waffle cushion while in chair.
  - Bed sheets should be kept dry and clean.
  - Pillows can be used to minimize bony prominences contact with bed.
- Reposition:
  - Patient should be turned every 2–4 h.
- Spinal cord injury population [19]:
  - Treat muscle spasm and extremity contracture.
  - Microclimate control.
  - Prophylactic electric stimulation.
- Patient and staff education:
  - Using pamphlets and ongoing training.

References

1. Mervis JS, Phillips TJ. Pressure ulcers: pathophysiology, epidemiology, risk factors, and presentation. J Am Acad Dermatol. 2019 Oct;81(4):881–90.
2. Harpin VA, Rutter N. Barrier properties of the newborn infant's skin. J Pediatr. 1983;102:419–25.
3. Mylene Baharestani M, Ratliff CR, Baharestani MM. Pressure ulcers in neonates and children: an NPUAP white paper original investigation. Adv Skin Wound Care. 2007;20:208–20.
4. Pittman J, Gillespie C. Medical device–related pressure injuries. In: Critical care nursing clinics of North America, vol. 32. W.B. Saunders; 2020. p. 533–42.
5. Moore Z, Patton D, Avsar P, McEvoy N, Curley G, Budri A, et al. Prevention of pressure ulcers among individuals cared for in the prone position: lessons for the COVID-19 emergency. J Wound Care. 2020;29(6):312.
6. Chaboyer WP, Thalib L, Harbeck EL, Coyer FM, Blot S, Bull CF, et al. Incidence and prevalence of pressure injuries in adult intensive care patients: a systematic review and meta-analysis. Crit Care Med. 2018;46(11):E1074–81.
7. Bergstrom N, Bennett M, Carlson C. Treatment of pressure ulcers. Clinical practice guideline, no. 15. 15th ed. Rockville: U.S Department of Health and Human Services, Agency for Health Care Policy and Research; 1994.

8. Delmore B, Cox J, Rolnitzky L, Chu A, Stolfi A. Differentiating a pressure ulcer from acute skin failure in the adult critical care patient C L I N I C A L M A N A G E M E N T extra [Internet]. Adv Skin Wound Care. 2015;28:514. Available from: http://cme.lww.com.
9. Jay R. Pressure and shear: their effects on support surface choice. Ostomy Wound Manage. 1995;41:36–8.
10. Langemo D, Parish LC. The past, present, and future of skin failure. Adv Skin Wound Care. 2022;35(2):81–3.
11. Lineback CB, Nkemngong CA, Wu ST, Li X, Teska PJ, Oliver HF. Hydrogen peroxide and sodium hypochlorite disinfectants are more effective against Staphylococcus aureus and Pseudomonas aeruginosa biofilms than quaternary ammonium compounds. Antimicrob Resist Infect Control. 2018;7(1):154.
12. Morin RJ, Tomaselli NL. Interactive dressings and topical agents. Clin Plast Surg. 2007;34:643–58.
13. Wurzer P, Winter R, Stemmer SO, Ivancic J, Lebo PB, Hundeshagen G, et al. Risk factors for recurrence of pressure ulcers after defect reconstruction. Wound Repair Regen. 2018;26(1):64–8.
14. Keys KA, Daniali LN, Warner KJ, Mathes DW. Multivariate predictors of failure after flap coverage of pressure ulcers. Plast Reconstr Surg. 2010;125(6):1725–34.
15. Cushing CA, Phillips LG. Evidence-based medicine: pressure sores. Plast Reconstr Surg. 2013;132(6):1720–32.
16. Marin J, Nixon J, Gorecki C. A systematic review of risk factors for the development and recurrence of pressure ulcers in people with spinal cord injuries, vol. 51. Spinal Cord; 2013. p. 522–7.
17. Kwok AC, Simpson AM, Willcockson J, Donato DP, Goodwin IA, Agarwal JP. Complications and their associations following the surgical repair of pressure ulcers. Am J Surg. 2018;216(6):1177–81.
18. McLaughlin JM, Tran JP, Hameed SA, Roach DE, Andersen CR, Zhu VZ, et al. Quality improvement intervention bundle using the PUPPIES acronym reduces pressure injury incidence in critically ill patients. Adv Skin Wound Care. 2022;35(2):102–8.
19. Tran JP, McLaughlin JM, Li RT, Phillips LG. Prevention of pressure ulcers in the acute care setting: new innovations and technologies. Plast Reconstr Surg. 2016;138(3):232S–40S.

Chapter 12
Head and Neck Anatomy/Function

Alice Yu, Josh Hwang, and Kristen Echanique

Anatomy and Function

- *General Principles*
  - Head and neck anatomy is complex as there are many different subsites within a relatively small area.
  - Learning the significance of important landmarks and their spatial relationship to other structures is key to understanding procedures in the head and neck region.
- *Face*
  - *Bones*
    - Comprised of 22 bones
    - *Skull*: Frontal, ethmoid, sphenoid, parietal (2), occipital, temporal (2)
    - *Face*: Vomer, inferior nasal conchae (2), nasal (2), palatine (2), mandible, maxilla (2), zygomatic (2), lacrimal (2) (Fig. 12.1)
  - *Muscles*
    - *Major muscles of facial expression* include the frontalis, corrugators, procerus, zygomaticus major and minor, nasalis, orbicularis oculi and orbicularis oris, depressor labii inferioris, and depressor anguli oris. All facial muscles are powered by branches of the facial nerve (Fig. 12.2).

A. Yu · J. Hwang · K. Echanique (✉)
Department of Head and Neck Surgery, David Geffen School of Medicine, Los Angeles, CA, USA
e-mail: alyu@mednet.ucla.edu; songhonhwang@mednet.ucla.edu; kechanique@mednet.ucla.edu

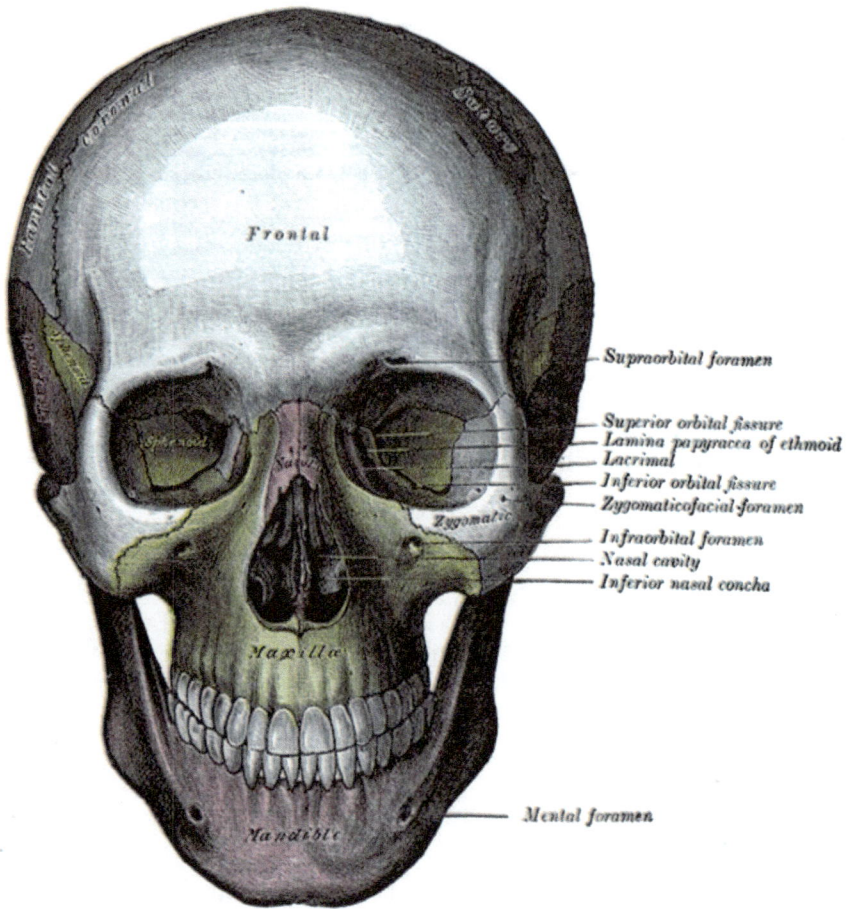

Fig. 12.1 Bony anatomy of the skull

- *Major muscles of mastication* include the temporalis, medial and lateral pterygoids, and masseters. These muscles are innervated by the mandibular branch of the trigeminal nerve (CN V3) (Fig. 12.3).
- Arteries
  - The *facial artery* supplies most of the face. It is a branch off of the external carotid artery and travels deep to the submandibular gland.
  - The *superficial temporal artery*, *occipital artery*, and *posterior auricular artery* supply blood to the scalp (Fig. 12.4).
- Veins
  - Within the parotid gland, the superficial temporal and maxillary veins merge to form the *retromandibular vein*, which splits into two portions.

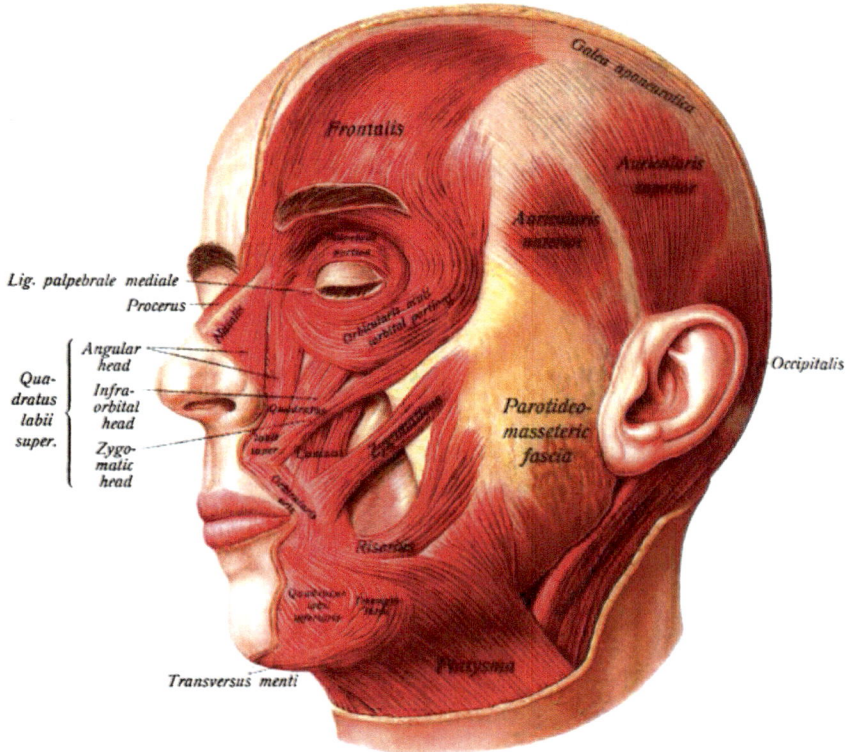

Fig. 12.2 Major muscles of the facial expression

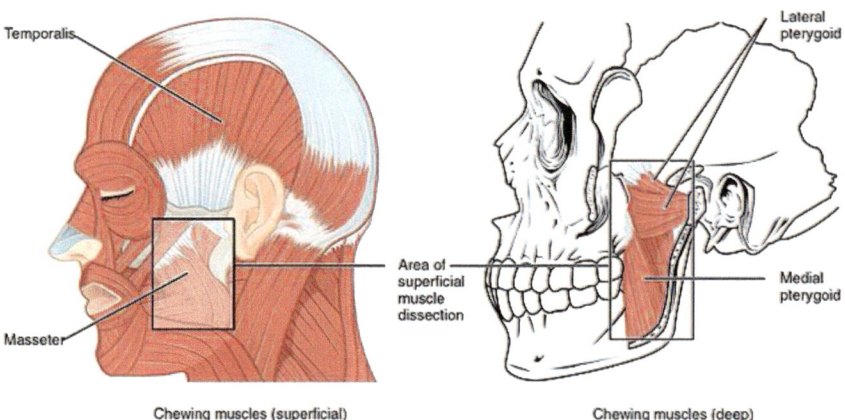

Fig. 12.3 Major muscles of mastication

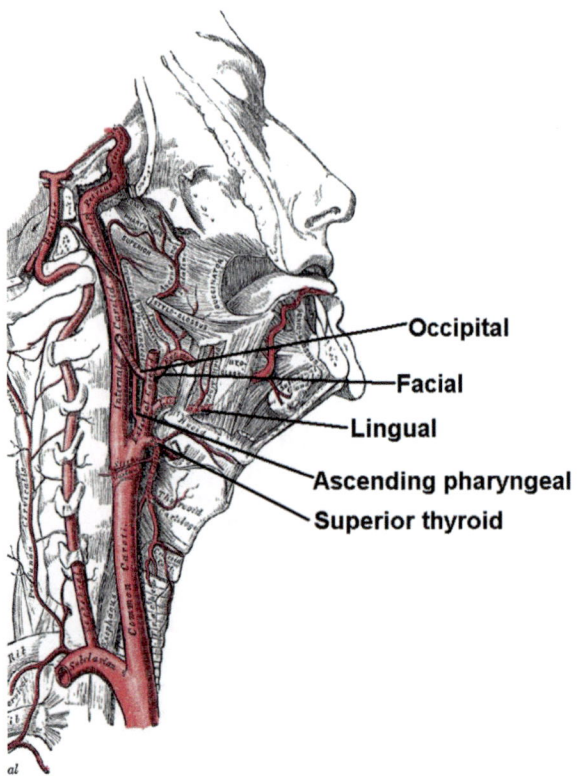

Fig. 12.4 Critical branches of the external carotid feeding the face

- The *anterior division of the retromandibular vein* merges with the *facial vein* to form the *common facial vein*, which drains into the *internal jugular vein*.
- The *posterior division of the retromandibular vein* joins the *posterior auricular vein* which drains into the *external jugular vein*, which ultimately drains into the *subclavian vein*.
- Nerves
  - Sensory innervation to the face
    - Through the *trigeminal nerve* (CN V1–3)
      - Ophthalmic division (CN V1)
        - Innervates the forehead, upper eyelids, skin overlying the nose
      - Maxillary division (CN V2)
        - Innervates the lower eyelid and upper lip to zygoma
      - Mandibular division (CN V3)

12 Head and Neck Anatomy/Function

- Innervates the lower face, scalp, and preauricular region (Fig. 12.5)
- Motor innervation to the face
  - Through the *facial nerve*, courses through the parotid gland and divides gland into superficial and deep lobes.
  - *Five main branches*: Temporal, zygomatic, buccal, marginal mandibular, and cervical (*To Zanzibar By Motor Car*).
  - Damage to the facial nerve along its course results in facial paralysis:
    - This is scored using the *House-Brackmann* scoring system, where 1/6 is normal facial nerve function and 6/6 is complete paralysis.
    - House-Brackmann scoring is subdivided between the five branches of the facial nerve (Fig. 12.6).
- Rough rule of thumb: Sensory nerves come medial to lateral; motor nerves come lateral to medial.
- Glands
  - *Parotid Gland*
    - Paired salivary gland that overlies the masseter muscle anteriorly and sternocleidomastoid muscle posteriorly.
    - Divided into superficial and deep lobes by the facial nerve, radiologically superficial and deep lobe separated by the retromandibular vein.

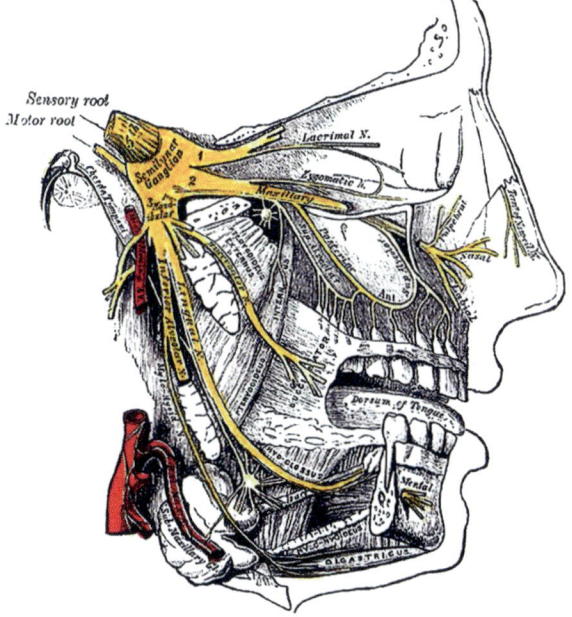

Fig. 12.5 Branching of the facial nerve

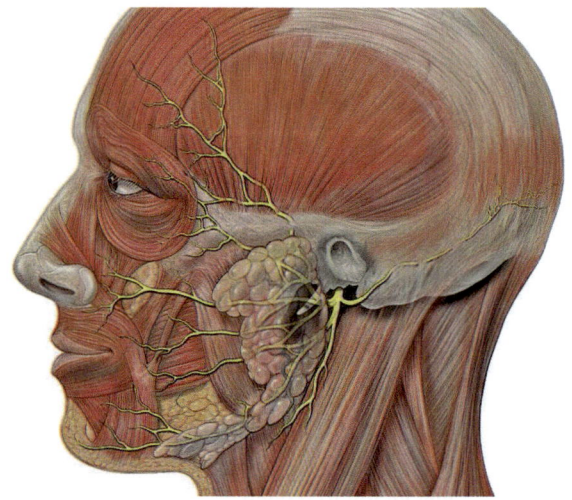

Fig. 12.6 Relationship of the facial nerve to the parotid

- *Stenson's duct* extends from gland to the buccal mucosa adjacent to the second upper molar to deliver saliva into the mouth
- Functional innervation from CN IX.
- Anatomic relationship to CN VII: Facial nerve is found between the lobes of the parotid and branches in that plane.

- *Submandibular and Sublingual Gland*
  - Submandibular gland (SMG):
    - Paired salivary glands found in the submandibular triangle.
    - Facial artery runs through the gland and exits into facial notch of the inferior mandible.
    - *Wharton's duct* extends from the gland to the floor of the mouth, opens posterior to incisors, lateral to the frenulum.
  - Sublingual gland:
    - Found in the floor of the mouth above mylohyoid muscle
    - Has multiple ducts
  - Both ducts are innervated by branches of CN VII via the lingual branch of V3.

- *Orbit*
  - *Bones*: Seven bones make up the orbit—sphenoid, frontal, lacrimal, zygoma, ethmoid, maxilla, and palatine.
  - *Muscles*:
    - The muscle inserting on the upper eyelid is the levator palpebrae superioris which elevates the eyelid.

- The muscles attaching to the sclera include the superior rectus, inferior rectus, medial rectus, lateral rectus, superior oblique, and inferior oblique.
- *Artery*: The main artery of the orbit is the ophthalmic branch of the internal carotid artery.
- *Vein*: The main venous supply of the orbit is the ophthalmic venous plexus.
  - It communicates with the facial vein, cavernous sinus, and the pterygoid venous plexus.
- *Nerves of the orbit*:
  - Sensory innervation
    - *Lacrimal nerve*
      - Sensation to the lateral eyelid
    - *Frontal nerve*
      - Divides into:
        - Supraorbital nerve
          - Sensation to the skin of the forehead lateral to supratrochlear territory
          - Sensation to frontal sinuses
        - Supratrochlear nerve
          - Sensation to the skin of the forehead
    - *Nasociliary nerve*
      - Sensation to the skin of the nose, sphenoid and ethmoid sinuses
  - Visual perception: *Optic nerve* (CN II)
    - Transmits visual information through fibers that decussate at optic chiasm→ send to optic tract on opposite side
    - Further detail beyond scope of this review
  - Motor innervation
    - CN III—*Oculomotor nerve*
      - Innervates levator palpebrae superioris, inferior oblique, superior rectus, inferior rectus, medial rectus
    - CN IV—*Trochlear nerve*
      - Innervates superior oblique
    - CN VI—*Abducens nerve*
      - Innervates lateral rectus

- *Oral Cavity*
    - The first part of the digestive system, the oral cavity plays an important role in the intake and digestion of food as well as in respiration and speech formation.
    - Boundaries:
        - Anterior: Lips
        - Posterior: Palatoglossal muscles
        - Superior: Hard and soft palate
        - Inferior: Mylohyoid muscle
        - Lateral: Buccinator muscles
    - The oral cavity is subdivided into an anterior and posterior part by the alveolar processes containing the teeth:
        - *Oral vestibule*: Region between the lips/cheek and the teeth
        - *Oral cavity proper*: Region behind the teeth, including the hard palate as well as the tongue
    - Subsites: oral tongue, buccal mucosa, hard palate floor of the mouth, retromolar trigone, lips, alveolar ridge
- *Tongue*
    - *Muscles*: Divided into extrinsic and intrinsic muscles. The intrinsic muscles make up the bulk of the tongue, while the extrinsic muscles help to move the tongue:
        - *Extrinsic*: Genioglossus, hyoglossus, styloglossus, and palatoglossus
        - *Intrinsic*: Transverse, vertical, superior, and inferior longitudinal muscles (Fig. 12.7)
    - *Innervation*
        - *Motor*: Motor innervation of all the intrinsic and extrinsic muscles of the tongue, except the palatoglossus, comes from the *hypoglossal nerve* (CN XII). The palatoglossus nerve is innervated by the *vagus nerve* (CN X).
        - *Sensory*: The anterior two-thirds receive general sensory innervation from the *lingual nerve*, a branch of CN V3, while taste sensation is via the *chorda tympani nerve*, a branch of the facial nerve (CN VII). The posterior one-third of the tongue receives both general and taste sensations via the *glossopharyngeal nerve* (CN IX).
    - *Vasculature*: Lingual artery, branch of the external carotid artery.
- *Hard Palate*
    - Composed of the palatal process of the maxilla and the horizontal process of the palatine bone which forms the roof of the mouth
    - Anterior to the soft palate

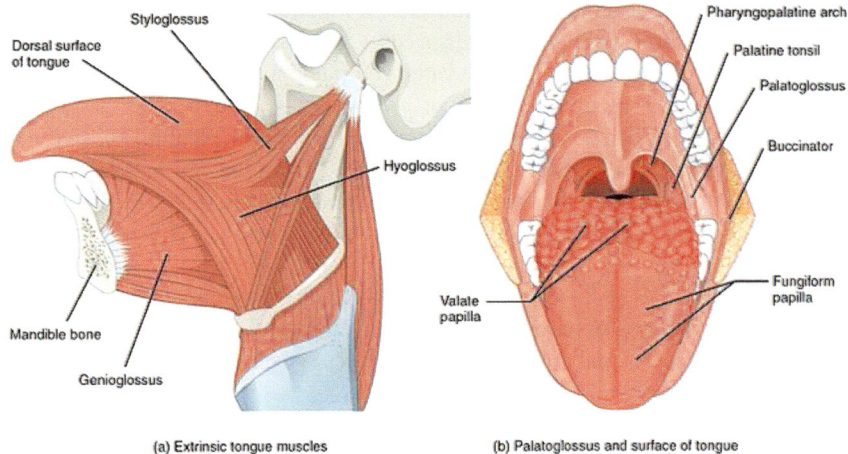

Fig. 12.7 Muscular structure of the tongue and palate

- *Innervation*: Greater palatine and nasopalatine nerves
- *Vasculature*: Greater palatine artery

- *Floor of the Mouth*: Helps to support the structures of the oral cavity. It also houses the deep submandibular glands and the sublingual gland:
  - *Muscles*: Mylohyoid, geniohyoid, genioglossus.
  - *Innervation*: The mylohyoid muscle is innervated by the inferior alveolar nerve (branch of V3); the genioglossus and geniohyoid are innervated by the hypoglossal nerve (CN XII). General sensation from the floor of the mouth is carried by the lingual branch of the mandibular nerve (CN V3).
  - *Vasculature*: Lingual artery and branches.

- *Oropharynx*
  - Connects the oral cavity to the hypopharynx and the nasopharynx to guide in food intake as well as play a role in respiration and speech
  - Boundaries:
    - Anterior: Circumvallate papillae, border of the hard and soft palate, and palatoglossus muscles
    - Posterior: Posterior pharyngeal wall
    - Superior: Soft palate
    - Inferior: Superior portion of the hyoid bone
    - Lateral: Tonsillar fossa/palatoglossus
  - Subsites: Soft palate, base of the tongue, posterior and lateral pharyngeal walls, tonsillar fossa, and palatine tonsils

- *Soft Palate*

- Composed of several different muscles; it functions to block the nasal airway during swallowing and facilitate speech.
- *Muscles*: Tensor veli palatini, levator veli palatini, palatoglossus, palatopharyngeus, and musculus uvulae.
- *Innervation*: All the muscles, except the tensor veli palatini, receive their innervation from the vagus nerve (CN X). The tensor veli palatini is innervated by the mandibular branch of the trigeminal nerve (CN V3).
- *Vasculature*: Ascending palatine artery, which is a branch of the facial artery

- *Lateral Pharyngeal Wall of the Oropharynx*
  - *Muscles*: Palatoglossus and palatopharyngeus muscles.
  - *Innervation*: The palatoglossus and palatopharyngeus muscles are innervated by the vagus nerve (CN X).
  - *Vasculature*: The palatoglossus muscle is supplied mainly by the lingual artery and by some branches of the facial artery. The palatopharyngeus muscle is supplied by branches of the facial, ascending pharyngeal, and internal maxillary artery.

- *Palatine Tonsils:* Collection of encapsulated lymphatic tissue that is bordered anteriorly and posteriorly by the palatoglossus and palatopharyngeus pillars, respectively
  - *Innervation*: Palatoglossus and palatopharyngeus muscle are innervated by the vagus nerve, and the superior constrictor is innervated by the glossopharyngeal and vagus nerve.
  - *Vasculature*: Ascending palatine and tonsillar arteries (branches of facial artery), ascending pharyngeal artery, greater palatine and descending palatine arteries (branches of internal maxillary artery), and the dorsal lingual branch of the lingual artery.
  - *Base of the Tongue*: Consists of the posterior third of the tongue behind the circumvallate papillae. The *lingual tonsils* reside here.

- *Hypopharynx*
  - The hypopharynx is the region surrounding the larynx that connects the oropharynx to the upper portion of the cervical esophagus.
  - *Boundaries*:
    - Anterior: Larynx
    - Posterior: Retropharyngeal space
    - Superior: Hyoid bone
    - Inferior: Cricopharyngeus muscle (upper esophageal sphincter)
  - *Subsites*: Piriform sinus, posterior pharyngeal wall, postcricoid region
    - *Piriform sinus*: Located lateral to the esophageal inlet on either side and medial to the thyroid cartilage, this sinus is shaped like an inverted pyra-

mid. Clinically, this subsite is important because it is the most common site for hypopharyngeal cancer. It is also a common place for food or other ingested foreign objects to become stuck.

- *Nose*
  - External nasal skin divided into subunits: nasal dorsum, nasal sidewalls (2), nasal tip, columella, nasal ala (2), soft tissue triangles
- *Nasal Cavity*
  - Boundaries:
  - Anterior: *nasal vestibule*
  - Posterior: *choanae* posteriorly
  - Medial: *septum*
  - Lateral: *lateral nasal walls* and *maxillary sinus antrum*
  - Superior: frontal, ethmoid, and sphenoid bones
  - Inferior: the palatine process of the maxilla and the horizontal plate of the palatine (Fig. 12.8)

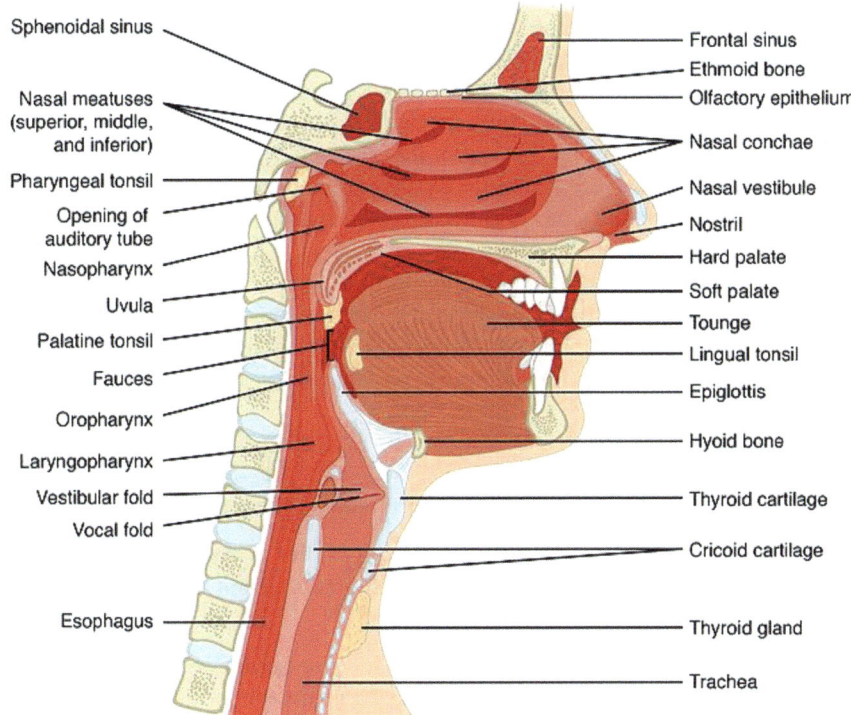

Fig. 12.8 Muscles of the nasopharynx and oropharynx

- *Lateral Nasal Wall*
  - *Turbinates (Conchae)*: paired bony projections covered in erectile mucosa that mainly functions to direct, humidify, and filter airflow
  - *Inferior Turbinate*: largest of the three turbinates, distinct
  - *Middle Turbinate*: Part of the ethmoid bone, may contain neuroepithelium and contribute to olfaction
  - *Superior Turbinate*: Part of the ethmoid bone, likely contains neuroepithelium and contributes to olfaction in the majority of people
  - *Meatuses*: Distinct air spaces underneath the turbinates
    - *Inferior Meatus*: Drains the nasolacrimal duct, location of Hasner's valve
    - *Middle Meatus*: Drains the frontal, anterior ethmoid, and maxillary sinuses
    - *Superior Meatus*: Drains the posterior ethmoid and sphenoid sinuses
- *Paranasal Sinuses*: Four, paired, air-filled spaces involving the different bones surrounding the nasal cavity. Thought to decrease the weight of the skull, to provide resonance for voice, and to buffer against facial trauma:
  - *Maxillary Sinus*: Located underneath the orbit and above the mouth and is the largest paranasal sinus.
  - *Frontal Sinus*: Located in the frontal bone, it is the anterior most sinus. It is divided into the right and left frontal sinus by the frontal septum. Embryologically is the last to develop. The anatomy of the frontal sinus is highly variable.
  - *Ethmoid Sinus*: Located between the eyes on both sides of the septum, the ethmoid cells make up the roof of the nasal cavity. Typically, there are three to four air cells present at birth. By adulthood, there are around 10–15 paired cells. The ethmoid sinus is divided into an anterior and posterior division by the *basal lamella of the middle turbinate*.
  - *Sphenoid Sinus*: Located centrally on the sphenoid bone, it is the posterior most sinus and is divided by the intersphenoid septum. It is typically not present at birth and matures by adolescence. It is in close proximity to several important structures, including the *carotid artery*, the *optic nerve*, and the *pituitary gland*.
- *Neck*
  - The neck is subdivided into the anterior and posterior triangles:
    - *Anterior Triangle*: Borders are inferior border of mandible, posterior border of SCM, and midline raphe of the neck. Comprised of four smaller triangles:
      - *Submandibular*: Boundaries are inferior border of mandible, anterior and posterior bellies of digastric. Contains submandibular gland, facial artery and vein, and CN XII
      - *Muscular*: Boundaries are superior omohyoid, midline of the neck, posterior border of SCM. Contains strap muscles

- *Carotid*: Superior omohyoid, posterior digastric muscle, posterior border of SCM. Contains carotid artery and IJV
- *Submental*: Anterior bellies of digastric and hyoid bone (Fig. 12.9)

- *Posterior Triangle*: Boundaries are posterior border of SCM, clavicle, and anterior border of trapezius muscle. Comprised of two smaller triangles:
  - *Occipital*: Boundaries are inferior omohyoid, anterior border of trapezius, and posterior border of SCM.
  - *Supraclavicular (subclavian)*: Boundaries are posterior border of SCM, clavicle, and inferior omohyoid.

- *Neck dissection levels*: Commonly, dissections of the neck are broken down into levels. Different cancers metastasize to different levels, and selective neck dissections for regional control of tumor spread may involve one or many of these levels:
  - 1A: *Submental*—between the anterior belly of the digastric. Superiorly bounded by mandible and inferiorly by hyoid.
  - 1B: *Submandibular*—between the anterior and posterior bellies of digastric and mandible.
  - II: *Upper jugular*—between the hyoid or carotid bifurcation and skull base. CN XI divides II into IIa (anterior to CN XI) and IIb (posterior to CN XI).
  - III: *Middle jugular*—between the cricoid or omohyoid to hyoid or carotid bifurcation.
  - IV: *Lower jugular*—between the clavicle and cricoid or omohyoid.

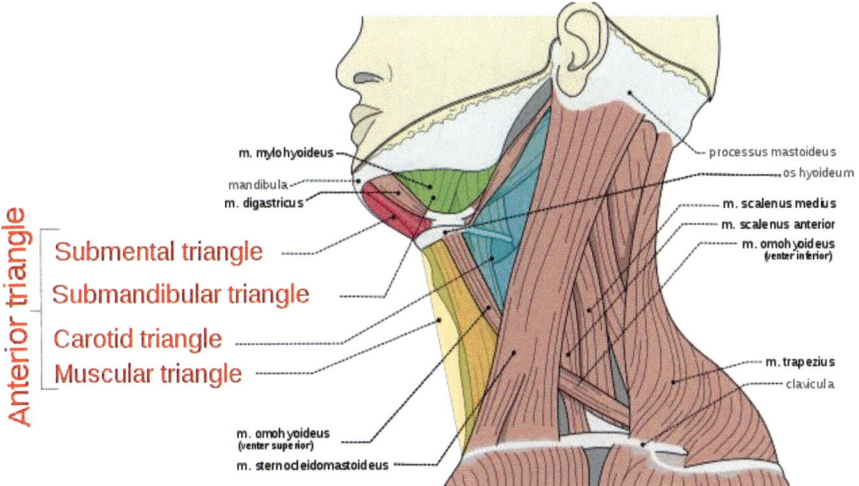

Fig. 12.9 Triangles of the neck

- V: *Posterior triangle*—between the posterior border of SCM, trapezius, and clavicle. Va is superior to omohyoid; Vb is inferior to omohyoid.
- VI: *Anterior neck/central compartment*—between carotid sheaths.
- VII: *Superior mediastinum* suprasternal notch to anterior mediastinum (Fig. 12.10).

– Highlighted Muscles of the Neck

- *Platysma*: Innervated by CN VII, the most superficial muscle in the neck, differentiate from SCM as it runs medial to lateral direction.
- *Sternocleidomastoid* (SCM): Innervated by CN XI. Fibers run lateral to medial, from mastoid tip to sternum and clavicular heads.
- *Infrahyoid strap muscles*: Innervated by ansa cervicalis

    – Mnemonic *TOSS*:

    - *T*hyrohyoid
    - *O*mohyoid
    - *S*ternohyoid
    - *S*ternothyroid

– Vasculature of the Neck

- Arteries

    – Common carotid artery divides into two main branches at carotid bifurcation:

    - The *external carotid artery* is the anterior branch of the common carotid artery:

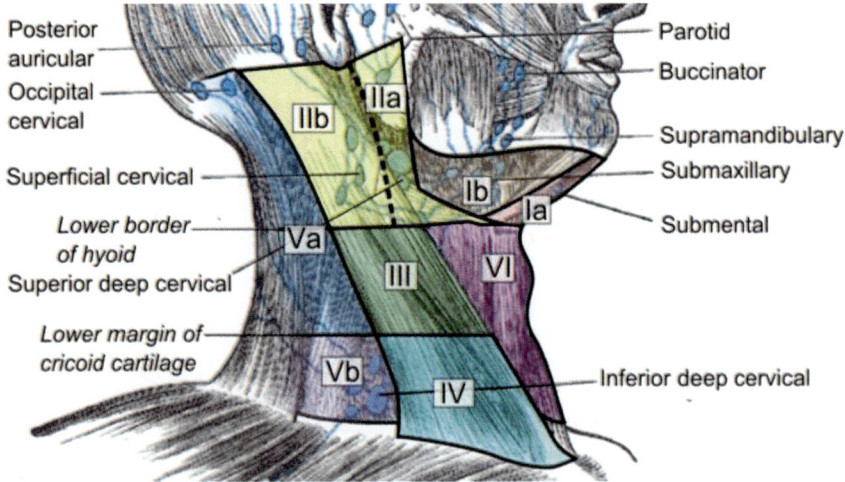

Fig. 12.10 Lymph node basins of the neck

- Branches: mnemonic SALFOPMS (Some Attendings Like Freaking Out Poor Medical Students)
- Branches in order from inferior to superior
- *S*uperior thyroid, *A*scending pharyngeal, *L*ingual, *F*acial, *O*ccipital, *P*osterior auricular, *M*axillary, and *S*uperficial temporal arteries
  - The *internal carotid artery* is the posterior branch of the common carotid artery:
    - No branches in the neck
- The *thyrocervical trunk* is a branch of the subclavian artery:
  - Gives off *inferior thyroid artery, suprascapular artery, ascending and transverse cervical arteries*
- *Subclavian artery*:
  - Gives off thyrocervical trunk
- Veins: Anterior jugular vein, external jugular vein, internal jugular vein, and subclavian vein
- *Major Nerves of the Neck*
  - *Ansa cervicalis*: innervates infrahyoid strap muscles, except the thyrohyoid
  - *Phrenic nerve*: innervate the diaphragm. From C3-C4-C5 (*3-4-5 keep the diaphragm alive*)
  - *Greater auricular nerve*: sensory innervation to the ear as well as skin over parotid and mastoid process
  - *Facial nerve (CN VII)*
    - Innervates muscles of facial expression, digastric, auricular muscles, platysma. Chorda tympani branch responsible for anterior $2/3$ of tongue taste
    - Mnemonic for main branches: *To Zanzibar By Motor Car (Temporal, Zygomatic, Buccal, Marginal Mandibular, Cervical)*
  - *Vagus nerve (CN X)*: vagus, travels within carotid sheath between IJ and carotid. Innervates many muscles, importantly gives off recurrent laryngeal nerve (RLN) to innervate the larynx, as well as innervates many muscles of the pharynx
  - *Spinal accessory nerve (CN XI)*: innervates SCM and trapezius
  - *Hypoglossal nerve (CN XII)*: innervates intrinsic and extrinsic tongue musculature, except palatoglossus
- *Thyroid gland*: Two lobes connected by the thyroid isthmus, which lies atop the second to fourth tracheal rings. It is tethered to the trachea on either side by *Berry's ligament*. Arteries: superior and inferior thyroid arteries. Veins: superior, middle, and inferior veins

- *Parathyroids*: Generally four, located posterior to the thyroid gland. Can present ectopically (esophagus, throughout the neck):
  - Superior parathyroid glands: deep to the RLN
  - Inferior glands: superficial to the RLN
- *Trachea*
  - Anterior: made up of cartilaginous rings (incomplete, C-shaped)
  - Posterior: trachealis muscle
- *Esophagus*
  - Divided into cervical esophagus, thoracic esophagus, abdominal esophagus
  - Arterial supply: inferior thyroid artery (upper third), esophageal branches off the thoracic aorta (middle third), branches off left gastric (lower third)
- *Larynx*
  - *Cartilages* (9): thyroid, cricoid, epiglottis, arytenoid (2), corniculate (2), cuneiform cartilages (2)
  - *Muscles*:
    - Abductor:
      - Posterior cricoarytenoid, the only abductor of the larynx
    - Adductors:
      - Thyroarytenoid, cricothyroid, posterior cricoarytenoid, transverse arytenoid/interarytenoid, vocalis muscle
  - *Nerves*: Recurrent laryngeal nerve (RLN) innervates all muscles of the larynx except for the cricothyroid, supplied by superior laryngeal nerve (SLN).
    - Injury to SLN during surgery results in difficulty tensing and elongating cords, producing high-pitch voice
- *Fascial Planes of the Face*
  - The entire body has deep and superficial fascial systems.
  - Superficial Fascia
    - Galea in the scalp -> temporoparietal fascia -> superficial muscular aponeurotic system/muscles of facial expression -> platysma
  - Deep Fascia
    - Periosteum in the scalp ->deep temporal fascia ->parotid/masseteric fascia->cervical fascia

- Highlighted Cranial Nerves
  - *V: Trigeminal nerve.* V1 (ophthalmic), V2 (maxillary), V3 (mandibular). These three branches emerge from the skull base through the three foramen: superior orbital fissure, rotundum, and ovale, respectively (*Standing Room Only*)
  - *VII: Facial nerve*
    - Mnemonic: *To Zanzibar By Motor Car (Temporal, Zygomatic, Buccal, Marginal Mandibular, Cervical)*
  - *X: Vagus nerve*
    - *Superior laryngeal nerve*: Supplies internal mucosa of the larynx and the *cricothyroid muscle* (tenses vocal folds to produce sound)
    - *Recurrent laryngeal nerve*: Innervates all muscles of the larynx except cricothyroid. Runs in tracheoesophageal groove. On the L side, wraps around the aortic arch while on the R side wraps around R subclavian vein. Most commonly damaged in thyroid surgery
  - *XI: Spinal accessory nerve.* Innervates SCM and trapezius muscles
  - *XII: Hypoglossal nerve*: Innervates intrinsic and extrinsic muscles of the tongue with exception of palatoglossus. Found under the digastric muscle and mylohyoid muscle

Suggested Reading

1. Bailey BJ. Head & neck surgery—otolaryngology. 4th ed. Philadelphia: Lippincott Williams & Wilkins; 2006.
2. Hansen JT, et al. Netter's clinical anatomy. 4th ed. Philadelphia: Elsevier; 2019.
3. Robbins KT, et al. Neck dissection classification update: revisions proposed by the American Head and Neck Society and the American Academy of Otolaryngology–Head and Neck Surgery. Arch Otolaryngol Head Neck Surg. 2002;128(7):751–8.
4. Lalwani AK. Current diagnosis & treatment otolaryngology—head and neck surgery. McGraw Hill; 2020.

Chapter 13
Cleft Lip and Palate

Brendan J. Cronin

Epidemiology

- Cleft lip with or without cleft palate (CLP) and isolated cleft palate (CP) are genetically, embryologically, and anatomically distinct entities.
- They have distinct patterns of etiology, incidence, racial/gender distributions, and associated genetic factors (Table 13.1).
- Identifying these differences is key for additional clinical workup, genetic counseling, and operative management.

B. J. Cronin (✉)
Division of Plastic and Reconstructive Surgery, University of California, Los Angeles, CA, USA

Table 13.1 Comparing the epidemiologic factors of cleft lip and palate with isolated cleft palate

	CLP	CP
Incidence	1/700	1/1500
Gender distribution	M:F = 2:1	F:M = 3:2
Incidence varies by ethnicity	Asian/white/black 4:2:1	No difference
Laterality	Left/right/bilateral 6:3:1	N/A
Syndromic?	15%	50%
Risk for future pregnancies		
One parent or child affected.	4%	2%
Two prior children affected.	9%	6%
One parent one child affected.	17%	15%

Pathogenesis

- *Environmental teratogens*
  - Intrauterine phenytoin exposure (x10 risk), maternal smoking (x2 risk), EtOH, retinoic acid
- *Genetic factors*
  - *Non-syndromic*—characterized by single defect or anomalies from single inciting event/malformation
    - Secondary to multiple gene interactions or gene-environment interactions
    - *Pierre Robin sequence* (micrognathia, glossoptosis, airway obstruction); frequently, also see *wide,* U-shaped cleft palate:
      - Cleft palate is *not* part of the diagnostic criteria for Pierre Robin.
  - *Syndromic*—defects across multiple developmental "fields".
    - Often due to mutations in specific named genes.
    - *Van der Woude*—IRF 22 gene, autosomal dominant, associated with CLP/CP and lip pits.
    - *Stickler*—mutation in collagen formation; cleft palate, ocular abnormalities, hearing loss.
    - *22q11—"DiGeorge" syndrome*: cleft palate, immunocompromised, hypocalcemia, cardiac abnormalities, velopharyngeal insufficiency (VPI)

13 Cleft Lip and Palate

Embryology

- *General Overview*
  - Facial structures are derived from the frontonasal prominences (comprised of medial and lateral nasal prominences), maxillary prominences, and mandibular prominences (Fig. 13.1):
    - Medial nasal prominence —> nasal tip, columella, philtrum.
    - Lateral nasal prominence —> nasal ala.
    - Maxillary prominences —> upper lip lateral to philtrum.
    - Mandibular prominences —> lower lip and mandible.
- *Lip formation*:
  - Upper lip—composite structure of the philtrum (fused medial nasal prominences) + lateral lip elements (maxillary prominences).
- *Palate formation*:
  - Primary palate—consists of the lip, nostril sill, alveolus, and hard palate anterior to the incisive foramen.
    - Formed from the fusion of the medial nasal prominences which gives rise to the outer *labial* element and bony *palatal* component.

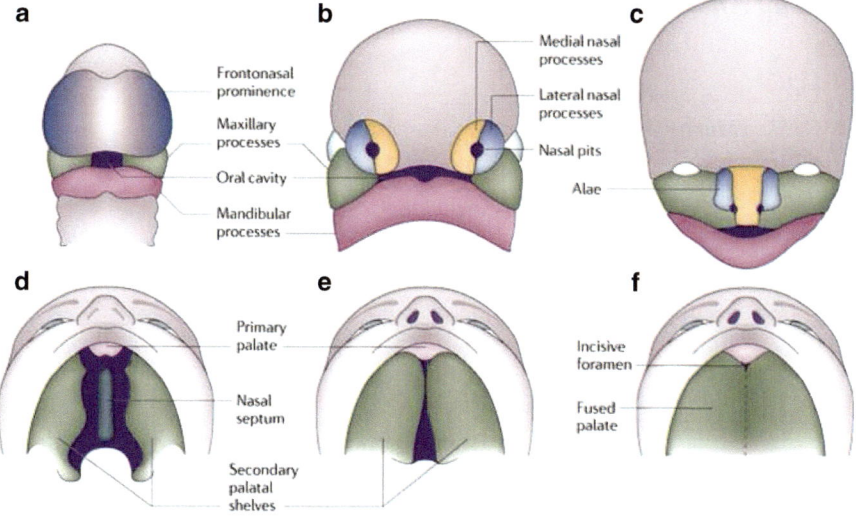

Fig. 13.1 Embryological origin of the upper lip and palate. (Dixon, M., Marazita, M., Beaty, T. et al. Cleft lip and palate: understanding genetic and environmental influences. *Nat Rev Genet* 12, 167–178 (2011). https://doi.org/10.1038/nrg2933. https://www.nature.com/articles/nrg2933. Permission license number: 5334481445012)

Table 13.2 Clefts resulting from failed fusion of facial structures

Failure to fuse (structures)	Result
Medial nasal prominences	Median cleft lip
Medial nasal prominence + maxillary prominence	Unilateral CL
Medial + lateral palatine processes	Primary cleft palate
Lateral palatine processes	Secondary cleft palate

- Secondary palate—consists of the hard palate posterior to the incisive foramen and soft palate:
  - Formed from fusion of outgrowths of the paired maxillary processes (these outgrowths are called the *lateral palatine shelves*).
  - Fuse in anterior to posterior fashion with the nasal septum to form the hard and subsequently soft palate.
- *Failure of fusion of certain structures and resulting clefts* (Table 13.2).

Anatomy

Normal Anatomy

- *Lip*.
  - *Skin/Mucosa*—see Fig. 13.2.
  - *Muscle*:
    - Orbicularis oris—two distinct components:
      - *Deep*—runs from modiolus to modiolus and acts as oral sphincter to maintain oral competence.
      - *Superficial*—has two components:
        - *Peripheralis*—runs obliquely and interdigitates with other muscles of facial expression:
          - Insertion into the dermis at the contralateral lip creates the vertical bulge of the philtral columns.
        - *Marginalis* (runs within dry vermilion, functions in lip eversion/tubercle formation).
    - Levator labii superioris:
      - Inserts onto white roll, defines the lateral element of peak of Cupid's bow, elevates the lip.

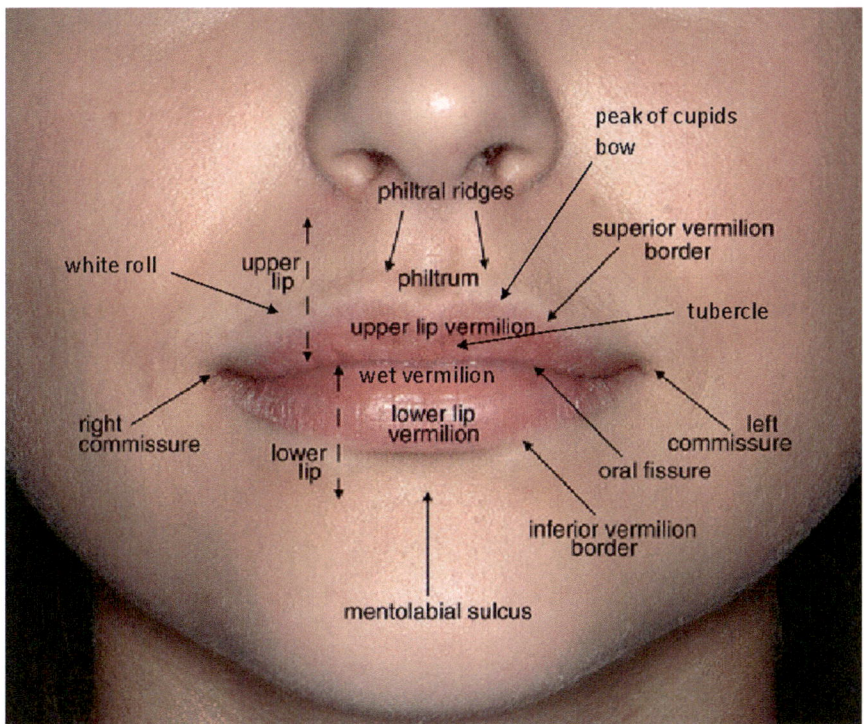

Fig. 13.2 Normal lip anatomy. (Modified from "von Arx T., Lozanoff S. (2017) Oral Fissure and Lips. In: Clinical Oral Anatomy. Springer, Cham. Figure 2.1. https://doi.org/10.1007/978-3-319-41993-0_2". Permissions: 5334490119079)

- *Blood supply*:
  - Labial artery—travels posterior to the orbicularis anterior to the mucosa.
- *Innervation*:
  - Sensory: V3 (lower lip) and V2 (upper lip).
  - Motor: CN VII (facial).
- Palate
  - *Hard palate*:
    - Primary palate—premaxillary portion of the maxilla.
    - Secondary palate—palatine processes of the maxilla and palatine bone.
  - *Soft palate*—Paired muscles function to elevate and depress the palate and seal off the nasopharynx for speech and swallowing (Fig. 13.3):
    - Levator veli palatini—elevates the palate (CN X).

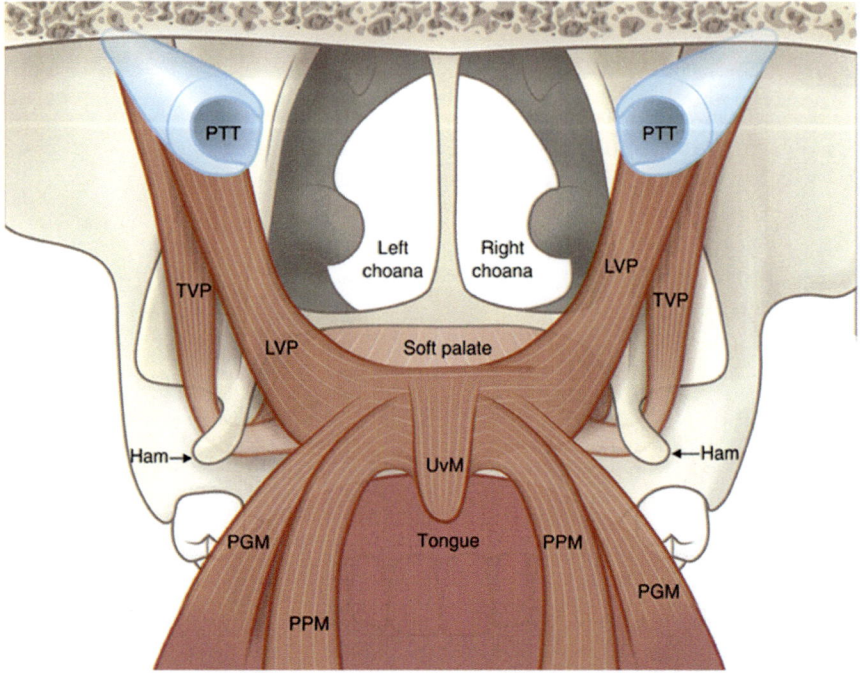

Fig. 13.3 Muscles of the velum. (von Arx T., Lozanoff S. (2017) Hard and Soft Palate. In: Clinical Oral Anatomy. Springer, Cham. https://doi.org/10.1007/978-3-319-41993-0_10. Permissions: 5333701236505)

- Tensor veli palatini—opens eustachian tube (CN V).
- Muscular uvulae—retracts and shortens uvula (CN X).
- Palatoglossus—depresses the palate (CN X).
- Palatopharyngeus—depresses the palate (CN X).
- Superior pharyngeal constrictor—causes inward movement of lateral pharyngeal walls (CN X).
- *Blood supply and innervation* (Fig. 13.4):
  - Blood supply.
    - Hard palate.
      - Paired greater palatine arteries (maxillary artery — > descending palatine artery).
      - Sphenopalatine artery.
    - Soft palate.
      - Lesser palatine arteries (maxillary), ascending pharyngeal artery (external carotid), ascending palatine branch of the facial artery.

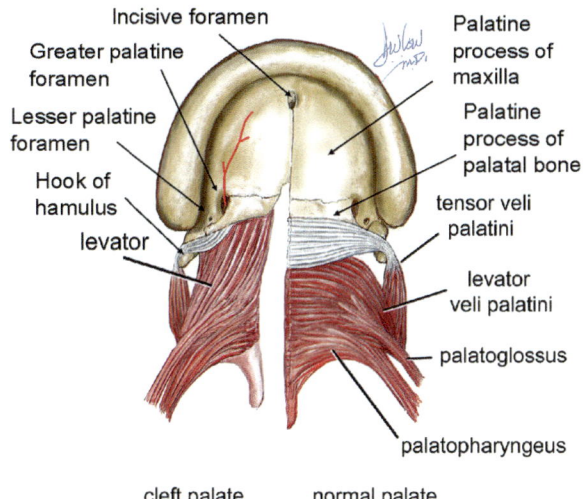

Fig. 13.4 Anatomy of the normal and cleft palate. (da Silva Freitas, R., Nasser, I.J.G., Zimmerman, C., Lupion, F.G. (2021). Patterns, Anatomy, and Classification of Clefts. In: Swanson, J.W. (eds) Global Cleft Care in Low-Resource Settings. Springer, Cham. Figure 5.11. https://doi.org/10.1007/978-3-030-59105-2_5. Permissions: 5334490410049)

- Innervation.
  - Premaxilla—nasopalatine nerve.
  - Hard palate—greater palatine nerve.
  - Soft palate—lesser palatine nerve.

Cleft Anatomy and Classifications

Key Anatomical Aberrances of the Cleft Lip

- *Lip*
  - Shortened vertical lip height, "cleft" or "lateral" element with transverse deficiency and hypoplastic orbicularis.
  - "Non-cleft" or "medial" element with trough and lateral peak of Cupid's bow, philtral column and philtral dimple
- *Orbicularis.*
  - Superficial fibers are disrupted and have abnormal insertions into philtral column ("non-cleft" side) and alar base ("cleft" side) that contribute to nasal deformity (below).
  - Deep fibers are disrupted but do not have abnormal insertions.

- Prolabium (bilateral cleft) contains no muscle fibers.
- *Alveolar cleft*
  - Unilateral vs bilateral, complete vs incomplete, wide vs narrow, collapse vs no collapse.
- *Spectrum of cleft lip deformity* (Table 13.3).
- *Cleft lip nasal deformity* (Fig. 13.5).
  - Aberrant insertion of orbicularis + hypoplastic ipsilateral maxillary segment and posteriorly displaced piriform rim on cleft side — > lateral and superior

Table 13.3 Spectrum of cleft lip

Deformity	Description and treatment
Mini-micro*	Disrupted vermilion cutaneous junction without elevation of cupid's bow peak; lenticular excision
Microform	<3 mm above cupid's bow peak; double z-plasty
Minor form	>3 mm above cupid's bow peak; rotation advancement
Simonart's band	Vertical separation of lip with *intact* vertical sill, rotation advancement (Rx the same as *complete* cleft lip, may actually be a more challenging repair)
Incomplete cleft lip	Cleft lip without Simonart's band but intact alveolar ridge; rotation advancement
Complete cleft lip	Cleft of the lip and alveolus; rotation advancement
Bilateral incomplete	Near normal nose, normally position premaxilla, *Simonart's bands across the nasal floors*, clefts involving only the lip; triangle flap approach in one- or -two-stage repair
Bilateral complete	Protruding/"flyaway" premaxilla, severely decreased nasal projection, columellar skin deficiency; treatment—NAM (expand columellar skin + optimizing alignment of premaxillary and maxillary segments) + delayed repair

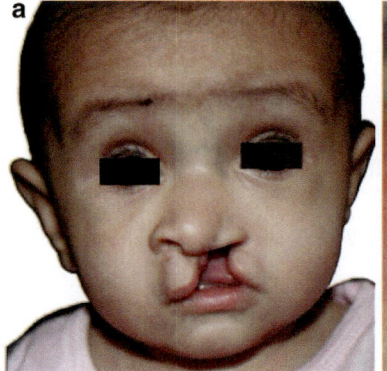
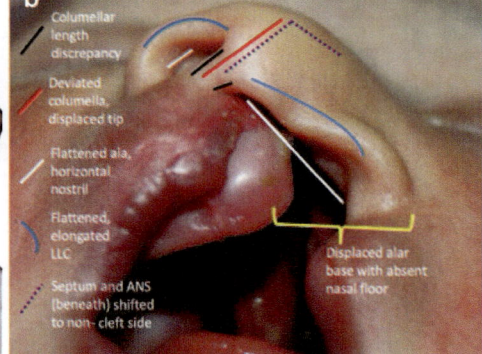

Fig. 13.5 Unilateral cleft lip nasal deformity. (Bonanthaya, K., Jalil, J. Management of the Nasal Deformity in the Unilateral Cleft of the Lip and Nose. *J. Maxillofac. Oral Surg.* 19, 332–341 (2020). Figure 1. https://doi.org/10.1007/s12663-020-01412-0. Permissions: 5334490587736)

displacement of the lateral crus of the alar base — > increased alar base width + separation of medial crus of the lower lateral cartilage from the nasal tip + concavity of the lateral crus — > decreased projection of the nasal tip and convexity of the lateral cartilage, caudal displacement of the lower lateral cartilage with alar hooding and deficient nasal lining, shortening of the columella.
- Caudal septum deviated to non-cleft side.
- Arguably more challenging to correct than the lip, often requires multiple revisions.

- *Cleft palate*
  - Primary palate—can involve any structures anterior to the incisive foramen.
    - Unilateral or bilateral and complete/incomplete.
  - Secondary palate—clefts of the hard palate posterior to incisive foramen +/− soft palate.
  - Unilateral or bilateral:
    - Nasal septum fused to non-cleft side in unilateral cleft, septum not fused to either palatal shelf in bilateral clefts.
    - Clefting results in abnormal insertion and orientation of the palatal muscles.
    - Levator—runs along cleft margin and inserts onto the posterior aspect of the hard palate (see Fig. 13.3).
- Veau classification (Fig. 13.6).
  - *Veau I*: cleft of soft palate.
  - *Veau II*: cleft of soft + hard palate.
  - *Veau III*: cleft of soft + hard palate + alveolus/lip.
  - *Veau IV*: bilateral cleft lip and palate.
  - *Submucous cleft*: no mucosal or hard palate cleft yet still have aberrant muscular insertions of the levator. Manifests as a (1) zona pellucida (white pallor of midline palatal mucosa due to the lack of muscle fibers crossing the midline); (2) notching of the hard palate (due to reactive bony protuberance of the hard palate in the areas of levator insertion, like the medial/lateral epicondyle); and (3) bifid uvula.

Treatment

Management Principles

- Standard of care includes treatment by multidisciplinary cleft care team:
  - Craniofacial orthodontist, pediatric dentist, speech pathologist, audiologist, pediatrician, genetic counselor, plastic surgeon, otolaryngologist.
- The goal is to optimize early outcomes and limit secondary surgeries (revision rhinoplasty, secondary alveolar bone grafting, maxillary/midface advancement).

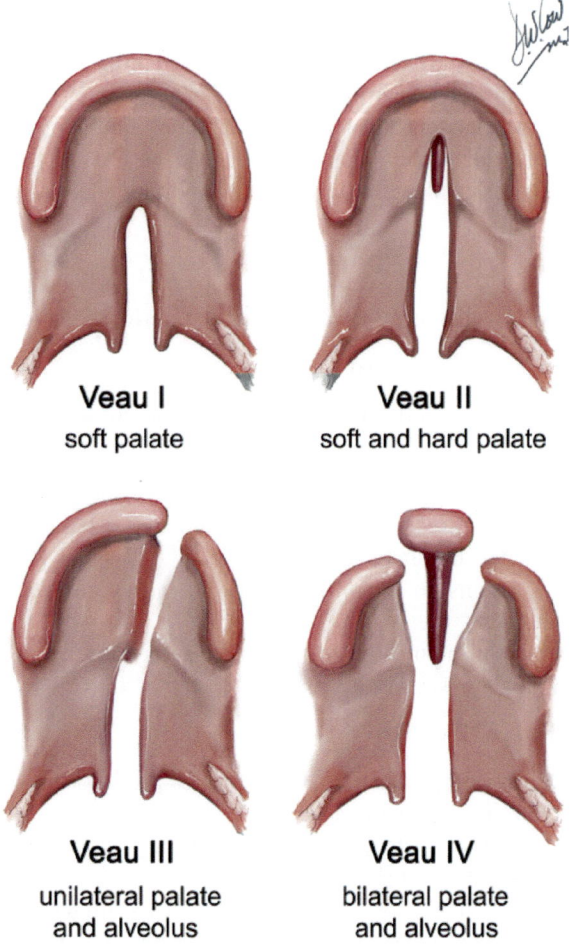

Fig. 13.6 Veau classification. (da Silva Freitas, R., Nasser, I.J.G., Zimmerman, C., Lupion, F.G. (2021). Patterns, Anatomy, and Classification of Clefts. In: Swanson, J.W. (eds) Global Cleft Care in Low-Resource Settings. Springer, Cham. Figure 5.3. https://doi.org/10.1007/978-3-030-59105-2_5. Permissions: 5334490410049)

13 Cleft Lip and Palate

Table 13.4 Sequence and timing of surgical interventions

Age	Treatment	Goal
0–3 Mons	Pre-surgical orthopedics (nasoalveolar molding/Latham device) Lip adhesion	Align maxillary segments and decrease cleft width, improve nasal form and symmetry, increase alar dome height, expand columellar skin, reposition "flyaway" premaxillary segment (bilateral clefts)
3–6 months	Cleft lip repair + primary tip rhinoplasty +/− gingivoperiosteoplasty	Restore continuity of orbicularis oris, correction of vertical lip height deficiency, correction of nasal deformity
1–2 years	Cleft palate repair	Restore velopharyngeal competence to facilitate speech development
3–4 years	VPI treatment (if present) Secondary palatal lengthening Pharyngoplasty	Ensure velopharyngeal competence (speech development, prevent oronasal reflux)
~8–12 years (mixed dentition)	Secondary alveolar bone grafting	Restore continuity of alveolar cleft to provide stable base for erupting adult dentition (lateral incisor or canine) "Primary" alveolar bone grafting is before 2 years of age
Skeletal maturity	LeFort I/midface advancement +/− orthognathic surgery	Correction of maxillary/midface hypoplasia or malocclusion
After puberty	Definitive open rhinoplasty	Correct residual cleft nasal deformity, increase nasal tip projection

Sequence and Timing of Procedures

- See Table 13.4.

Cleft Lip Repair: Goals and Techniques

Unilateral

Goals.

- Restore vertical lip height:
  - Borrow transverse length to restore vertical height.
- Reapproximate orbicularis.
- Create symmetric Cupid's bow and wet/dry vermilion.
- Correct nasal deformity.
  - *Techniques.*
  - *Straight line.*

- Edges of cleft margin are excised and reapproximated in straight-line closure; it fails to correct lip height deficiency.
- Has a limited role in correction of mini-microform clefts.
  - *Millard*
    - Rotation advancement flap (Fig. 13.7).
    - Most common repair in the USA:
      - Superior z-plasty adds lip length, and scar is placed along philtral column and preserves Cupid's bow.
    - "C" flap: columella flap, rotates to provide additional columellar skin and permits improved nasal tip projection, can also be used for creation of nasal sill
    - "A" flap: advancement flap (cleft side)
    - "R" flap: rotation flap (medial lip is rotated downward, non-cleft side)
    - "M" flap: mucosal flap used to recreate gingivolabial sulcus and nasal floor back to the incisive foramen
    - "L" flap: used to create nasal lining/nasal floor

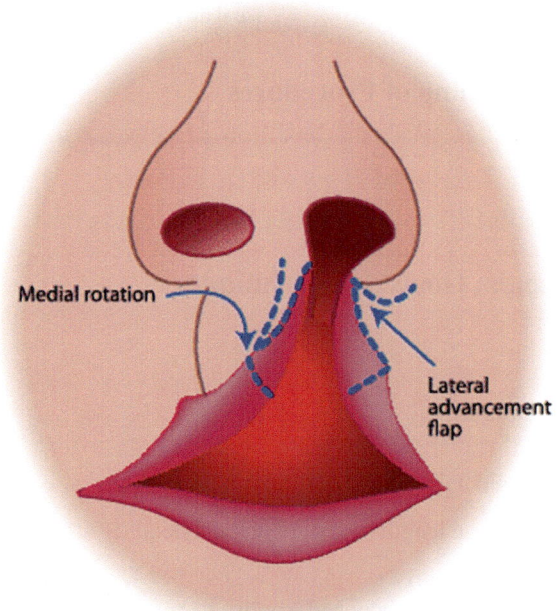

Fig. 13.7 Rotation advancement repair of the unilateral cleft lip. (Raine P.A.M. (2013) B3 Cleft Lip and Palate. In: Carachi R., Agarwala S., Bradnock T.J., Lim Tan H., Cascio S. (eds) Basic Techniques in Pediatric Surgery. Springer, Berlin, Heidelberg. Figure 1. https://doi.org/10.1007/978-3-642-20641-2_35. Permissions: 5334490683053)

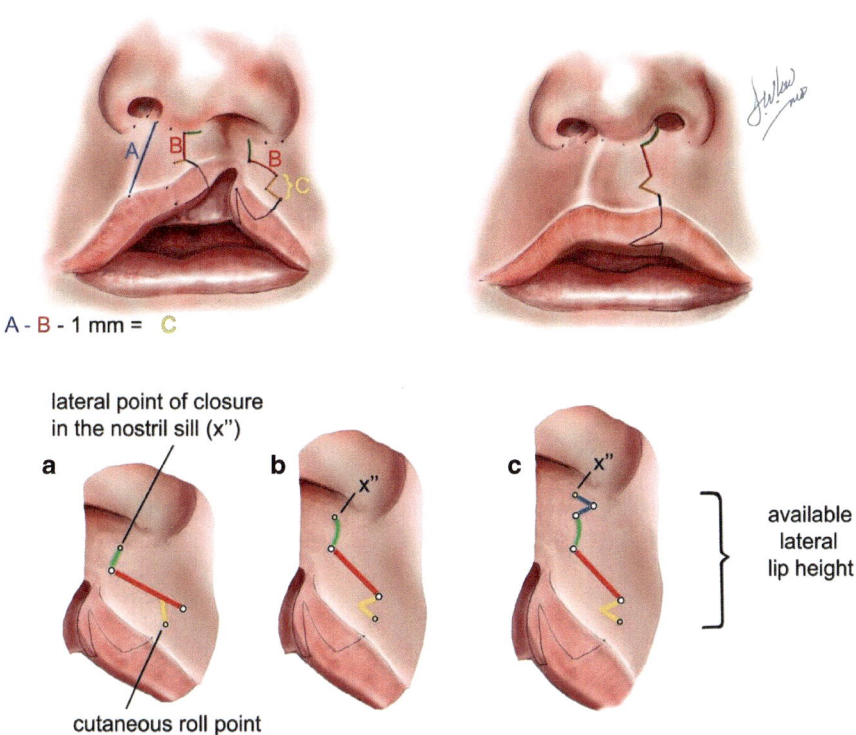

Fig. 13.8 Anatomical subunit repair (Fisher). (Tse R.W., Fisher D.M. (2021) Unilateral Cleft Lip Repair: Anatomic Subunit Approximation Technique. In: Swanson J.W. (eds) Global Cleft Care in Low-Resource Settings. Springer, Cham. Figure 13.3. https://doi.org/10.1007/978-3-030-59105-2_13. Permissions: 5334490790546)

- *Fisher*
  - Anatomical subunit repair (Fig. 13.8).
  - Incorporates a dry vermilion and cutaneous triangle from the lateral lip element that are inserted into backcuts on the medial lip element to augment lip height.
  - Height of triangle is calculated by finding the difference between the preserved philtral column and the cleft side philtral column.

Bilateral

- Goals.
  - Restore symmetric philtral columns (prolabium) and recreate Cupid's bow/tubercle.

- Reconstitute orbicularis oris across premaxilla.
- Correct nasal deformity.

Technique

- Millard (Fig. 13.9).
  - Ten-mm-tall prolabium consisting of only skin is created from the premaxillary segment:
    - Mucosa is discarded because it lacks minor salivary glands that will lead to permanently chapped lips if incorporated into repair.
  - Cupid's bow and tubercle are constructed from bilateral rotation advancement of the lateral lip elements.
  - Symmetric nasal sill wedge excisions narrow the alar base and enable reapproximation of the cleft margins.

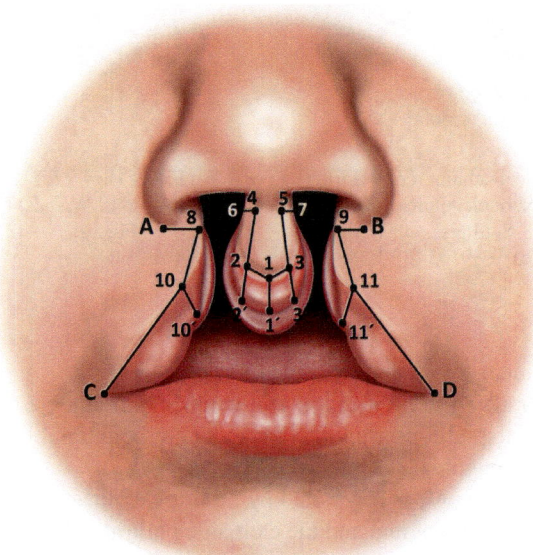

Fig. 13.9 Bilateral cleft Lip Repair. (Rossell-Perry P. (2020) Bilateral Cleft Lip Repair. In: Atlas of Operative Techniques in Primary Cleft Lip and Palate Repair. Springer, Cham. Figure 6.7. https://doi.org/10.1007/978-3-030-44681-9_6. Permissions: 5334490996016)

Cleft Palate Repair: Goals and Techniques

- *Goals.*
  - *Closure of cleft to establish velopharyngeal competence and enable normal speech*:
    - Abnormal speech pathology is intrinsic to cleft deformity due to shortened palatal length and poor palatal excursion that impair velopharyngeal closure.
    - Infants start forming first words ~13 months, repair prior to this milestone.
    - Closure of cleft involves soft tissues; there is no bony closure of the cleft.
  - *Minimize impairment of craniofacial growth*:
    - Scar from dissection during the lip/alveolus/vomer and hard palate repair leads to significant facial growth restriction (soft palate repair does not affect growth).
    - Optimal timing of repair is controversial—have to balance onset of speech and delaying dissection/scarring that impairs facial growth:
      - Typically, benefit of speech outweighs impaired facial growth as this can be corrected with orthognathic and secondary procedures later in life.
  - *Facilitate normal hearing*:
    - Incidence of hearing loss in CP is 50% secondary to eustachian tube dysfunction and recurrent otitis media, reduced with early cleft palate repair.
    - Often, children with cleft palate will require pressure equalizing tympanostomy tubes from head and neck surgeons.

Hard Palate Techniques

- *Von Langenbeck palatoplasty* (Fig. 13.10)
  - Bilateral bi-pedicled mucoperiosteal flaps:
    - Anterior pedicle: sphenopalatine artery.
    - Posterior pedicle: greater palatine artery.
  - Requires lateral relaxing incisions, which are left to heal by secondary intention.
  - Can lead to maxillary growth restriction, poor speech outcomes unless intravelar veloplasty is also performed.

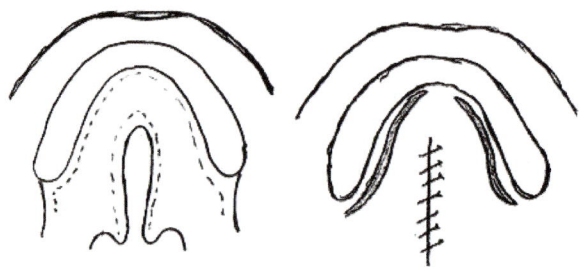

Fig. 13.10 Von Langenbeck palatoplasty. (Gwanmesia I., Griffiths M., Simmons J. (2012) Cleft Lip and Palate. In: P. Hettiaratchy S., Griffiths M., Ali F., Simmons J. (eds) Plastic Surgery. Springer, London. Figure 8.3. https://doi.org/10.1007/978-1-84882-116-3_8. Permissions: 5334491159928)

Von-Langenbeck Palatoplasty

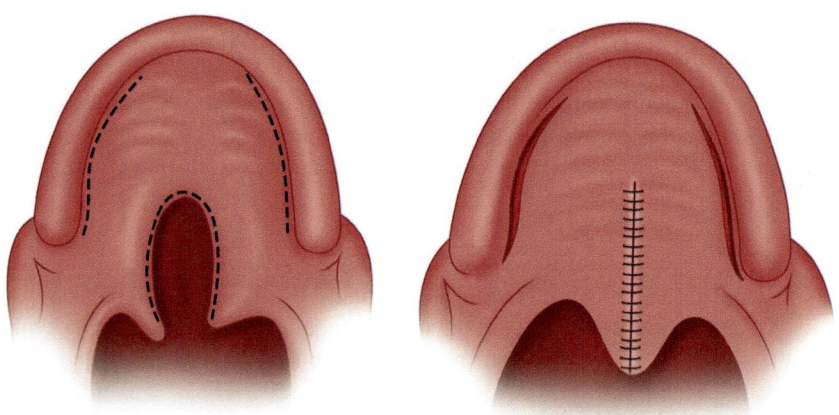

Fig. 13.11 Two-flap palatoplasty. (Morris, H.L., Bardach, J., VanDemark, D.R. et al. Results of two-flap palatoplasty with regard to speech production. *Eur. J. Plast. Surg.* 12, 19–24 (1989). https://doi.org/10.1007/BF02892640. Permissions: 5334491255944)

- *V-Y pushback*
  - Posteriorly based mucoperiosteal palatal flaps are advanced in a V-Y fashion anteriorly to add palatal length, associated with better speech outcomes.
  - Lateral areas left to heal by secondary intention, can lead to maxillary growth impairment.
- *Two-flap palatoplasty* (Fig. 13.11)
  - Most common technique.
  - Mucoperiosteal flaps are raised bilaterally as islandized flaps based posteriorly on the greater palatine arteries:

- Requires elevation of the entire palate.
- Lateral relaxing incisions allow medial advancement for cleft obliteration:
  - Good for wide clefts.
  - Can cause maxillary growth restriction.

Soft Palate Techniques

- *Intravelar veloplasty (IVV)*:
  - Dissection of abnormal levator insertion + reorientation across midline in the posterior aspect in transverse fashion to recreate the levator sling, closure of nasal and oral lining in separate layers.
- *Double-opposing z-plasty (Furlow palatoplasty)* (Fig. 13.12):
  - A two-layered z-plasty that serves to add palatal length (lengthening effect of z-plasty) and transposes muscles to recreate levator sling.
    - Z-plasty leads to shortening in transverse dimension which limits utility in wide clefts.
  - Each z-plasty contains one mucosal and one musculo-mucosal flap:
    - Anteriorly based flaps contain only mucosa; posteriorly based flaps contain muscle + mucosa.

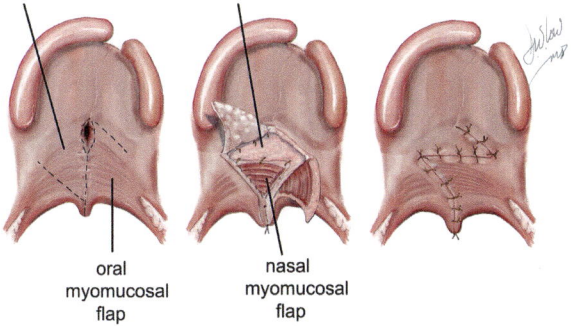

Fig. 13.12 Double-opposing z-plasty ("Furlow palatoplasty"). (Jackson O.A., Mehendale F.V. (2021) Speech Surgery and Treatment of Velopharyngeal Insufficiency. In: Swanson J.W. (eds) Global Cleft Care in Low-Resource Settings. Springer, Cham. Figure 20.9. https://doi.org/10.1007/978-3-030-59105-2_20. Permissions: 5334491365260)

Treatment Algorithm [Tse Paper]

Veau I — > Furlow palatoplasty
Veau II — > Von Langenbeck palatoplasty + IVVP
Veau III — > Two-flap palatoplasty + IVVP
Veau IV — > "Two-flap repair" + IVVP

Complications

- *Acute*: airway compromise, bleeding
- *Fistula*
- Incidence 5%
- 50% involve hard palate
- Indications for repair: VPI, oronasal reflux
- Options for repair: need to provide both *nasal and oral* lining

  - Nasal lining: "book" flaps, FAMM flap, buccal myomucosal flaps
  - Oral lining: tongue flap, alloderm, FAMM flap

- *Impaired craniofacial growth*
- Extensive palatal/maxillary dissection and scarring — > facial growth impairment — > class III occlusion with midface retrusion
- Address at the age of skeletal maturity with LeFort I advancement

- *VPI.*

  - Presents as oronasal regurgitation, hypernasal speech
  - Diagnose with nasoendoscopy
  - Treat with fat grafting, pharyngoplasty, or palatal obturator

References

1. Tse R, Lien S. Unilateral cleft lip repair using the anatomical subunit approximation: modifications and analysis of early results in 100 consecutive cases. Plast Reconstr Surg. 2015 Jul;136(1):119–30. https://doi.org/10.1097/PRS.0000000000001369.
2. Losee JE, Kirschner RE. Comprehensive cleft care. New York: McGraw-Hill Medical; 2009. Print.
3. Thorne CH, Chung KC, Gosain AK, Gurtner GC, Mehrara BJ, Rubin JP, Spear SL. *Grabb and smith's plastic surgery: seventh edition*. Wolters Kluwer Health Adis (ESP); 2013.
4. Fisher DM, Sommerlad BC. Cleft lip, cleft palate, and velopharyngeal insufficiency. Plast Reconstr Surg. 2011;128(4):342e–60e. https://doi.org/10.1097/PRS.0b013e3182268e1b.
5. Gosman AA. Selected readings in plastic surgery; vol 10, issue 16. Cleft lip and palate II: surgical management. Dallas: Southwestern; 2007.

Chapter 14
Velopharyngeal Dysfunction

Brendan J. Cronin

Background and Epidemiology

- *What is velopharyngeal competence?*
  - Velopharyngeal competence is the ability to separate the oropharyngeal and nasopharyngeal compartments.
  - Achieved by elevation of the velum and contraction of the lateral and posterior pharyngeal musculature to create a "valve" or "sphincter" to control passage of air (speech) and food (swallowing).
  - Enables phonation, prevents oronasal regurgitation, facilitates swallowing.
- *What is velopharyngeal dysfunction?*
  - Velopharyngeal dysfunction is the inability to create this adequate sphincter or valve function due to [Hopper, CME article]:
    - Velopharyngeal insufficiency (insufficient tissue or mechanical restriction).
    - Velopharyngeal incompetence (lack of neuromotor competency).
    - Velopharyngeal mislearning (maladaptive articulatory habits).
    - Oronasal fistula.
- *Why does it happen?* (Table 14.1)
  - Most commonly, VPI is due to an unrepaired cleft palate or inadequate palatal motion or length following cleft palate repair.
  - Can be due to congenital/acquired and structural or dynamic abnormalities [Gosain].

B. J. Cronin (✉)
Division of Plastic and Reconstructive Surgery, University of California, Los Angeles, CA, USA

Table 14.1 Etiologies of velopharyngeal dysfunction

Mechanism	Congenital	Acquired
Structural abnormalities		
Palatopharyngeal disproportion	Short soft palate	Following tonsillectomy/adenoidectomy
Abnormal levator anatomy	Unrepaired cleft palate, submucous cleft, cleft repair without levator reconstruction or palatal pushback	–
Dynamic abnormalities		
Upper motor neuron	Cerebral palsy, dystonias	CVA, meningitis/encephalitis, brain tumors
Nuclear	Facial paralysis	SMA, polio, AML
Muscular abnormality	Hypoplasia Repaired cleft palate. Moebius syndrome.	Muscular dystrophy, collagen diseases (scleroderma), polymyositis

- *How often do we see it?*
    - In pts. with unrepaired clefts—~100%.
    - Following cleft palate repair—20–30% [Losee CME paper, Gosain paper]:
        - Due to (1) inadequate palatal lengthening, (2) abnormal levator function (inadequate transposition on initial repair), and (3) cicatricial contracture of the velum [Gosain].
        - Depends on technique (higher rates in two-stage palate and Von-Langenbeck repairs) [Tache et al], age of repair (more VPI with early repair), presence of palatal fistula.
    - Submucous cleft—1–9% [Gosain submucous paper].
    - 22q11—up to 65% [Nature review paper]

Anatomy

Table 14.2: *Muscle of the velum* (Fig. 14.1).

Clinical Presentation

- *What symptoms do patients with VPI have?*
    - Nasal air emissions
    - Hypernasality

14 Velopharyngeal Dysfunction

Table 14.2 Muscles of the velum

Muscle	Origin	Insertion	Innervation	Function
Levator veli palatini	Petrous portion of the temporal bone (cranial base)	*Normal*: Middle 1/3 of the soft palate, fuses to contralateral muscle at midline to form levator sling *Cleft*: Posterior aspect of hard palate	CN X	Elevate the palate
Superior pharyngeal constrictor	Median raphe (posterior pharyngeal midline)	Medial pterygoid Pterygomandibular raphe	CN X	Lateral wall motion
Palatopharyngeus	Posterior and lateral pharyngeal walls	Velum via posterior tonsillar pillar	CN X	Mostly lateral wall motion, depresses palate
Tensor veli palatini	Membranous wall of eustachian tube	Pterygoid hamulus, midline aponeurosis spans the anterior 1/3 of soft palate	CN V	Opens eustachian tube
Palatoglossus muscle	Tongue	Anterior velum	CN X	Depresses palate
Muscular uvulae	Posterior velum	Mucous membrane of the uvula	CN X	Upward movement and shortening of the uvula

- Oro-nasal reflux
- Speech misarticulations—difficulty with plosives:
  - Plosives are speech sounds created by stopping airflow using teeth/lips or palate followed by sudden release of air (e.g., *d, g, b* and *t, k, p*).

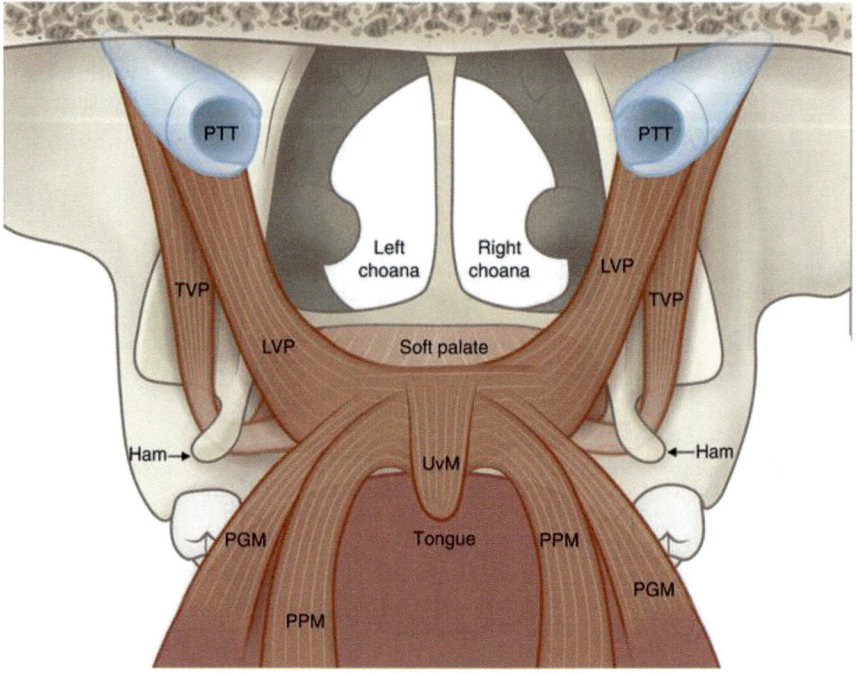

Fig. 14.1 Muscles of the velum. (von Arx T., Lozanoff S. (2017) Hard and Soft Palate. In: Clinical Oral Anatomy. Springer, Cham. Figure 10.26 https://doi.org/10.1007/978-3-319-41993-0_10. Permissions license number: 5333701236505)

Diagnosis

- *How can we diagnose patients with VPI?*
    - *Clinical history*—onset of speech abnormalities, hx of cleft lip/palate, hx tonsil/adenoid surgeries, hx neurologic disorders
    - *Speech evaluation*—evaluation by speech pathologist
        - Nasal air emissions—audible, inaudible (place mirror under nares, present if mirror fogs with vowel production), consistent, turbulent
        - Facial grimace—yes/no
        - Hypernasality/resonance—mild, moderate, severe
        - Phonation—hoarse, reduced in volume
        - Articulation—errors with plosives, nasal substitutions for pressure sounds (glottal stops, pharyngeal fricatives)
    - *Instrumental evaluation*
        - *Video nasopharyngeal endoscopy*

- Endoscope inserted through middle meatus to the posterior pharynx to visualize velopharyngeal mechanism during patient phonation of speech sample
- Enables visualization of size of opening and contribution of palatal and later/posterior pharyngeal musculature
- Also enables visualization of submucous clefts, fistula, scarring

- *Multi-view Videofluoroscopy*
  - Evaluate the same speech sample through multiple views—lateral and anteroposterior to assess contributions of velum and lateral/posterior pharyngeal muscles to closure
  - Can be useful in conjunction with nasoendoscopy or in children who don't tolerate nasoendoscopy
- *MRI*—emerging technique
- *Nasometry*—provides objective assessment of acoustic energy emitted from nasal vs nasal + oropharyngeal compartments

– What aspects are helpful for determining treatment methodology/surgical planning (Fig. 14.2)?

- *Closure pattern*—pattern of closure indicates
  - which muscles are functioning and which are inadequate
  - where the area of insufficiency is to better target with surgery

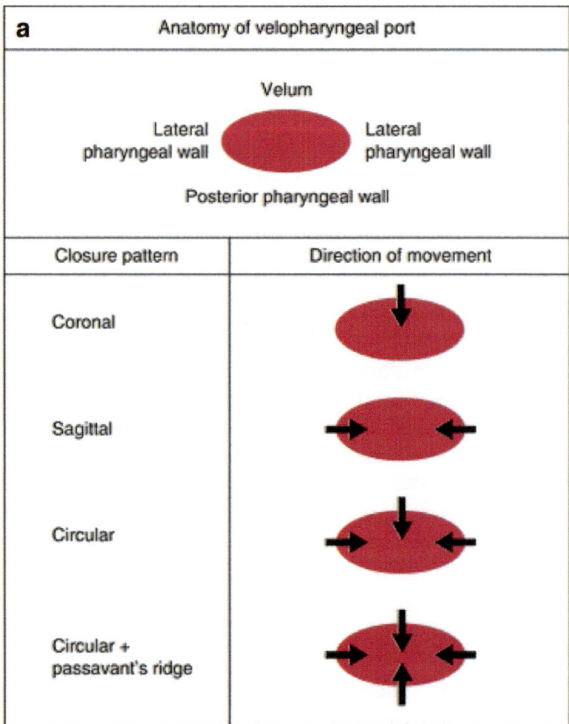
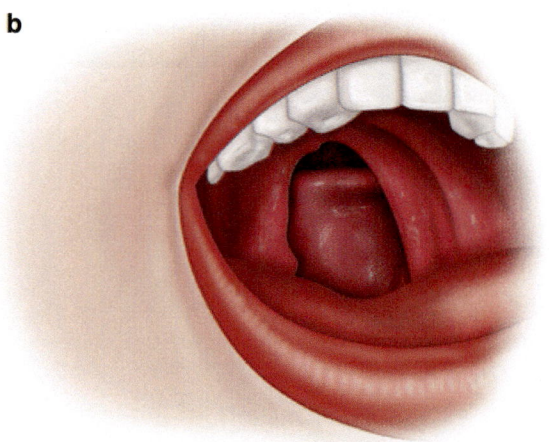

Fig. 14.2 Velopharyngeal port anatomy and closure patterns. (Alonso N., Lima J.E., Jenny H.E. (2018) Velopharyngeal Insufficiency: Etiopathology and Treatment. In: Alonso N., Raposo-Amaral C. (eds) Cleft Lip and Palate Treatment. Springer, Cham. https://doi.org/10.1007/978-3-319-63290-2_12)

Management

Nonoperative

Palatal Obturators and Lift Devices

- Temporary or permanent solutions for nonsurgical candidates.
- Palatal lift—aids sphincteric function by pushing the palate cranially, used for hypomobility or paresis
- Obturators—used to occlude unrepaired clefts or oronasal fistulas.

Speech Therapy

- The sole treatment for velopharyngeal *mislearning*
- Adjunctive postoperative treatment for patients with insufficiency to help them adapt to their "new" anatomy

Operative

Secondary palatal lengthening—both narrow the velopharyngeal sphincter and reposition the levator veli palatini

- *Furlow palatoplasty* (Fig. 14.3)
    - A two-layered "opposing" z-plasty:
        - Each z-plasty contains one mucosal and one musculomucosal flap.
        - Anteriorly based flaps contain only mucosa; posteriorly based flaps contain muscle + mucosa.

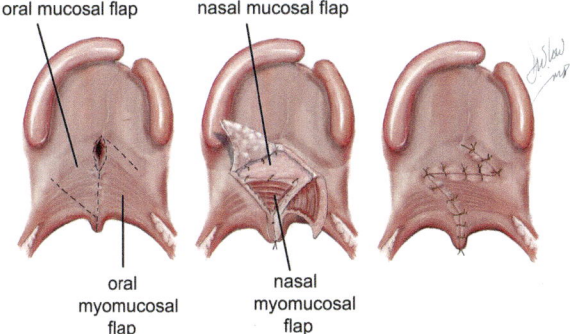

Fig. 14.3 Double opposing z-plasty ("furlow palatoplasty")Jackson O.A., Mehendale F.V. (2021) Speech Surgery and Treatment of Velopharyngeal Insufficiency. In: Swanson J.W. (eds) Global Cleft Care in Low-Resource Settings. Springer, Cham. Figure 20.9. https://link.springer.com/chapter/10.1007/978-3-030-59105-2_20. Permissions license number: 5333701495903)

- Threefold benefit for treating VPI:
  - Adds palatal length (lengthening effect of z-plasty).
  - Transposes muscles to recreate levator sling.
  - Z-plasty leads to shortening in transverse dimension (narrowing of the velopharyngeal port).
- *V-Y pushback (with intravelar veloplasty).*
  - Posteriorly based mucoperiosteal palatal flaps are advanced in a V-Y fashion anteriorly to add palatal length.
  - Combination with aggressive intravelar veloplasty and excision of levator scar recreates levator orientation.

Techniques to Narrow the Velopharyngeal Port

- *Posterior pharyngeal flap* (Fig. 14.4).
  - One of oldest and most frequently used techniques, first described by Passavant and Schoenborn in the 1860s/1870s with additional modifications by Hogan.
  - *Indications*: Sagittal closure patterns with large defects.
  - *Technique*: *Musculomucosal posterior* pharyngeal flap is raised and secured to the posterior aspect of the soft palate.
    - Creates musculomucosal bridge between the posterior pharynx and palate that divides velopharyngeal aperture into two:
      - Creates *static* central obstruction to compensate for anteroposterior deficiency seen with poor velar excursion (most commonly seen deficiency after cleft lip repair).
      - Relies on intact lateral wall motion to close two lateral ports.
      - Flap width = key to outcome:

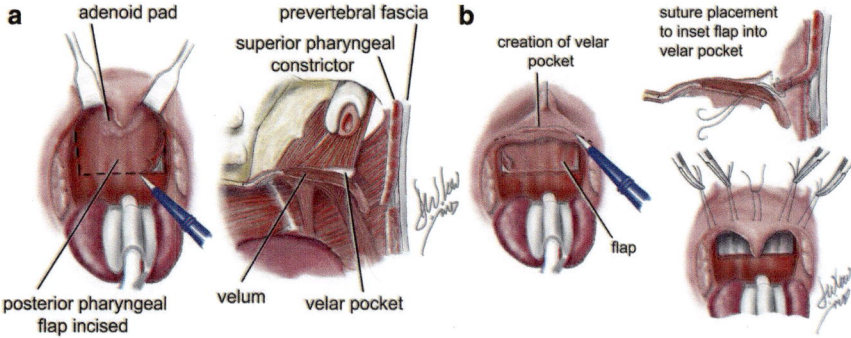

Fig. 14.4 Posterior pharyngeal flap. (Jackson O.A., Mehendale F.V. (2021) Speech Surgery and Treatment of Velopharyngeal Insufficiency. In: Swanson J.W. (eds) Global Cleft Care in Low-Resource Settings. Springer, Cham. Figure 20.14. https://doi.org/10.1007/978-3-030-59105-2_20. Permissions license number: 5333701495903)

- Determined via lateral wall excursion on nasoendoscopy.
- Too wide = OSA, airflow obstruction, hyponasality.
- Too narrow = persistent VPI symptoms.

• Can use superior or inferiorly based flap:

- **Palpate posterior pharynx to rule out *medialized carotid arteries (patients with 22q11 deletion)* prior to raising flap.**
- Superior extent of flap is 1–2 cm above tubercle of C1 (atlas).

• *Complications*:

- Postoperative airway obstruction—Keep overnight for observation, place tongue stitch, postoperative corticosteroid use, frequent intraoperative Dingman retractor release.
- OSA—Counsel parents on high risk of developing OSA.

• *Sphincter pharyngoplasty (Fig. 14.5)*:

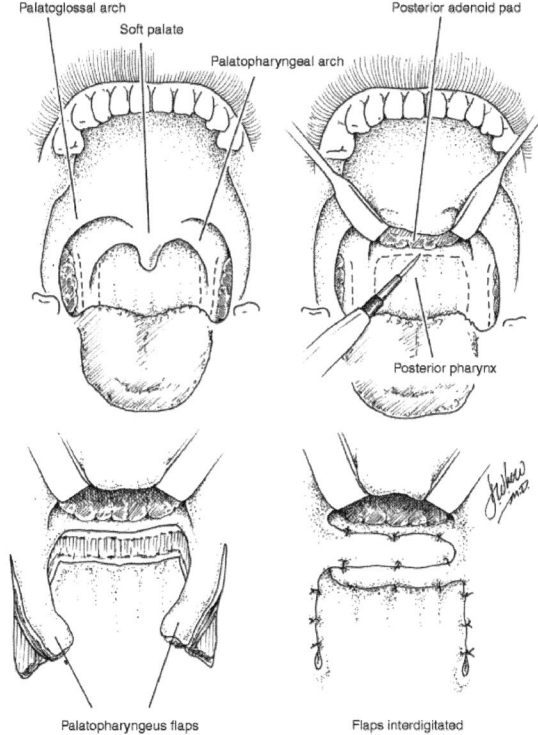

Fig. 14.5 Sphincter pharyngoplasty. (Kirschner R.E., Kirschner R.E., Kirschner R.E., Baylis A.L., Baylis A.L. (2013) Surgical Management of Velopharyngeal Dysfunction. In: Berkowitz S. (eds) Cleft Lip and Palate. Springer, Berlin, Heidelberg. Figure 35.6. https://doi.org/10.1007/978-3-642-30770-6_35. Permissions license number: 5333710267601)

- Undergone multiple modifications over time:
    - Initially described by Orticochea.
    - Subsequent modifications focused on higher inset of the flaps to better oppose the posterior velum with resultant improved speech outcomes.
- *"Indications"*: *poor "lateral wall motion (coronal closure pattern)" with a "small defect"*
- *Technique*: elevation of posterior pharyngeal musculomucosal pillars and transposition at 90 degree angles to create dynamic sphincter along the posterior pharyngeal wall.
    - Inset at level of tubercle of atlas.
    - Inclusion of muscle may add dynamic element to static obstruction.
- *Complications*:
    - Upper airway obstruction and OSA: less common than posterior pharyngeal flaps but still possible.
- *Posterior pharyngeal wall augmentation:*
    - Injection of filler substance behind pharyngeal mucosa to augment posterior pharyngeal contact with the posterior velum:
        - Pharyngeal fat grafting is most common.
    - Static obstruction.
    - Easy with minimal/no donor site morbidity, however, limited data on long-term outcomes.

References

1. Hopper RA, Tse R, Smartt J, Swanson J, Kinter S. Cleft palate repair and velopharyngeal dysfunction. Plast Reconstr Surg. 2014;133(6):852e–64e. https://doi.org/10.1097/PRS.0000000000000184.
2. Gart MS, Gosain AK. Surgical management of velopharyngeal insufficiency. Clin Plast Surg. 2014;41(2):253–70. https://doi.org/10.1016/j.cps.2013.12.010.
3. Tache A, Maryn Y, Mommaerts MY. Need for velopharyngeal surgery after primary palatoplasty in cleft patients. A retrospective cohort study and review of literature. Ann Med Surg (Lond). 2021;12(69):102707. https://doi.org/10.1016/j.amsu.2021.102707. PMID: 34429961; PMCID: PMC8371190
4. Gosain AK, Conley SF, Marks S, Larson DL. Submucous cleft palate: diagnostic methods and outcomes of surgical treatment. Plast Reconstr Surg. 1996;97(7):1497–509. https://doi.org/10.1097/00006534-199606000-00032.
5. McDonald-McGinn DM, Sullivan KE, Marino B, Philip N, Swillen A, Vorstman JA, Zackai EH, Emanuel BS, Vermeesch JR, Morrow BE, Scambler PJ, Bassett AS. 22q11.2 deletion syndrome. Nat Rev Dis Primers. 2015;19(1):15071. https://doi.org/10.1038/nrdp.2015.71. PMID: 27189754; PMCID: PMC4900471

Chapter 15
Craniofacial Microsomia

Brendan J. Cronin

Background and Epidemiology

- Craniofacial microsomia: variable hypoplasia of the skeleton + overlying soft tissue.
  - Second most common congenital syndrome of the head and neck region.
  - Incidence 1:3500 births.
  - No clear difference in incidence between M and F.
  - Can be unilateral or bilateral.
- Differential includes

Treacher Collins	*Symmetrical pathology* (microsomia is not) *Absence of medial lower eyelashes + antegonial notching of the mandible*
Micrognathia (developmental or posttraumatic)	*Underdevelopment restricted to the mandible no evidence of facial paralysis, ear anomalies, or soft tissue hypoplasia of the cheeks*
Goldenhar syndrome	*Unilateral microsomia Dermoids or other growths around the eye Spinal deformities*

B. J. Cronin (✉)
Division of Plastic and Reconstructive Surgery, University of California, Los Angeles, CA, USA

Etiology

- Hypoplasia manifesting: in *any* of the structures from the *first and second branchial arches*.
    - As the first and second branchial arches develop into a wide variety of structures, this can lead to a *wide spectrum of deformity*.
- Vascular insult theory.
    - Varying degrees of vascular insult in early embryogenesis leads to varying degrees of damage and subsequent malformation in structures of the developing first and second branchial arches.
    - Teratogen exposure.
        - Rat study demonstrated hemorrhage of the stapedial artery in those exposed to thalidomide.
        - Human study showed increased incidence of craniofacial microsomia in mothers exposed to thalidomide during pregnancy.

Presentation/Clinical Features

- *OMENS+ criteria* [1]
    - Most popular "classification system" to define clinical features of microsomia.
    - *O*rbit, *M*andible, *E*ar, *N*erve, *S*oft tissues.
    - (+) = renal agenesis, vertebral anomalies, GERD, VSD
- *Mandibular deformity (mandibular hypoplasia)*
    - Pruzansky classifications (Fig. 15.1).
        - Describes varying degrees of mandibular and TMJ dysplasia.
        - Degree of deformity informs management.
        - *Type I: Small but intact.*
            - Mild hypoplasia of the ramus +/− body of the mandible; all structures still present and have normal form.
        - *Type IIa: Small with abnormal but functional TMJ.*
            - Decreased height of the ramus and the TMJ is hypoplastic but identifiable and functioning.
        - *Type IIb: Small with "absence" of the TMJ.*
            - Hypoplasia of the ramus and condyle; condyle is shortened and medially displaced (but still present).
            - Patients have restricted ipsilateral jaw opening.

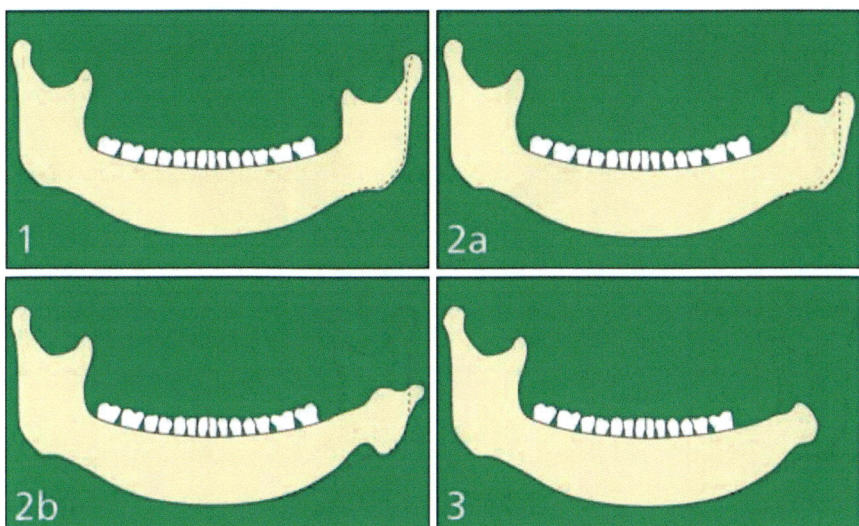

Fig. 15.1 Pruzansky classification of mandibular deformity. (Pruzansky classification of mandibular hypoplasia is shown above. Type I mandibles have mild hypoplasia of the ramus +/− body of the mandible; all structures still present and have normal form. Type IIa is characterized by decreased vertical height of the ramus and a hypoplastic but normally functioning TMJ. Type IIb mandibles demonstrate hypoplasia of the ramus and condyle. The TMJ is absent but the ramus is present. Type III mandibles *have an* absent or incredibly diminutive ramus, no condyle and no TMJ. https://www.nature.com/articles/sj.bdj.2015.48. Akram, A., McKnight, M., Bellardie, H. et al. Craniofacial malformations and the orthodontist. *Br Dent J* 218, 129–141 (2015). https://doi.org/10.1038/sj.bdj.2015.48. Permissions license number: 5333691119162)

- *Type III*: *Small with "absence" of TMJ and ramus.*
  - Absent or incredibly diminutive ramus, no condyle.
  - Absent TMJ.
- Other bony abnormalities *(Fig. 15.2)*
  - Maxilla can have a deformity with a cant corresponding to the degree of mandibular deformity.
  - Hypoplastic zygomatic arch and overlying soft tissue:
    - Leads to reduced distance between the tragus and oral commissure on affected side.
  - Hypoplastic temporal bone (mastoid, styloid process, petrous portion unaffected).
  - Small orbit.
  - Canal atresia (*temporal bone*).
  - Vertebrae malformations (hemivertebrae, fused vertebrae).
- *Muscles of mastication*

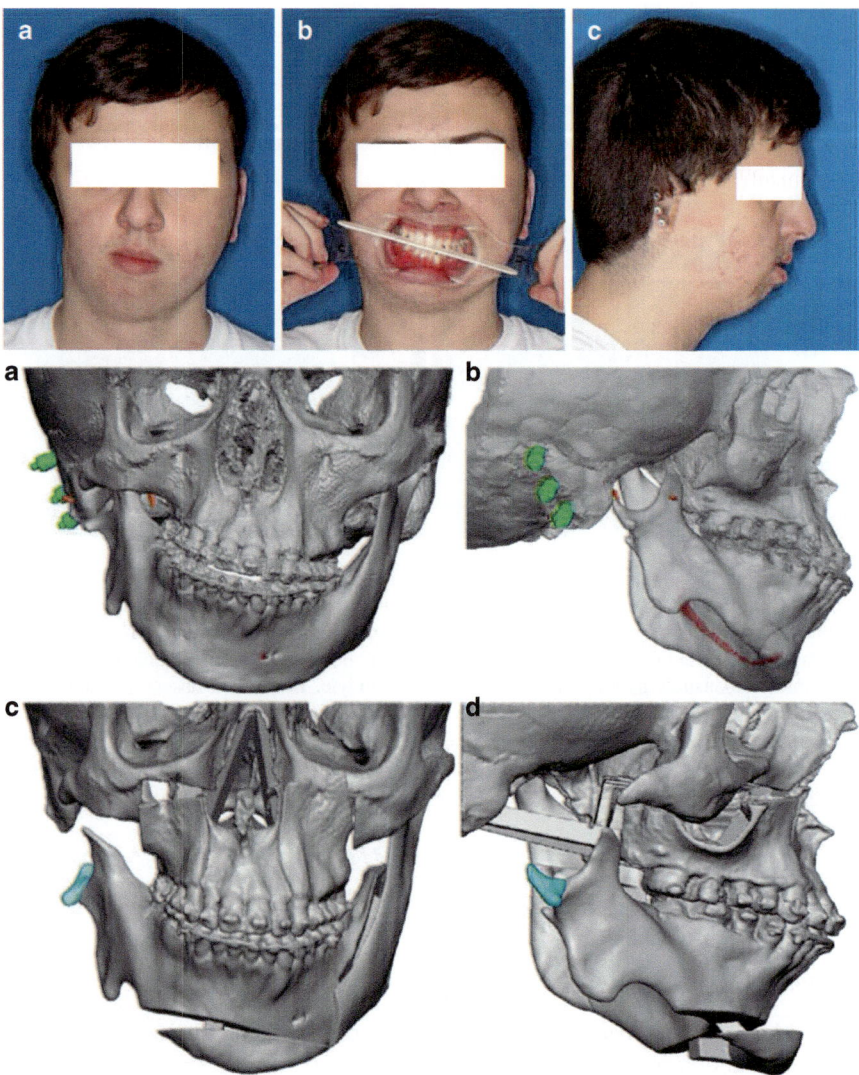

Fig. 15.2 Clinical manifestations of craniofacial microsomia. The OMEN criteria are evident in this patient with craniofacial microsomia. He demonstrates orbital dystopia, mandibular hypoplasia with marked canting of the occlusal plane, microtia and atrophy of the soft tissues of the cheek with a laterally displaced commissure, and temporal bone malformation. The hypoplastic mandible with a diminutive malformed condyle and right-sided zygomatic arch absence and maxillary hypoplasia are visible on the 3D reconstruction. https://link.springer.com/chapter/10.1007/978-3-030-84733-3_6. Wolford, L.M. (2022). Surgical Management of Hemifacial Microsomia with Temporomandibular Joint Malformation. In: Yates, D.M., Markiewicz, M.R. (eds) Craniofacial Microsomia and Treacher Collins Syndrome. Springer, Cham. https://doi.org/10.1007/978-3-030-84733-3_6. Permissions license number: 5333690907958)

- Hypoplastic:
  - Interestingly, not always correlated with the degree of mandibular hypoplasia.
- Can have hemi-palatal hypotonia and higher risk of velopharyngeal insufficiency.
- Diminutive ipsilateral lateral pterygoid (or absent TMJ) leads to deviation of the chin toward the affected side with mouth opening.

– *Ears* [2]
  - "Meurman" classification—ranges from smaller than normal to near complete absence:
    - Grade 1: small malformed ear with all anatomical components present.
    - Grade 2: complete atresia of the EAC, only small vertical remnant of the ear skin and cartilage.
    - Grade 3: only soft tissue lobule, otherwise structures absent.
  - Tanzer classification.
    - I: Loss of helix.
    - IIA: Loss of helix and scapha, without the need of supplemental skin.
    - IIB: Loss of helix and scapha with the need for supplemental skin.
    - III: Extreme.
  - Microtia classification (based on remnant tissue).
    - Anotia.
    - Lobule type.
    - Conchal type.
    - Small conchal type.
    - Atypical.

– *Nervous system*
  - Facial palsy (due to absent facial nerve or agenesis of facial muscles).
    - Usually minimal and *incomplete*—does not require facial reanimation.
    - Most commonly involves marginal mandibular nerve (25% of patients).

– *Soft tissue*
  - Preauricular skin tags:
    - Cartilage remnants.
  - Hypoplasia of the cheek skin/soft tissues.
  - +/− hypoplasia of the muscles and parotid gland.
  - Macrostomia (lateral cheek *cleft*) is also a common finding:
    - Equivalent to Tessier Cleft 7.
  - Cleft of the soft palate occurs in 25% of patients.

- *Associated syndromes*
  - *Goldenhar syndrome (oculo-auriculo-vertebral syndrome):*
  - *Presentation*:
    - A severe form of hemifacial microsomia with accessory auricles (chondrocutaneous remnants) (100% of patients) and heart and kidney defects.
  - *Ocular abnormalities*:
    - Epibulbar dermoid cyst.
    - Colobomas (eyelid and optic nerve, disruptions of circular shape of the eye).
      - Colobomas can be asymptomatic (affecting the iris alone), can lead to exposure keratopathy (in the case of eyelid colobomas), or can lead to visual disturbances (optic disc/nerve coloboma), such as visual field deficits or amblyopia.
  - *Auricular abnormalities*:
    - Deafness.
    - Chondrocutaneous remnants.

Preoperative Workup

- 3D CT +/− lateral cephalogram and panorex (Fig. 15.2)
- Renal U/S (renal agenesis).
- Spine radiographs (vertebral anomalies).
- ECHO (VSD).

Management [4]

- *Younger than two*:
  - Hearing issues (*conductive* hearing loss):
    - Newborn hearing test, bone conduction hearing aid immediately.
    - Perform canaloplasty or bone-anchored hearing aid placement at the time of ear reconstruction.
  - Excision of preauricular skin tags + cartilage remnants.
  - Correct of macrostomia (commissuroplasty).
  - If *severe* retrusion of the supraorbital bar, perform fronto-orbital advancement.
  - Mandibular distraction for newborns/infants with OSA.

- *2–6 years:*

  - Mild deformity (Pruzansky type I mandible and horizontal occlusal plane) — > *no surgical treatment recommended.*
  - Severe reduction of height of mandibular ramus (Pruzansky types I and II) — > *distraction osteogenesis* at age 2 [3].
    - Lengthens ramus (bone) but ALSO the overlying soft tissues and muscle.
    - Distracted ramus/condyle assume a more anatomic size, shape, and position.
  - Pruzansky type III (absence of the ramus, condyle, and glenoid fossa) — > *costochondral rib graft* at age 4.

- *6–15 years:*

  - Ear reconstruction (see Chap. 21).
  - Free flap soft tissue augmentation of facial contour.

- *>15 years (skeletal maturity):*

  - Consider any additional procedures not previously performed to address residual or recurrent skeletal deformity:
    - Bone grafting-deficient portions of craniofacial skeleton.
    - Mandibular advancement in those with micrognathia.
    - Le Fort I, BSSO, and genioplasty.
    - Microvascular free flap augmentation of soft tissues.

References

1. Vento AR, LaBrie RA, Mulliken JB. The OMENS classification of hemifacial microsomia. Cleft Palate Craniofac J. 1991;28(1):68–76.
2. Keogh IJ, Troulis MJ, Monroy AA, Eavey RD, Kaban LB. Isolated Microtia as a marker for unsuspected Hemifacial Microsomia. Arch Otolaryngol Head Neck Surg. 2007;133(10):997–1001. https://doi.org/10.1001/archotol.133.10.997.
3. Molina F, Ortiz-Monasterio F. Mandibular elongation and remodeling by distraction: a farewell to major osteotomies. Plast Reconstr Surg. 1995;96:825.
4. Mulliken JB, Kaban LB. Analysis and treatment of hemifacial microsomia in childhood. Clin Plast Surg. 1987;14:91.

Chapter 16
Congenital Melanocytic Nevi

Brendan J. Cronin

Background

- *Definition*
  - Abnormal collection of melanocytes of neuroectodermal origin in an ectopic location.
  - Melanocytic nevi can be divided into lesions present at birth (congenital melanocytic nevi) or those that develop after birth (acquired melanocytic nevi):
    - Congenital melanocytic nevi are "always" present at birth, but some may have variable degrees of pigmentation which may increase over time ("tardive nevi").
- *Categorization.*
  - *Small*: <1.5 cm in diameter.
  - *Medium*: 1.5–20 cm in diameter.
  - *Giant*: >20 cm in diameter (adult) or will grow to be >20 cm diameter (9 cm head and 6 cm trunk lesions in an infant).
    - Many definitions used across the literature:
      - >1% TBSA (head and neck) or > 2% TBSA (trunk)
      - >100cm^2
      - Unable to be excised in a single stage.

B. J. Cronin (✉)
Division of Plastic and Reconstructive Surgery, University of California, Los Angeles, CA, USA

- *Pathophysiology*
  - Congenital nevi thought to arise from disruption of normal growth, migration, and development of melanoblasts:
    - Arise during weeks 5–25 of development.
    - Normal development involves migrations of melanoblast cells from neural crest to various areas of the body (skin, mucous membranes, leptomeninges, mesentery, eyes, ears) where they differentiate into melanocytes.
    - Most nevi are acquired nevi, which migrate to their intended destination without issue and develop from melanoblasts into nevi later in life.
    - Congenital melanocytic nevi result from dysregulated growth during neuroectodermal development at any time during migration or differentiation.
  - Genetics.
    - Poorly understood.
    - Possibly related to excess expression of *hepatic growth factor/scatter factor* (this factor regulates development and migration of neuroectodermal cells).
- *Epidemiology*
  - Congenital melanocytic nevus—1% of children.
  - *Giant congenital melanocytic nevi*—1,20:000 births.
- *Histology*
  - *Characteristics of congenital melanocytic nevi (compared to acquired nevi).*
    - Nevus cells present in lower two-thirds of the dermis.
    - Nevus cells extending between collagen bundles of the reticular dermis as cords or bundles.
    - Nevus extension into surrounding hair follicles, sebaceous/eccrine glands, blood vessels, and nerves.
    - Infiltration into erector pili muscles.
    - Perivascular/perifollicular nevus cell infiltration with inflammatory reaction.
    - *Giant congenital melanocytic nevi can have cells that extend beyond the subcutaneous tissue into the fascia or muscle.
  - Atypical features
    - Dysplasia of intraepidermal nevus cells, pagetoid spread of nevus cells, proliferative dermal nodules.
  - Features indicative of malignant transformation
    - High mitotic rate, high-grade atypia, inflammatory infiltrate, necrosis, and perineural invasion.

Clinical Presentation [1, 3]

- *Distribution*
  - Most commonly located on the trunk, followed by the extremities and then the head and neck.
- *Clinical features and natural course*
  - Begin as flat, hairless, pale brown lesions.
  - Evolve to have various degrees of verrucosity, hypertrichosis, hyperpigmentation, erosions/ulcerations, and nodularity (indicative of neurotization of the lesion).
  - Expand *in proportion* to body growth.
  - 80% of patients with giant congenital melanocytic nevi will have satellite lesions
- *Melanoma*
  - Clinical features of malignant degeneration:
    - Ulceration, tenderness, bleeding, dark pigmentation, pruritus/pain.
  - Risk of malignant degeneration [4]:
    - Can have malignant degeneration of cells into *cutaneous and non-cutaneous melanoma*:
      - Non-cutaneous sites include GI tract mucosa, retroperitoneal, and deposits of neurocutaneous melanosis.
    - Historically, the risk of malignant transformation in the literature ranged from 1to 40%:
      - Recent prospective data suggests the risk of transformation is closer to 4–6%.
      - 17x higher risk than the general population.
      - 50% arise in the first 3 years of life, 60% by childhood, and 70% by puberty.
  - Risk factors
    - Multiple lesions (>3).
    - >20 cm diameter
    - Young age (age 3–5 years):
      - *As a result, surgical excision is best performed "early" in life to decrease this risk of malignant transformation.*

- *Neurocutaneous Melanosis.*
  - *Definition/background:*
    - Rare syndrome associated with congenital melanocytic nevi.
    - <100 cases reported in the literature
    - Caused by abnormal proliferation and migration of melanoblasts.
    - Leads to abnormal benign and/or malignant melanocytic proliferations in the central nervous system (brain or spinal cord).
  - *Risk factors:*
    - >20 lesions
    - Large lesions located over the midline trunk and skull.
    - *Patients with these risk factors should undergo screening MRI of the brain and spinal cord at age 4–6 mons (before myelination of the brain which obscures visualization of melanocytic deposits)
  - *Presentation:*
    - Hydrocephalus, seizures, developmental delay, cranial nerve palsies, tethered spinal cord:
      - Symptoms present regardless of malignant transformation.
    - Bimodal distribution of presentation:
      - Age 2–3 years: increase ICP, hydrocephalus, or developmental delay.
      - 20–30 years: space-occupying lesions, increased ICP, spinal cord compression
  - *Management*:
    - Should obtain a brain MRI if suspected.
    - Multidisciplinary and may include VP shunt placement, surgical excision, radiation therapy, or immune modulation.
    - Poor prognosis: usually die within 2–3 years of diagnosis.

Treatment [2]

- *Rationale*
  - Treatment in early childhood recommended due to the risk of malignant transformation (50% by age 3), psychological benefit (operations completed before school years), and patient tolerance of reconstruction (especially with tissue expansion).

- *Indications*
  - Excision in diagnosis of melanoma.
  - Prophylactic excision to decrease the risk of malignant transformation.
  - Psychosocial well-being.
- *Treatment options*
  - *Noninvasive*
    - *Dermabrasion*—risks hypertrophic scarring.
    - *Curettage*—limited available evidence.
    - *Laser*—typically carbon dioxide laser (ablative), risks hypertrophic scarring.
    - *Noninvasive techniques do "not" eliminate the risk of malignant transformation—highest density of remaining nevi cells is located in the deep dermis following these techniques, which is clinically challenging to surveil.
  - *Surgical management*
    - *Serial excision.*
      - Recommended if complete excision able to be achieved in <3 procedures.
      - Less complications than tissue expansion.
      - Recommend 6 months between excisions.
    - *Tissue expansion.*
      - Recommended for lesions not amenable to serial excision.
      - Can be used to create expanded local flaps, full-thickness skin grafts or free flaps.
      - Overfill expanders by 75–100%.
      - Associated skeletal deformities (i.e., on the skull) rapidly remodel with growth without permanent deformity.
      - If lesion requires multiple expansions to excise, wait 3–6 months for scar maturation and healing prior to next expander placement.
      - Complications: infection, extrusion, rupture, flap ischemia.
    - *Skin grafting.*
      - Options include split-thickness, full-thickness, expanded full-thickness grafts.
      - Full-thickness grafts preferred due to better color/thickness/texture match and better hair growth/sweat gland content.
    - *Free tissue transfer.*

References

1. Arneja JS, Gosain AK. Giant congenital melanocytic nevi. Plast Reconstr Surg. 2007;120(2):26e–40e.
2. Gosain AK, Santoro TD, Larson DL, et al. Giant congenital nevi: a 20-year experience and an algorithm for their management. Plast Reconstr Surg. 2001;108:622.
3. Lanier VC, Pickrell KL, Georgiade NG. Congenital giant nevi: clinical and pathological considerations. Plast Reconstr Surg. 1976;58:48.
4. Marghoob AA, Schoenbach SP, Kopf AW, et al. Large congenital melanocytic nevi and the risk for the development of malignant melanoma: a prospective study. Arch Dermatol. 1996;132:170.

Chapter 17
Vascular Malformations

Shervin Etemad

Pathogenesis [1]

- Vasculogenesis gives rise to the heart and primitive vascular plexus. Angiogenesis is characterized by endothelial cell migration, proliferation, and tube formation leading to vascular network development.
- Errors in vasculogenesis and angiogenesis lead to vascular anomalies. Molecular pathways involving tyrosine kinase signaling, RAS, PI3K, and VEGF have been implicated in vascular anomalies and represent potential therapeutic targets.

Evaluation

History and physical examination alone may be sufficient to establish a diagnosis. Radiologic evaluation can aid in defining the pathology and extent of disease. Pathologic diagnosis remains the gold standard.

S. Etemad (✉)
Keck Medicine of USC, Resident in Plastic and Reconstructive Surgery, University of Southern California, Los Angeles, CA, USA

Patient History

- Vascular tumors: present after birth but may be present at birth (i.e., congenital hemangioma).
  - These typically regress.
- Vascular malformations: always present at birth but may not be clinically apparent until later in life. They grow in proportion with the body and do not regress.

Radiologic Evaluation

- Ultrasound with Doppler may demonstrate low- versus high-flow characteristics of malformations and aid in the initial evaluation.
- MRI is the preferred imaging modality as it demonstrates the extent of the anomaly and adjacent soft tissue structures.

Classification and Specific Anomalies [2]

The International Society for the Study of Vascular Anomalies has created a classification scheme, summarized in Table 17.1. In this text, we will only focus on the major ones seen in plastic surgery clinics: benign and aggressive vascular tumors and simple vascular malformations.

Table 17.1 Differentiation of vascular tumors and malformations with classifications

Tumors	Malformations			
Benign Infantile hemangioma Congenital hemangioma Pyogenic granuloma	Simple Capillary Lymphatic Venous Arteriovenous	Combined malformations that involve capillary, lymphatic, venous, and arteriovenous components	Malformations of other major named vessels: Aneurysm, atresia, ectasia, and stenosis	Malformations associated with other anomalies
Locally aggressive Kaposiform hemangioendothelioma				
Malignant Angiosarcoma				

Vascular Tumors

- Infantile hemangiomas (Fig. 17.1).
  - Benign proliferation of endothelial cells, most common in the head/neck.
  - Glut-1-positive (beta blockers effective).
  - High flow.
  - Typically go through three phases:
    - Proliferation (0–12 months).
    - Involuting (1–8 years).
    - Involuted (> 8 years).
  - Diagnose based on history—grows out of proportion with patient) and ultrasound.
  - Treatment can be observational if not in area of critical importance.
  - Indications for treatment include bleeding, ulceration, obstruction of critical structures (eye—amblyopia—lip, throat), cosmetics.
  - Initial treatment with beta blocker, steroids.
  - Resect if functionally impaired or ulcerated during proliferative phase.
  - Can often delay resection to involuted phase.

Fig. 17.1 Infantile hemangioma

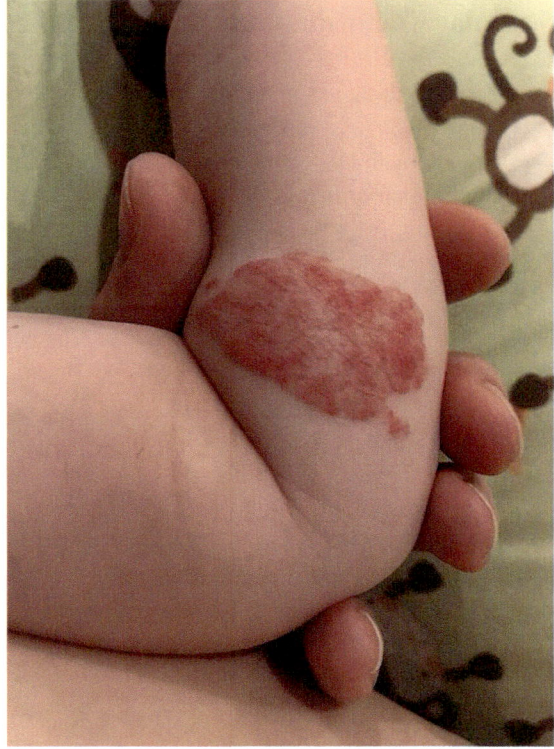

- Congenital Hemangioma.
    - Rapidly involuting congenital hemangiomas (RICH) involute after birth, with 50% involution by 7 months and complete involution by 14 years.
    - Non-involuting congenital hemangiomas (NICH) persist and may require surgical excision.
    - High flow.
    - *Not* Glut-1-positive (beta blockers not effective).
- Pyogenic Granuloma.
    - Painless, benign proliferation of capillary blood vessels often presenting on digits. Treatment includes topical therapy, cryotherapy, or surgical excision.
- Kaposiform hemangioepithelioma.
    - Locally aggressive hemangioma.
    - Can be life-threatening: associated with Kasabach-Merritt syndrome (thrombocytopenia).
    - Carries malignant potential.
    - Needs resection +/- vincristine or sirolimus.

Vascular Malformations (Figs. 17.2, 17.3, and 17.4)

- Presents at birth.
- Do not grow out of proportion with the body.
- Diagnosis with Doppler US or MRI.
- Capillary malformation.
    - Slow flow lesion.
    - Dilated capillaries in the superficial dermis that may present as a port-wine stain or telangiectasias.
    - Darken over time and may be associated with deeper vascular malformations.
    - Manage with observation or PDL.
    - Surgical excision may be last line.
    - Lymphatic Malformation.
        - Slow flow.
        - Malformed lymphatic channels leading to microcystic, macrocystic, or combined malformations.
        - May have associated bony overgrowth.
        - MRI and US findings include multiloculated fluid filled spaces with septations.
        - May lead to recurrent infections, bleeding, and pain.

Fig. 17.2 Port-wine stain

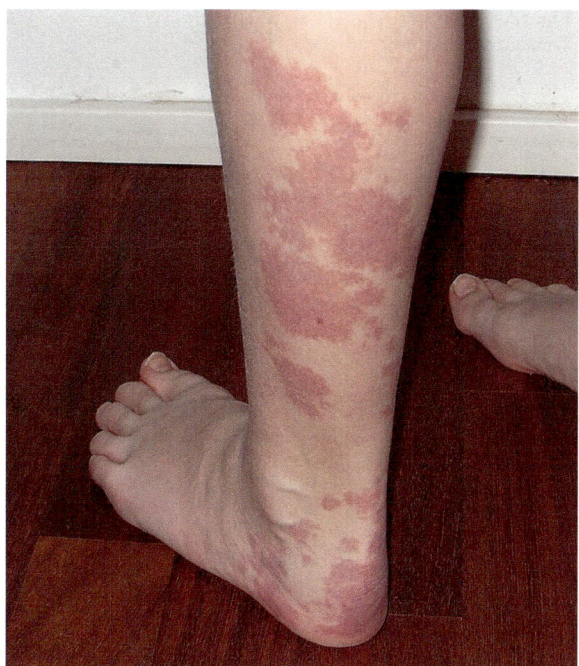

Fig. 17.3 Lymphangioma

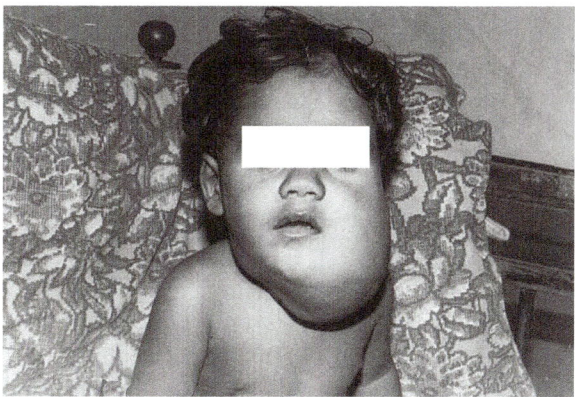

- Treatment includes sclerotherapy, compression, and excision:
    - Macrocystic lesions act as venous malformation and responds to sclerotherapy with doxycycline and ethanol.
    - Microcystic acts as capillary malformations, treated with laser.
- Venous Malformations.
- Slow flow lesion.

Fig. 17.4 Klippel-Trenaunay syndrome

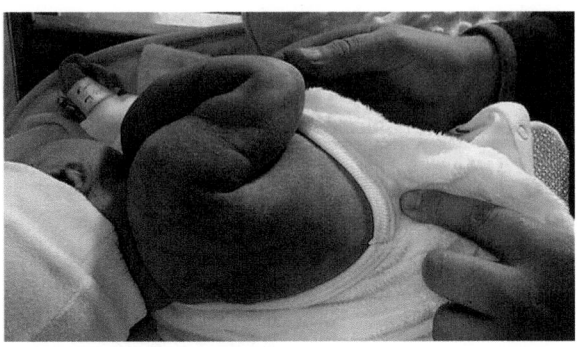

Table 17.2 Schobinger clinical staging system [4]

Stage I	Quiescent	No clinical symptoms
Stage II	Expansion	Enlarged, pulsatile, and palpable
Stage III	Destruction	Ulceration, pain, hemorrhage, lytic bone lesions
Stage IV	Decompensation	Increased cardiac output and cardiac failure

- Bluish and compressible.
- Changes in size with hormonal changes.
- Engorge and increase in size in dependent positions.
- Treatment options include compression anticoagulation to prevent thrombosis, sclerotherapy, and surgical excision.
- Arteriovenous malformations.
  - High flow
  - Errors in vasculogenesis leading to shunting of blood directly from an artery into a venous system.
  - Characterized by warmth, pain, palpable thrill.
  - Clinical spectrum ranging from quiescent to decompensation (Tables 17.2 and 17.3).
  - Management includes a combination of embolization and resection.

Table 17.3 Surgical principles in the treatment of vascular malformations

1. Evaluate imaging
2. Plan extent of resection
3. Place incisions thoughtfully
4. Use magnification
5. Consider vascularity
6. Avoid intraneural dissection
7. Avoid partial dissection
8. Replace abnormal skin
9. Consider postoperative bleeding
10. Immobilize the operated extremity
11. Avoid sacrificing normal anatomy
12. Be prepared to amputate
13. Follow patients long term

Commonly Associated Syndromes

Parkes-Weber Syndrome

– Combined CM and AVM with associated soft tissue overgrowth.

Maffucci Syndrome

– VM and associated enchondromatosis, with risk of chondrosarcoma.

Sturge-Weber Syndrome

– Port-wine stain in trigeminal nerve distribution.
– Associated with glaucoma, seizures, developmental delay.

Osler-Weber-Rendu Syndrome

– Hereditary hemorrhagic telangiectasias.
– Mucocutaneous telangiectasias and AVMs.

Spina Bifida Occulta

– Lumbar hemangioma.

PHACES

– Acronym for posterior fossa abnormalities, hemangiomas, cardiac anomalies, eye abnormalities, sternal cleft.

Von Hippel-Lindau

– Retinal hemangiomas, hemangioblastomas of cerebellum, visceral cysts, mental disability.

Klippel-Trenaunay Syndrome

– Capillary malformation and/or lymphatic-venous malformation.
– Skeletal and soft tissue hypertrophy.

References

1. Taghinia AH, Upton J. Vascular anomalies. J Hand Surg Am. 2018;43(12):1113–21. https://doi.org/10.1016/j.jhsa.2018.03.046. Epub 2018 Jun 12
2. Issva.org. 2022. Classification | International Society for the Study of Vascular Anomalies. [online] Available at: https://www.issva.org/classification. Accessed 27 July 2022.
3. Cox JA, Bartlett E, Lee EI. Vascular malformations: a review. Semin Plast Surg. 2014;28(2):58–63. https://doi.org/10.1055/s-0034-1376263. PMID: 25045330; PMCID: PMC4078214
4. Gilbert P, Dubois J, Giroux MF, Soulez G. New treatment approaches to arteriovenous malformations. Semin Intervent Radiol. 2017;34(3):258–71. https://doi.org/10.1055/s-0037-1604299. Epub 2017 Sep 11. PMID: 28955115; PMCID: PMC5615391

Chapter 18
Craniosynostosis

Sumun Khetpal

Overview

- Occurring in 1 in 2000–2500 live births, craniosynostosis is defined as the premature fusion of cranial sutures [1].
- Fusion of the sagittal suture is most common (40–55%), followed by coronal (20–25%), metopic (5–15%), and lambdoid (1–5%) sutures.
- Premature suture fusion results in compensatory skull growth parallel to the fused suture and a decreased growth perpendicular to the suture (Virchow's law).
- The diagnosis, management, and treatment of craniosynostosis often require interdisciplinary collaboration between professionals including but not limited to craniofacial surgery, neurosurgery, genetics, ophthalmology, orthodontics, pediatrics, dentistry, prosthodontics, social work, psychiatry, speech therapy, audiology, otorhinolaryngology, and hand surgery [1].
- Craniosynostosis may be classified into non-syndromic or syndromic forms. Common craniofacial syndromes and relevant details are listed in Table 18.1.

S. Khetpal (✉)
Division of Plastic and Reconstructive Surgery, University of California, Los Angeles, CA, USA
e-mail: SKhetpal@mednet.ucla.edu

Table 18.1 Overview of syndromic craniosynostosis forms with key features [2]

Syndrome	Associated gene	Inheritance pattern	Key features
Apert	FGFR-2	Autosomal dominant	Exorbitism, midface hypoplasia, and symmetric syndactyly of both hands and feet Coronal sutures
Pfeiffer	FGFR-1, FGFR-2	Autosomal dominant	Exorbitism, maxillary hypoplasia, broad thumbs, and great toes Coronal sutures
Crouzon	FGFR-2	Autosomal dominant	Midface hypoplasia, shallow orbits, ocular proptosis Coronal, sagittal, metopic sutures
Saethre-Chotzen	TWIST-1	Autosomal dominant	Brachycephalic skull, a low-set frontal hairline, prominent crus helicis extending through the Conchal bowl, facial asymmetry, and ptosis of the eyelids Unicoronal, bicoronal sutures
Muenke	FGFR-3	Autosomal dominant	Hearing loss, developmental delay, thimble-like middle phalanges Unicoronal, bicoronal sutures
Antley-Bixler	FGFR2, POR	Autosomal recessive	Radioulnar synostosis, dysplastic ears, midface hypoplasia, bowed femora
Carpenter	RAB23	Autosomal recessive	Syndactyly, intellectual disability Multisuture craniosynostosis

Pathogenesis

- There are three theories regarding the pathogenesis of craniosynostosis: [1] fate of cranial sutures was entirely independent of the surrounding neurocranial environment (Virchow, 1851), [2] craniosynostosis is caused by a defect in the cranial suture mesenchymal blastema which leads to premature suture fusion (Park and Powers, 1920), and [3] dura mater acted as a conduit or functional matrix for cranial base biomechanical forces, including suture fusion (Van der Klaauw, 1946; Moss, 1959) [1–5].

Evaluation

- Physical examination includes assessment of suture ridging along implicated sutures, overall skull and facial configuration, age-appropriate neurological examination, concurrent torticollis, and evidence of papilledema.
- Deformational plagiocephaly, or asymmetric flattening, has become more prevalent due to the American Academy of Pediatrics 1992 "Back to Sleep Campaign," launched to reduce the incidence of sudden infant death syndrome. This condition resembles posterior synostotic plagiocephaly but can be distinguished by occipital flatness, ipsilateral anterior ear shear, and forehead bossing. Treatment may be helmet therapy or physical therapy.
- Relevant physical examination findings associated with various types of synostoses are listed in Table 18.2, Fig. 18.1.

18 Craniosynostosis

Table 18.2 Key physical examination findings associated with types of synostosis

Type of synostosis	Time of typical suture fusing	Key features
Metopic (trigonocephaly)	3–9 months	Keel-shaped deformity (triangular head), small, flat frontal bones, hypotelorism, lateral orbital rim posteriorly displaced and hypoplastic, flattened profile of squamosal bone, biparietal widening of the skull
Sagittal (scaphocephaly)	20 years	Increased anteroposterior length and decreased width (boat-like)
Bilateral coronal (brachycephaly)	24 years	Bilateral retrusion of the frontal bone and supraorbital rims, bilateral lateral bulge of squamous temporal bones, increased biparietal diameter
Unilateral coronal (anterior plagiocephaly)	24 years	Shortening of ipsilateral palpebral fissure, superior and posterior displacement of ipsilateral orbital rim and eyebrow (harlequin), flattened ipsilateral forehead, contralateral forehead bossing
Lambdoid (posterior plagiocephaly)	22 years	Ipsilateral occipital flattening, posterior/inferior displacement of the ipsilateral ear, bossing of the ipsilateral mastoid, and decreased height of the cranial vertex on affected side

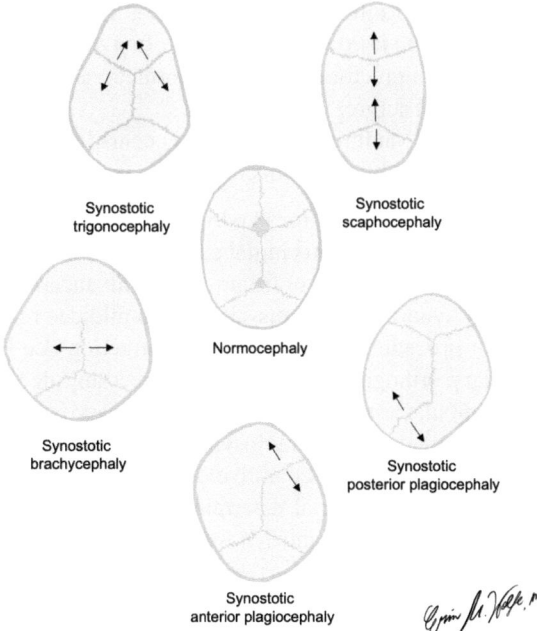

Fig. 18.1 Craniosynostosis types

Imaging

- The most definitive study for diagnosis for craniosynostosis is CT scan, which may demonstrate fusion of cranial suture. Skull radiographs may also be utilized to assess for fusion of sutures.

Treatment and Additional Considerations

- Goals of treatment are to resolve increased intracranial pressure and prevent neurocognitive impairment that could arise from compression and to create a normal aesthetic-appearing calvarium for the patient.
- There is great variation within the treatment of non-syndromic craniosynostosis, including the use of endoscopic-assisted extended craniectomies with postoperative cranial orthosis, springs, distraction devices, and open partial or total cranial vault remodeling procedures. Individualized treatment plan is dependent on factors including patient's age, number and location of sutures, severity of pathology, and presence of associated syndrome:
  - Typically, the affected suture is excised to restore the ability for the calvarium to grow perpendicular.
  - Cranial vault remodeling involves removal of much of the calvarium and replacing it in a corrected (and often overcorrected) configuration.
  - Pure suturectomy can be performed earlier in life ~3–6 months for isolated sagittal suture.
  - Cranial vault remodeling often occurs later in life 12 months or late and often requires blood transfusions due to the large volume loss in a small child.
- On the other hand, for syndromic craniosynostosis, the current surgical treatment approach entails initial early posterior cranial vault distraction (to augment intracranial volume) or fronto-orbital advancement and cranial vault remodeling.
- Many syndromic patients suffer from midface retrusion, and a midface advancement procedure with or without distraction (Le Fort III or monobloc) and secondary orthognathic surgery to correct any dentofacial deformities (Le Fort I, mandibular osteotomies) may be necessary [1].
- Proper treatment of craniosynostosis is important, as several studies have cited the long-term neurocognitive deficits and psychosocial consequences of inadequate care [6]. Social determinants of health have also been implicated in the care pathway for craniosynostosis [7–8].

References

1. Rogers GF, Warren SM. Single suture craniosynostosis and deformational plagiocephaly. In: Thorne CH, editor. Grabb and smith's plastic surgery. Lippincott Williams & Wilkins; 2014. p. 221–31.
2. Sawh-Martinez R, Steinbacher DM. Syndromic craniosynostosis. Clin Plast Surg. 2019;46(2):141–55.
3. Bartlett SP, Derderian CA. Craniosynostosis syndromes. In: Thorne CH, editor. *Grabb and Smith's plastic surgery*. Lippincott Williams & Wilkins; 2014. p. 232–40.
4. Forrest CR, Hopper RA. Craniofacial syndromes and surgery. Plast Reconstr Surg. 2013;131(1):86e–109e.
5. Persing JA, Jane JA, Shaffrey M. Virchow and the pathogenesis of craniosynostosis: a translation of his original work. Plast Reconstr Surg. 1989;83(4):738–42.
6. Chandler L, Allam O, Park KE, et al. Spring-assisted strip Craniectomy versus cranial vault remodeling: long-term psychological, behavioral, and executive function outcomes. J Craniofac Surg. 2020;31(7):2101–5.
7. Hauc SC, Junn A, Dinis J, et al. Disparities in Craniosynostosis outcomes by race and insurance status. J Craniofac Surg. 2022;33(1):121–4.
8. Lin Y, Pan IW, Harris DA. The impact of insurance, race, ethnicity on age at surgical intervention among children with nonsyndromic Craniosynostosis. J Pediatr. 2015;166(5):1289–96.

Chapter 19
Orthognathic Surgery

Mia Joseph

Introduction to Dental Malocclusion

- Dental malocclusions are highly prevalent and most often corrected through orthodontics. However, orthodontic treatment is limited to correction of tooth position within the alveolus.
- Malocclusions caused by abnormal alignment or growth of the jaws typically require extensive movements not possible through orthodontics alone. Additionally, orthognathic surgery may be necessary in addition to orthodontics to restore balance of the facial skeleton, to improve airway patency, or to treat temporomandibular joint (TMJ) disorders [1, 2].
- While approximately 20% of the population in the United States has a malocclusion, 2% of the population has a dentofacial deformity severe enough to require surgical correction [3].
- The relationship between the maxillary and mandibular teeth influences masticatory function and force distribution, adequate access for oral hygiene, periodontal stability, speech phonetics, and facial esthetics [4].

Occlusal Relationships

- Dentofacial deformities and malocclusions are assessed within the anterior-posterior, vertical, and transverse planes.
- The permanent dentition consists of 32 teeth including 3 molars, 2 premolars, 1 canine, and 2 incisors in each quadrant (Fig. 19.1).

M. Joseph (✉)
School of Dentistry, University of California, Los Angeles, CA, USA
e-mail: mia.joseph@ucla.edu

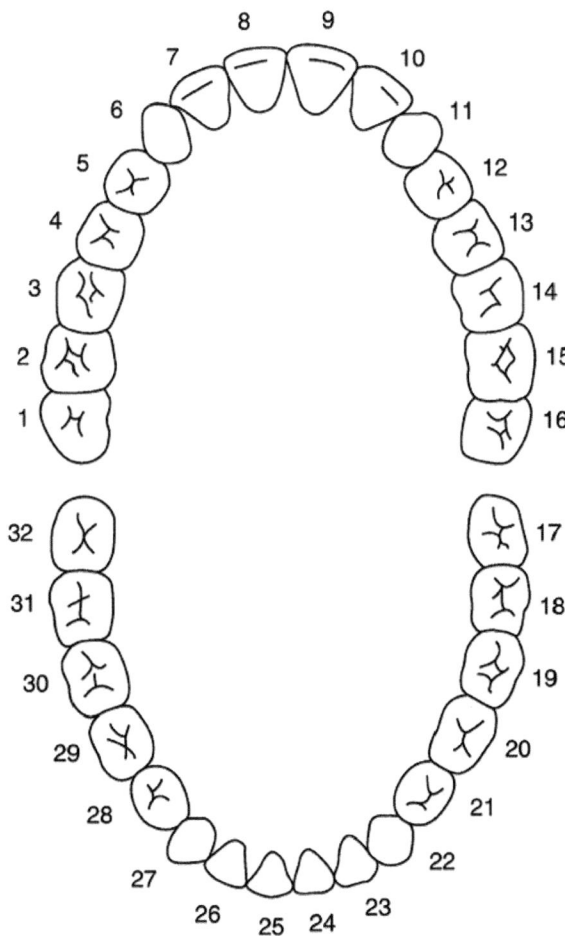

Fig. 19.1 Diagram of adult dentition with corresponding numbering system used in the United States [5, 6]

- In dentistry, the surfaces and directions are described as:
  - Mesial: toward the midline.
  - Distal: away from the midline.
  - Buccal/Facial/Labial: toward the frontal aspect of the tooth.
  - Lingual/Palatal: posterior aspect of the tooth, toward the tongue or palate.
- Overjet: horizontal relationship, or overlap, between the upper and lower incisors. Two to three mm of overjet is typical. In an anterior crossbite, the mandibular incisors are anterior to the maxillary incisors, producing a negative overjet (Fig. 19.2).
- Overbite: vertical relationship, or overlap, between the upper and lower incisors. Ideal overbite is 1–2 mm. In an anterior open bite, there is vertical separation between the upper and lower incisors and a negative overbite (Fig. 19.2).

Fig. 19.2 Illustration of overbite and overjet [7]

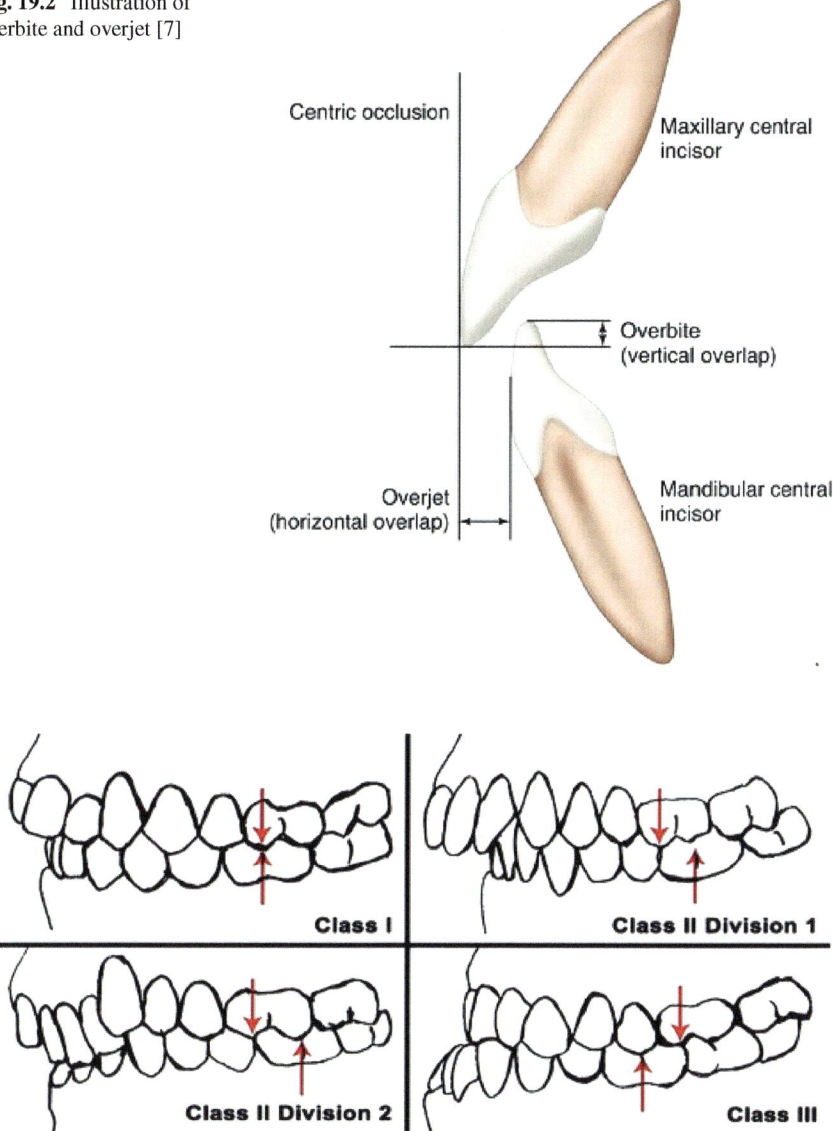

Fig. 19.3 Angle's classification of malocclusion [10]

- Angle's classification of malocclusion is defined by the relationship between the maxillary and mandibular first permanent molars (Fig. 19.3):
  - Class I: Normal molar relationship, occlusion of the mesiobuccal (MB) cusp of the maxillary first molar aligns with the mesiobuccal groove of the mandibular first molar.

- Class II: Mesiobuccal cusp of the maxillary first molar occludes mesial to the MB groove of the mandibular first molar.
  - Division 1: In addition to the molar relationship, the incisors display excessive overjet and anterior proclination.
  - Division 2: Retroclined maxillary incisors produce increased overbite and minimal overjet.
  - Facial features include convex facial profile (Fig. 19.3). Class II Division 2 cases are characterized by deficient lip support with a thin vermillion border, as well as a prominent nose and chin.
  - Skeletal causes may be maxillary prognathism or mandibular retrognathism (Fig. 19.4). Habits including thumb sucking and mouth breathing in children have been reported as causal factors of class II malocclusion [8].
- Class III: Mesiobuccal cusp of the maxillary first molar occludes distal to the MB groove of the mandibular first molar.
  - Facial features include a concave facial profile (Fig. 19.5). Mandibular prognathism can create a prominent chin, while maxillary retrognathism can lead to inadequate lip support.
  - Skeletal causes include mandibular hyperplasia or prognathism or maxillary hypoplasia or retrognathism (Fig. 19.4). Acromegaly may lead to excess mandibular growth and result in a class III malocclusion [9].

Imaging

- Panoramic radiograph provides broad anatomical information of both jaws. Gross pathology of the maxilla or mandible or TMJ may be assessed.
- Cephalometric imaging is useful for observation of facial growth patterns and dental relationships. Cephalometric radiographs may be superimposed to visualize growth of structures throughout development or to study progression of treatment.
- Cephalometric analysis utilizes various facial landmarks. The coordinates of these structures and points are used in a digital model that calculates numerous facial relationships (i.e., incisor inclination, mandibular plane angle, nasolabial angle) that provide information on facial form and deviations from a reference standard (Fig. 19.6).
- Cone beam computed tomography (CBCT) has gained popularity as a 3D imaging technique in dentistry and oral surgery as it incurs less radiation exposure than traditional medical CT scans and allows surgeons to plan precise three-dimensional surgical movements. A CBCT scan is taken of the patient and imported to a software program to formulate a final surgical plan. 3D-printed customized splints, fixation plates, or cutting guides are fabricated and used intraoperatively to accurately reposition and fixate the bony segments.

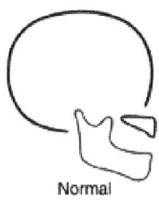

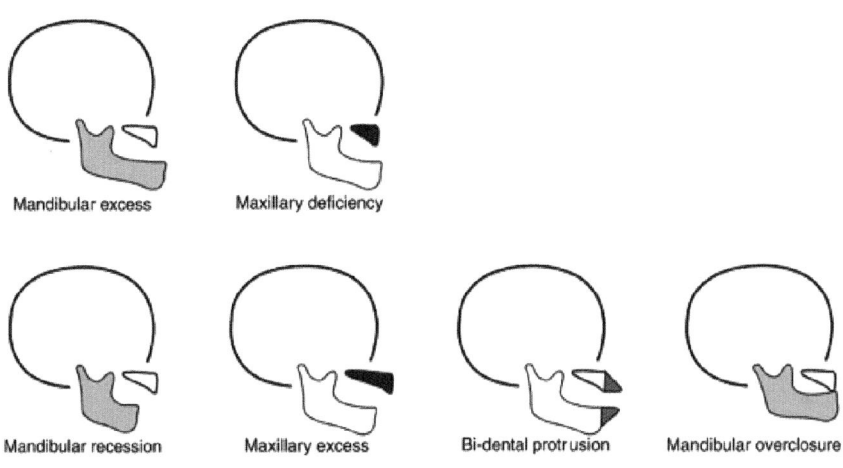

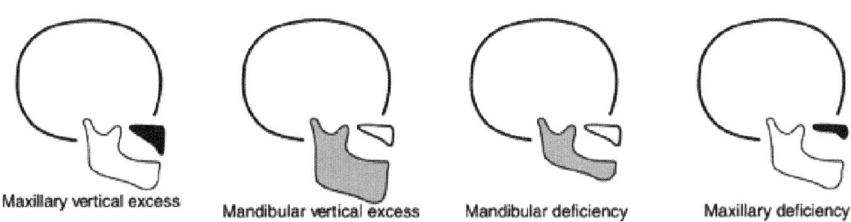

Fig. 19.4 Illustration of antero-posterior and vertical abnormalities in dentofacial deformities [11]

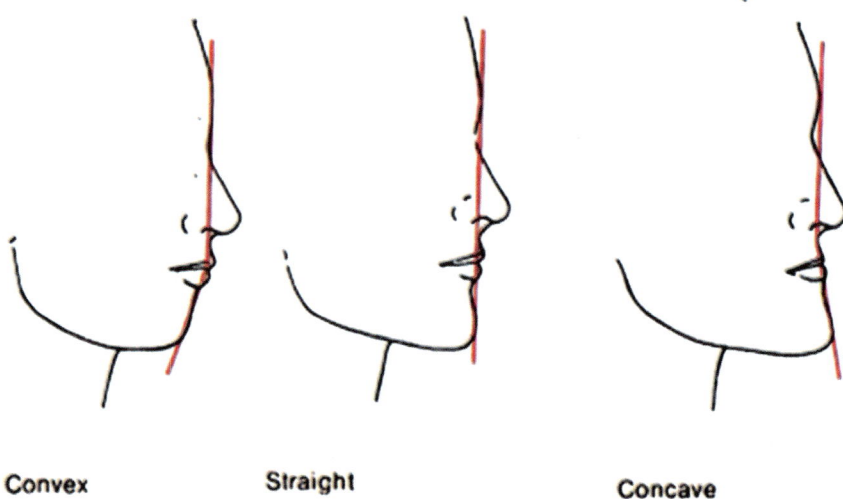

Fig. 19.5 Illustration of facial profiles [12]

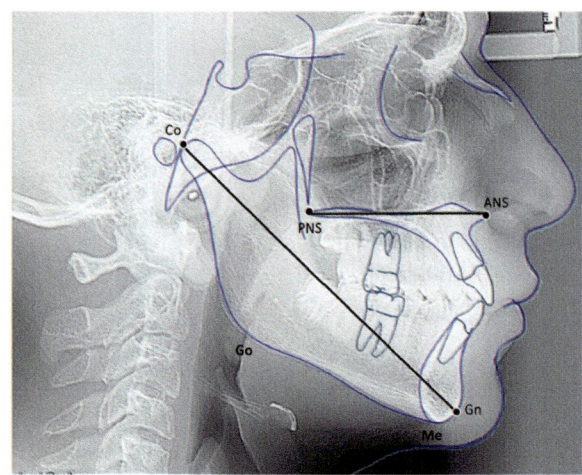

Fig. 19.6 Lateral cephalogram with hard and soft tissue tracings. Landmarks labelled include ANS, anterior nasal spine; Co, condylion; Gn, gnathion; Go, gonion; Me, menton; PNS, posterior nasal spine [13]

Specifics of Orthognathic Surgical Evaluation

- Oral Examination
  - Assess occlusion, cant
  - Ideal incisal show 2–4 mm
- Cephalometrics
  - Key anatomic points:
    - Sella

- Nasion
- A point (maxilla)
- B point (mandible)
- Measure SNA and SNB angles:
  - If angle is acute, then the bone is depressed
- Patterns of Diagnosis
  - Vertical maxillary excess
    - "Gummy smile" with long face and excessive incisor show
    - Class II
    - Decreased SNA/SNB
  - Vertical maxillary deficiency
    - No incisor show
    - Class III
    - Increased angles
  - Maxillary retrusion
    - Flat face with depressed nose
    - Decreased SNA, normal SNB
  - Retrognathia
    - Depressed mandible with obtuse cervicomental angle
    - Eversion of lip
    - SNB decreased
    - Class II
  - Prognathia
    - Protruding mandible
    - SNA normal but SNB obtuse
    - Class III

Orthodontic Decompensation

- In Class II or Class III patients, the incisors compensate for the malocclusion by tipping labially or lingually.
- Presurgical orthodontics align, level, and decompensate the occlusion in preparation for surgical movement. This often results in an exaggeration of the existing malocclusion. Postsurgical orthodontic treatment is also necessary to restore and stabilize the corrected occlusion [14].

Orthognathic Surgical Procedures

- Most often the Le Fort I osteotomy of the maxilla and the bilateral sagittal split osteotomy (BSSO) of the mandibular ramus:
  - These procedures involved cutting the bone and repositioning and stabilizing it to allow it to heal in an improved location.
  - Larger movements (usually >1 cm) may require distraction osteogenesis rather than single-stage advancement.
  - Maxillary procedures are based on the Le Fort fracture schema, but typically a Le Fort I is used for isolated occlusal problems. Le Fort II or III is used for higher midface deficits that may be present in syndromic patients.
- These procedures must be performed under general anesthesia in the operating room setting. A nasotracheal tube is utilized for intubation as occlusion must be assessed throughout the procedure.
- Patients undergoing orthognathic surgery should demonstrate cessation of facial skeletal growth, which typically occurs around age 15 in females and 17 in males. The gold standard to evaluate the cessation of facial skeletal growth is serial cephalometric superimposition [15, 16].
- Certain dentofacial deformities with severe psychosocial impact or those due to deficient growth may be treated early (skeletal Class II deformities). Dentofacial deformities related to excessive growth, such as mandibular hyperplasia (skeletal class III deformities), should not be treated early due to risk of relapse [17].
- Advancements in rigid fixation techniques have shortened the necessary duration of postoperative jaw immobilization. Orthodontic elastics are utilized to guide and stabilize the occlusion, and patients are restricted to a soft diet for 6–8 weeks following the procedure. Patients typically return to normal activity within 3 months [18].

Le Fort I Osteotomy [19]

- The maxilla may be advanced, setback, or repositioned vertically with the Le Fort I osteotomy. Segmentation of the maxilla in two or three pieces allows for more complex surgical movements.
- Maxilla is exposed intraorally with dissection extending from first molar to first molar and superiorly to the infraorbital foramina.
- The osteotomy extends horizontally from the piriform rim to the lateral maxillary buttresses with caution to avoid the apices of the maxillary teeth. Osteotomes are used to separate the maxilla from the nasal septum, nasal floor, and pterygomaxillary junction (Fig. 19.7).

- In cases of large movements, bone grafts may be necessary using local bone from the osteotomy. The maxilla is secured in the planned position with the surgical splint and fixated with plates and screws.

- Bilateral sagittal split osteotomy:
  - The BSSO is the most common surgical technique to reposition the mandible and correct for asymmetries, prognathism, or retrognathism. In cases that require extensive movements, the inverted-L osteotomy may be indicated [21].
  - The incision exposes the anterior ramus and body of the mandible as well as the medial ramus above the lingula.
  - The osteotomy is prepared horizontally through the medial ramus of the mandible, sagittally along the anterior ramus, and vertically to the inferior border of the mandible. Upon separation of the two segments, the inferior alveolar nerve is protected and remains in the distal segment. The mandibular condyles remain in the proximal segments (Fig. 19.8).
  - Rigid internal fixation is performed with screws or plates.

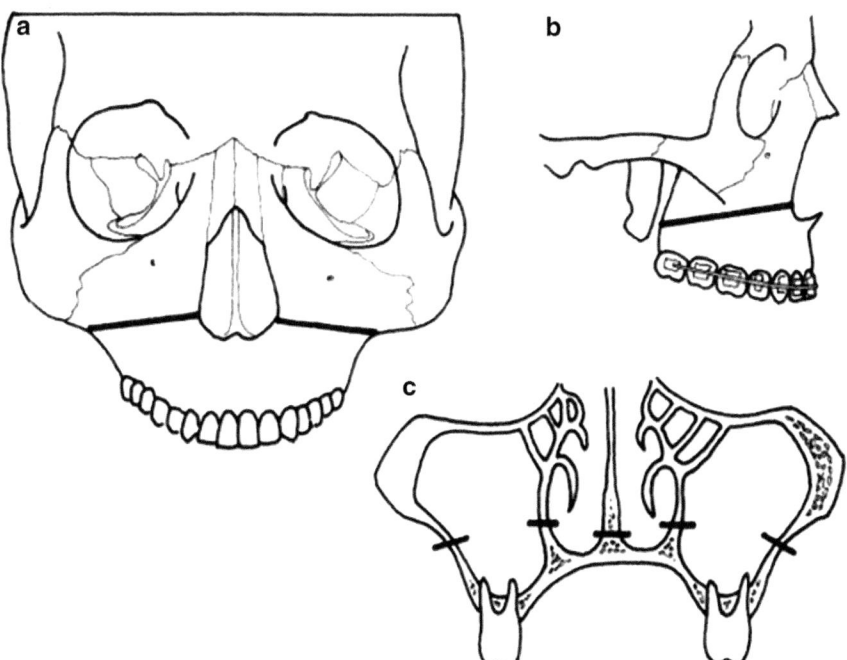

Fig. 19.7 Illustration of Le Fort I osteotomy. (**a**) Frontal view, (**b**) lateral view, (**c**) coronal section [20]

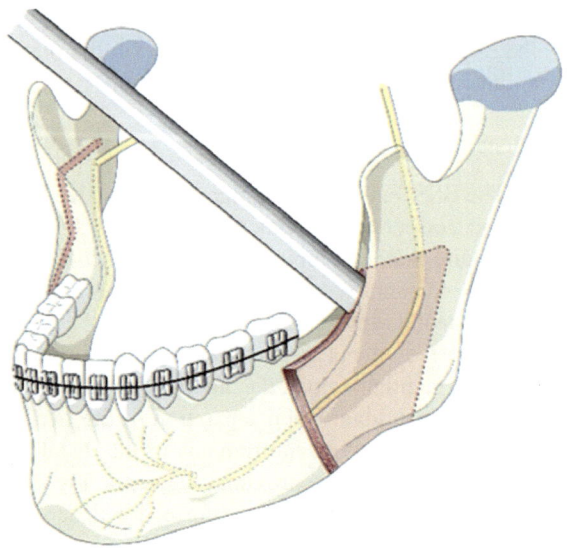

Fig. 19.8 Illustration of the bilateral sagittal split osteotomy [22]

- Complications [23–26]:
  - Infection.
  - Hemorrhage.
  - Development of a temporomandibular joint disorder.
  - Airway compromise.
  - Mechanical issues such as deformation or failure of hardware leading to nonunion of the osteotomy.
  - Dental relapse requiring additional orthodontics or surgical correction.
  - BSSO.
    - Hemorrhage from inferior alveolar or facial vessels.
    - Damage to the inferior alveolar nerve is the most common complication; approximately one-third of patients demonstrate neurosensory deficit at 1 year follow-up [27].
    - Unfavorable fractures due to inadequate osteotomy of the inferior border of the mandible. Reported association with the presence of impacted mandibular third molars [28].
    - Postoperative malocclusion due to failure of fixation hardware or intraoperative malposition of the condyles.
    - A significant percentage of patients report improvement in TMJ symptoms following surgery; however, worsening of symptoms is a rare complication [29].

- Le Fort I.
  - Higher risk of complications in patients that require extensive movements >9 mm or patients with anatomic irregularities such as orofacial clefts or vascular anomalies [19].
  - Tooth necrosis.
  - Hemorrhage from the internal maxillary artery, descending palatine artery, or pterygoid venous plexus.
  - Infraorbital nerve damage causing midface insensitivity.
  - Maxillary sinusitis or abscess.
  - Avascular necrosis of the maxilla is rare but may lead to bone resorption, periodontal defects, and pulpal necrosis.

References

1. Boyd SB. Management of obstructive sleep Apnea by Maxillomandibular advancement. Oral Maxillofac Surg Clin North Am. 2009;21:447–57.
2. Ploder O, Sigron G, Adekunle A, Burger-Krebes L, Haller B, Kolk A. The effect of Orthognathic surgery on temporomandibular joint function and symptoms: what are the risk factors? A longitudinal analysis of 375 patients. J Oral Maxillofac Surg. 2021;79:763–73.
3. Proffit WR, Fields HW Jr, Moray LJ. Prevalence of malocclusion and orthodontic treatment need in the United States: estimates from the NHANES III survey. Int J Adult Orthodon Orthognath Surg. 1998;13:97–106.
4. Gandedkar NH, Darendeliler MA. Combined orthodontic-surgical treatment may be an effective choice to improve oral health—related quality of life for individuals affected with severe dentofacial deformities. J Evid Based Dent Pract. 2020;20:101462.
5. Ghali GE, Meram AT, Garrett BC. Dental injury: anatomy, pathogenesis, and anesthesia considerations and implications. In: Fox IIIC, Cornett E, Ghali G, editors. Catastrophic perioperative complications and management. Cham: Springer; 2019. p. 83–94.
6. Türp JC, Alt KW. Anatomy and morphology of human teeth. Dent Anthropol. 1998:71–94.
7. Attaie AB, Ahmed MK. Oral anatomy. In: Ferraro's fundamentals of maxillofacial surgery. New York: Springer; 2015. p. 49–63.
8. Saghiri MA, Eid J, Tang CK, Freag P. Factors influencing different types of malocclusion and arch form – a review. J Stomatol Oral Maxillofac Surg. 2021;122:185–91.
9. Belmehdi A, Chbicheb S. Oral disorders related to acromegaly case report. Pan Afr Med J. 2019;34:96.
10. Sedeño Iii EJ, Alfonso M, Dolce C, Sedeño EJ. Orthodontics. In: The dental reference manual. Cham: Springer; 2017. p. 343–71.
11. Tashima A, Mackay DR. Orthognathic surgery. In: Tips and tricks in plastic surgery. Springer; 2022. p. 487–509.
12. Samizadeh S. Aesthetic assessment of the face. In: Non-surgical rejuvenation of asian faces. Cham: Springer; 2022. p. 107–21.
13. Hamdan A-L. Fundamental frequency and dentofacial anomalies. In: Dentofacial anomalies. Cham: Springer; 2021. p. 133–41.
14. Wolford LM. Comprehensive post Orthognathic surgery orthodontics: complications, misconceptions, and management. Oral Maxillofac Surg Clin North Am. 2020;32:135–51.
15. Caplin J, Han MD, Miloro M, Allareddy V, Markiewicz MR. Interceptive Dentofacial orthopedics (growth modification). Oral Maxillofac Surg Clin North Am. 2020;32:39–51.

16. Weaver N, Glover K, Major P, Varnhagen C, Grace M. Age limitation on provision of orthopedic therapy and orthognathic surgery. Am J Orthod Dentofacial Orthop. 1998;113:156. https://doi.org/10.1016/S0889-5406(98)70287-2.
17. Juan Alberto O'Ryan S. Surgical management of growing patients through orthognathic surgery: a review. Res Rep Oral Maxillofac Surg. 2020;4:029. https://doi.org/10.23937/2643-3907/1710029.
18. Wolford LM, Rodrigues DB, Limoeiro E. Orthognathic and TMJ surgery: postsurgical patient management. J Oral Maxillofac Surg. 2011;69:2893–903.
19. Buchanan EP, Hyman CH. LeFort I Osteotomy. Semin Plast Surg. 2013;27:149. https://doi.org/10.1055/s-0033-1357112.
20. Greenberg AM, Aziz SR. Maxillary osteotomies. In: Craniomaxillofacial reconstructive and corrective bone surgery; 2019. p. 575–602.
21. Franco PB, Farrell BB. Inverted L osteotomy: a new approach via intraoral access through the advances of virtual surgical planning and custom fixation. Oral Maxillofac Surg Cases. 2016;2:1–9.
22. Choi J-W, Lee JY. Update on Orthognathic surgical techniques. In: The surgery-first orthognathic approach. Singapore: Springer; 2021. p. 149–58.
23. Robl MT, Farrell BB, Tucker MR. Complications in orthognathic surgery: a report of 1000 cases. Oral Maxillofac Surg Clin North Am. 2014;26:599–609.
24. Verweij JP, Houppermans PNWJ, Gooris P, Mensink G, van Merkesteyn JPR. Risk factors for common complications associated with bilateral sagittal split osteotomy: a literature review and meta-analysis. J Craniofac Surg. 2016;44:1170–80.
25. Kotaniemi KVM, Suojanen J, Palotie T. Peri- and postoperative complications in Le fort I osteotomies. J Craniofac Surg. 2021;49:789–98.
26. Zaroni FM, Cavalcante RC, João da Costa D, Kluppel LE, Scariot R, Rebellato NLB. Complications associated with orthognathic surgery: a retrospective study of 485 cases. J Craniofac Surg. 2019;47:1855–60.
27. Bays RA, Bouloux GF. Complications of orthognathic surgery. Oral Maxillofac Surg Clin North Am. 2003;15:229–42.
28. Verweij JP, Mensink G, Fiocco M, van Merkesteyn JPR. Presence of mandibular third molars during bilateral sagittal split osteotomy increases the possibility of bad split but not the risk of other post-operative complications. J Craniofac Surg. 2014;42:e359–63.
29. Dujoncquoy JP, Ferri J, Raoul G, Kleinheinz J. Temporomandibular joint dysfunction and orthognathic surgery: a retrospective study. Head Face Med. 2010;6:27.

Chapter 20
Facial Clefts and Hypertelorism

Brendan J. Cronin

Background and Epidemiology

- *Congenital craniofacial clefts*
    - Anatomic distortions of the face and cranium with deficiencies or excesses of tissue in a linear pattern.
    - Occur along predictable embryologic lines.
    - Incredibly disfiguring.
- *Tessier classification.*
    - Originally proposed by Tessier derived from clinical observation + study of 3D CT scans; reinforced by newer neuroembryologic theories of developmental zones of the face.
- Clefts are numbered from 0 to 14 *depending on the relationship to the orbit (Fig. 20.1)*:
    - *The orbit* divides the face into upper and lower hemispheres and *separates the cranial clefts from the facial clefts.*
    - Numbered so that the facial component of the cleft + cranial component always add to 14.
    - The soft tissue and skeletal components of a cleft are seldom affected to the same extent.

B. J. Cronin (✉)
Division of Plastic and Reconstructive Surgery, University of California, Los Angeles, CA, USA

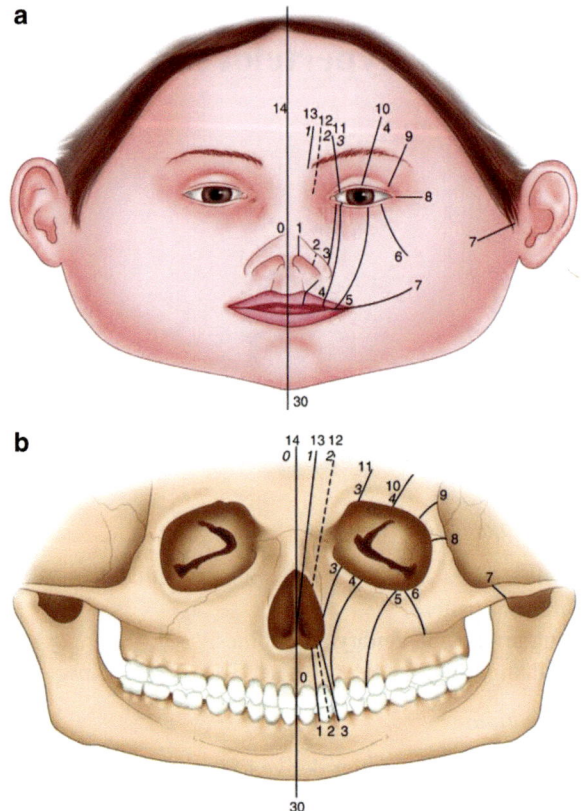

Fig. 20.1 Tessier classification of craniofacial clefts. (https://link.springer.com/chapter/10.1007/978-3-319-63290-2_21. Raposo-Amaral, C.E., Jarrahy, R., Lim, R., Alonso, N. (2018). The Rare Facial Cleft. In: Alonso, N., Raposo-Amaral, C. (eds) Cleft Lip and Palate Treatment. Springer, Cham. https://doi.org/10.1007/978-3-319-63290-2_21. Permissions license number: 5333700474781)

Craniofacial Clefts

- *Number 0.*
  - Unique because these clefts can present as either *tissue excess* or *tissue deficiency*.
  - *Deficiencies*—hypoplasia or agenesis of soft tissue structures of the midline.
    - Soft tissue deficiencies.
      - *Midline facial cleft*, including the lip and nose, can extend up into nasal floor causing complete lack of columella with depressed nasal tip and vestigial caudal septum.

20 Facial Clefts and Hypertelorism

- Skeletal deficiencies.
  - Range from separation of central incisors to absent premaxilla with cleft palate.
  - Deficient or absent nasal bones and septal cartilage, diminutive ethmoid sinus (can cause hypotelorism), possible encephalocele.
- *Excess*—widening or duplication of midline structures.
  - Soft tissue excess.
    - Broad philtral column, bifid nasal tip.
  - Skeletal excess.
    - Structures are broad or duplicated and displaced from midline.
      - Duplicate nasal spine and nasal septum.
      - Broad/flattened/laterally displaced nasal bones and upper/lower lateral cartilages.
      - Widening ethmoid and sphenoid sinuses leads to widened anterior cranial fossa which causes hypertelorism.
      - Widened crista galli/cribiform plate.
      - Broadened sphenoid body with lateral pterygoid plate displacement.

– *Number 1*
  - *Soft tissue*
    - Passes through Cupid's bow and alar rim causing *notching of the soft triangle of the nose* and septal deviation away from the cleft.
  - *Skeletal*
    - Alveolar cleft is rare (would pass between central and lateral incisor).
    - Passes through nasal floor just lateral to the nasal spine and can extend posteriorly as complete cleft palate.
    - Cephalad extension passes through junction of nasal bone and frontal process of the maxilla (broad flat nasal bones) and can cause hypertelorism due to ethmoidal expansion.

– *Number 2*
  - *Soft tissue*
    - Cupid's bow/cleft lip, hypoplasia of middle alar 1/3 (compared to *notching* seen in No. 1 cleft).
    - *No* eyelid involvement, passes *medial* to palpebral fissure.
    - Displaced medial canthus but *no* disruption of lacrimal apparatus.

- *Skeletal*
  - Cleft traverse the alveolus across lateral incisor.
  - Aperture lateral to septum and medial to maxillary sinus, can cause cleft of hard/soft palate.
  - Cephalad extension passes through junction of the nasal bone and frontal process of the maxilla (broad flat nasal bones) and can cause hypertelorism due to ethmoidal expansion.
- Number 3
  - *Oronasal-ocular cleft = most common Tessier cleft.*
  - *Soft tissue*
    - Passes through Cupid's bow and alar rim causing lateral alar base displacement, continues between medial canthus and inferior lacrimal punctum *disrupting the lacrimal apparatus (*can cause epiphora).
    - Lower eyelid colobomas (medial to lacrimal punctum).
      - May be the only soft tissue evidence of this cleft*.
  - *Skeletal*
    - Involves orbit.
    - Causes direct communication of oral, nasal, and orbital cavities.
    - Between lateral incisor and canine through frontal process of the maxilla into lacrimal groove disrupting the orbital floor.
- Number 4
  - *Soft tissue*
    - Begins *lateral* to the Cupid's bow (unlike clefts 0–3) and passes lateral to the alar rim (unlike cleft 3) onto the cheek and curves onto the lower eyelid (lateral to inferior punctum; lacrimal duct is *normal*).
      - Globe typically normal, however, can cause anophthalmia or epiphora.
  - *Skeletal*
    - Between lateral incisor and canine ☐ lateral to piriform aperture, involving maxillary sinus (medial wall is intact).
      - Oral cavity, maxillary sinus, and orbit are in continuity but "not" the nasal cavity.
    - Passes *medial* to the infraorbital foramen (cleft 5 passes *lateral* to the foramen) and terminates at medial aspect of inferior orbital rim.
- Number 5
  - *Extremely rare*
  - *Soft tissue*

20 Facial Clefts and Hypertelorism

- Begins just medial to oral commissure and passes along the cheek lateral to alar rim, terminates in lateral border of the lower eyelid.
- *Skeletal*
  - Lateral to canine (near premolars) ☐ "lateral" to infraorbital foramen ☐ lateral aspect of the orbital rim and floor.
  - Orbital contents can prolapse through lateral floor defect into maxillary sinus and cause vertical orbital dystopia.

- *Number 6*
  - *Seen in Treacher Collins and Nager syndromes.*
  - *Soft tissue*
    - Vertical furrow of hypoplasia running from angle of the mandible through zygomatic eminence to the lateral palpebral fissure.
    - Inferior displacement of the lateral canthus ☐ down-slanting palpebral fissure ☐ appearance of severe lower lid ectropion.
    - Lateral lower eyelid colobomas.
  - *Skeletal*
    - Cleft along the zygomaticomaxillary suture (cleft Nos. 8 and 9 pass along zygomaticotemporal and zygomaticofrontal suture, respectively) passes into lateral orbit and connects with inferior orbital fissure:
      - No alveolar cleft but posterior maxilla can be shortened.
    - Choanal atresia.
    - Hypoplastic zygoma but intact arch.

- *Number 7*
  - *Common cleft*—seen in craniofacial microsomia and Treacher Collins syndrome.
  - *Unpaired (no cranial extension).*
  - *Soft tissue.*
    - Begins at oral commissure—ranges from slight widening of oral commissure with preauricular skin tag to complete fissure and microtia.
    - Can have absence of the parotid gland, facial nerve weakness, possible weakness/hypoplasia of the ipsilateral palate and tongue.
  - *Skeletal*
    - Cleft passes through pterygomaxillary junction, centered around the zygomaticotemporal suture.
    - Hypoplastic ramus and posterior maxilla can lead to loss of posterior facial height and an up-slanting occlusal plane.

- Hypoplastic condyle can cause anterior open bite.
- Hypoplastic zygoma can have complete absence of the arch with residual zygomatic stump.

- *Number 8*
  - *Soft tissue.*
    - Divides the facial and cranial clefts.
    - Passes directly lateral from lateral canthus to the temporal region.
    - Presents as a true lateral commissure coloboma ("dermatocele") with an absent lateral canthus.
    - +/− epibulbar dermoids (associated with Goldenhar syndrome)
  - *Skeletal.*
    - Cleft through the zygomaticofrontal suture.
    - Lack of underlying zygoma to support the lateral canthus leads to draping of the lateral canthus region from the greater wing of the sphenoid alone and presents with down-slanting palpebra.
    - Presence of this cleft creates soft tissue continuity of the orbit and the temporal fossa.

- *Number 9*
  - *Rarest cleft*
  - *Soft tissue*
    - Marked by abnormalities of the *lateral 1/3* of the upper eyelid and eyebrow.
    - Can have microphthalmia (small globe) and superolaterally displaced globe (from upper orbit bony defect).
    - Extends into temporoparietal hairline causing anterior hairline displacement.
    - Can have frontal branch of CN VII abnormalities.
  - *Skeletal*
    - Cleft extends through superolateral orbit.
    - Causes hypoplasia of greater wing of sphenoid and outward and posterior rotation of the orbit and globe.
    - May present with abnormalities of squamosal part of temporal bone and parietal bones.

- *Number 10*
  - *Soft tissue*
    - Middle third of the upper eyelid and eyebrow.
    - Elongated palpebral fissure with inferolaterally displaced amblyopic eye due to herniation of soft tissue through fronto-orbital defect.
    - Can have complete upper eyelid absence in severe forms ("ablepharia").

- **Skeletal**
  - Involves middle part of supraorbital rim just *lateral* to the supraorbital foramen.
  - Gap in the frontal bone can lead to the presence of fronto-orbital *encephalocele*.
- Number 11
  - **Soft tissue**
    - Medial one-third of the upper eyelid +/− coloboma.
  - **Skeletal**
    - Cleft in medial one-third of supraorbital rim.
    - Can involve ethmoid and cause hypertelorism.
- Number 12
  - **Soft tissue**
    - Lies medial to medial canthus; coloboma can extend to include medial root of the eyebrow.
    - Causes lateral displacement of the medial canthus.
    - *No* upper eyelid notching.
  - **Skeletal**
    - Passes through the frontal process of the maxilla and then causes a widening of the ethmoid air cells that results in lateral displacement and rotation of the orbit/globe and telecanthus.
    - Located lateral to the olfactory groove—cribriform plate is *normal*.
    - *No* risk of encephalocele.
- Number 13
  - **Soft tissue**
    - Encephalocele (between frontal process of the maxilla and the nasal bone).
    - Soft tissue cleft, if any notable, is medial to the eyelid and eyebrow but can cause inferior displacement of the medial brow.
  - **Skeletal**
    - Classic finding is widening of the cribriform plate:
      - Can be displaced inferiorly leading to orbital dystopia.
      - Can have widening of the ethmoid sinus and hypertelorism.
    - Severe hypertelorism (most significant of any Tessier cleft) can be seen with bilateral No. 13 clefts.

- *Number 14*
  - *Like its counterpart cleft No. 0, can present with tissue excess or deficiency.*
    - Degree of facial deformity parallels degree of cranial/brain deformity and chances of neurological viability.
  - *Soft tissue*
    - *Deficiencies*—present with *hypotelorism*, on the *holoprosencephaly* spectrum (cyclopia, cebocephaly).
    - *Excess*—present with *hyper*telorism; encephalocele (frontonasal or midline frontal), glabellar flattening, and *extreme* lateral displacement of medial canthi.
  - *Skeletal*
    - Flattened caudal frontal bones leads to wide bossed forehead with midline furrow, depressed nasal root, and flaring of the lateral forehead.
    - Typically find widened olfactory grooves, inferiorly displaced cribriform plates, enlarged ethmoids.
    - Bifid crista gali and perpendicular plate of the ethmoid.
- *Number 30*
  - *Median cleft of the lower jaw.*
    - Caudal extension of cleft 14 and 0.
  - *Soft tissue.*
    - Spectrum ranging from notching of the midline lower lip to complete the lower lip and chin midline cleft with bifid mandible and tongue or even complete absence of the tongue.
  - *Skeletal.*
    - Cleft beginning between the central incisors (due to failure of formation of first branchial arch).
    - Neck abnormalities (due to failure of fusion of fourth branchial arch) including absent hyoid bone and diminutive thyroid cartilage and atrophic strap muscles.
- *Hypertelorism*
  - *Telecanthus (soft tissue)*: increased distance between the medial canthi (can have telecanthus with or without orbital hypertelorism).
  - *Orbital hypertelorism (bone)*: increased distance between the medial most aspect of the orbital rims ("interdacryon distance").
    - Normal, 32–34 mm; moderate, 45–39 mm; severe >40 mm.
    - *In children: >25 mm = abnormal

- Can be seen with Tessier clefts 10–14.
  - Due to widening of ethmoid bone/air cells.
- *Causes orbital dystopia, which can be vertical or horizontal.*
  - *Horizontal*: laterally displaced orbits (orbital hypertelorism) or medially displaced (hypotelorism).
    - Seen in No. 14 clefts.
  - *Vertical*: vertical orbital displacement.
    - Seen in clefts 10–13.
- *Management.*
  - Facial bipartition or box osteotomy.
    - Both correct vertical/horizontal orbital dystopia, but facial bipartition can also widen a constricted upper palate, while orbital box osteotomies have no effect on the dentition/palate.

Management

- *Timing of surgical intervention*
  - Degree of deformity
    - Mild deformity? Delay surgery.
    - Severe deformity or functional issues (ocular exposure, speech abnormalities)? Perform early surgery.
  - General guiding principles
    - *3–12 months of age*: cranial defects and soft tissue clefts
    - *6–9 years of age*: midface reconstruction and bone grafting
    - *Skeletal maturity*: orthognathic procedures.
- *Reconstructive procedures are tailored to anatomical regions*
  - *Nose* (clefts 0–3)
    - Cleft tissue is excised, cartilage reconstructed with grafts and the skin with local flaps.
    - Cantilever bone grafts can be used as needed for more severe deformities.
  - *Upper lip* (clefts 0–5)
    - Repaired with similar principles to the classic cleft lip/palate.
      - Vermilion and orbicularis are reapproximated.
      - If lateral to the philtral column, tissue is simply excised.

- Lateral commissure cleft closed in a straight line fashion.
- Lower lip clefts closed with V-excision.
- *Mandible* (clefts 6–8, microsomia, Treacher Collins)
  - *Mild deformity*: mandibular distraction (6–8 years old).
  - *Severe deformity*: costochondral grafts.
  - *Maxilla*: Le Fort I at skeletal maturity.
- *Periorbita*
  - *Eyelid:*
    - Requires urgent reconstruction in cases of orbital exposure to prevent blindness from corneal ulceration, however, have to maintain enough eyelid opening to prevent deprivation amblyopia.
    - Lid switch flaps for skin/muscle deficiencies.
  - *Medial canthus:* can be repositioned with transnasal wiring.
  - *Lateral canthus:* reposition as needed with lateral canthopexy.
  - *Lacrimal apparatus:* often disrupted, can be corrected with silastic stent placement or dacryocystorhinostomy.
  - *Orbit:* bone grafting to correct dystopia or restore orbital continuity.
    - *Orbital dystopia: corrected with facial bipartition* vs *box osteotomy* vs *subcranial Le Fort III.*

References

1. Kawamoto HK Jr. The kaleidoscopic world of rare craniofacial clefts: order out of chaos (Tessier classification). Clin Plast Surg. 1976;3(4):529–72.
2. Tessier P. Anatomical classification facial, cranio-facial and latero-facial clefts. J Maxillofac Surg. 1976;4(2):69–92.
3. da Silva FR, Alonso N, Shin JH, Busato L, Ono MC, Cruz GA. Surgical correction of Tessier number 0 cleft. J Craniofac Surg. 2008;19(5):1348–52.
4. Raposo-Amaral CE, Jarrahy R, Lim R, Alonso N. The Rare Facial Cleft. In: Alonso N, Raposo-Amaral C, editors. Cleft Lip and Palate Treatment. Cham: Springer; 2018. https://doi.org/10.1007/978-3-319-63290-2_21.

Chapter 21
Ear Reconstruction and Otoplasty

Brendan J. Cronin

Embryology

- *Auricle.*
    - Ear derived from six hillocks on the *first* and *second* branchial arches (Fig. 21.1)
        - Hillocks 1–3 (first branchial arch) give rise to the tragus, helical root, and helical crus.
        - Hillocks 4–6 (second branchial arch) give rise to the antihelix, antitragus, and lobule.
    - Forms in the lower neck and migrates posterolaterally during development—arrested growth □ low set ears (seen in many craniofacial syndromes).
- *External auditory canal (EAC).*
    - Ectodermal cells from *first* branchial cleft form a plug which then degenerates to create a patent canal—lack of degeneration of plug □ congenital aural atresia or stenosis.
    - Canal is 2/3 bone (inner part) and 1/3 fibrocartilaginous tissue (outer segment).
- *Tympanic membrane.*
    - Trilaminar structure of the epithelium (ectoderm), middle fibrous layer (mesoderm), and inner mucosal layer (endoderm).

B. J. Cronin (✉)
Division of Plastic and Reconstructive Surgery, University of California, Los Angeles, CA, USA

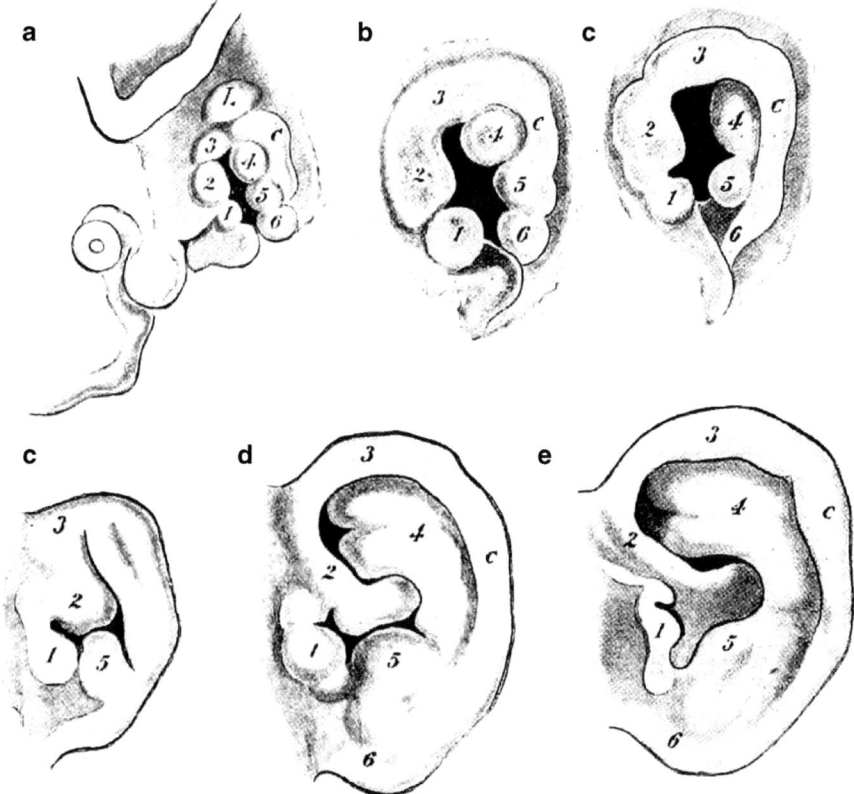

Fig. 21.1 The development of the ear from the first and second branchial arches as well as the first branchial cleft is shown above. The tragus, root of the helix, and apex of the helical rim are derived from the first branchial arch, helical rim, scapha, antitragus and lobule from the second and the external auditory canal from the first branchial cleft. (Prentiss, Charles William. "A laboratory manual and text-book of embryology" (1915). Philadelphia, London, W. B. Saunders. CC0 1.0 Universal (CC0 1.0). Public Domain Dedication. https://www.flickr.com/photos/internetarchivebookimages/20546648349/)

Anatomy

- *Ear topography* (Fig. 21.2).
- *Innervation* (Fig. 21.3).
  - *Greater auricular nerve (C2/C3)*—lower half of the ear (anterior + posterior).
    - *Injury leads to permanent numbness of the lower half of the ear*—must avoid injury during facelift/neck dissection.
    - Emerges at *Erb's point* (6.5 cm below tragus or 1/3 distance from mastoid to clavicular insertion of SCM at the posterior edge of the SCM).

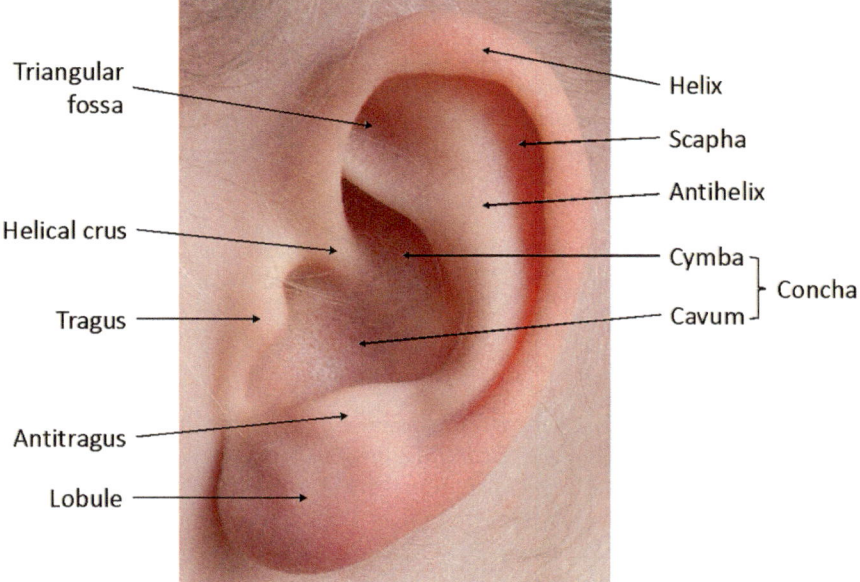

Fig. 21.2 Anatomy of the ear. (Brendan Cronin, MD. Own work)

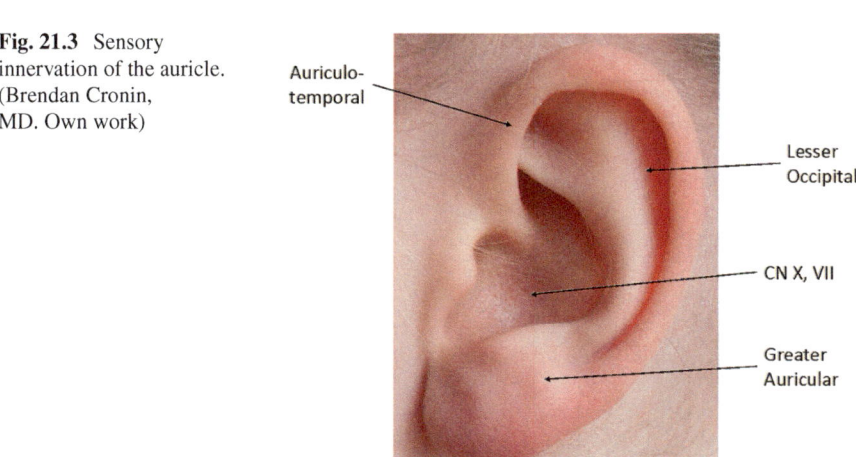

Fig. 21.3 Sensory innervation of the auricle. (Brendan Cronin, MD. Own work)

- *Lesser occipital nerve (C2/C3)*—posterior upper half of anterior and posterior surface of the ear.
- *Auriculotemporal nerve (V3)*—anterior upper half of anterior surface of the ear + anterior EAC.
- *Auricular branch of the vagus nerve (X)*—concha + posterior aspect of EAC.

- *Blood supply.*
  - *Posterior auricular artery*—dominant blood supply to both posterior *and* anterior aspects of the ear (via perforating branches).
  - *Superficial temporal artery*—supplies anterior surface and forms interconnections with posterior auricular artery perforating branches.
- *Lymphatics*: parallels embryologic development.
  - Tragus/helical root/helical crus (first arch) ☐ preauricular basin.
  - Antihelix, antitragus, lobule ☐ retro/infra-auricular nodal basins.
- *Clinical measurements and angles of the ear.*
  - *Position:*
    - Located 6 cm (one ear's worth) posterior to the lateral orbital rim, the normal ear spans from the level of the brow to the nasal ala with a main axis that is 20 degrees retroclined from vertical.
    - Normal projection (relative to the skull): 10–12 mm (upper third), 16–18 mm (middle third), 20–22 mm (lobule).
  - *Angles:*
    - *Auriculocephalic angle*—from bird's eye view, the angle formed by the mastoid and the line tangent to the midpoint of the helix. Normally 20–30 degrees.
    - *Scaphoconchal angle*—angle formed between the scapha and concha, normally <90 degrees.

Ear Deformities

- *Congenital*
  - *Prominent Ear.*
    - *Deformity*—can have prominence of the upper, mid, and lower thirds of the ear.
      - *Upper*—due to effacement of the antihelical fold.
        - Inadequate folding of the helix ☐ protrusion of the scapha and helical rim (normal angle is <90 degrees).
        - *Most common cause of prominent ear.*
      - *Mid*—due to excessively deep concha (>1.5 cm) or excess conchomastoidal angle.
      - *Lower*—due to a protruding earlobe.

- *Management—Otoplasty* [4].
  - *Timing*—6–7 years of age.
  - *Upper Third*—scaphoconchal sutures ("Mustarde" sutures) +/− cartilage scoring (Stenstrom technique).
    - The cartilage bends away from scored surfaces due to contraction of perichondrocytes on the intact side.
  - *Middle Third*—conchal resection (excessive depth) or "Furnas" conchomastoidal sutures (excess angle).
  - *Lower Third*—reduction of the ear lobe +/− inferior aspect of the conchal bowl.
- *Complications.*
  - Hematoma (needs to be immediately evacuated to prevent cauliflower ear).
  - Infection (cellulitis—rare but IV Abx are necessary to prevent chondritis which requires debridement and can be disfiguring).
  - Suture complications—protrusion of sutures through the skin (monofilament) and granuloma formation (braided suture).
  - *Overcorrection* (*most common* significant complication).
- *Macrotia.*
  - *Deformity*—excessively large (different than prominent) ears.
  - *Management*—Excise a semilunar strip of scapha and a small wedge of helical rim.
- *Constricted Ear—"Cup" or "Lop" Ear Deformity.*
  - *Deformity.*
    - Range of deformity from folding of the superior aspect of the helical rim (lop) to a deficiency of helical rim skin and cartilage that creates a tight and constricted upper ear.
  - *Management.*
    - Helical crus is advanced out of the concha and into the helical rim to replace deficient length +/− scaphoconchal sutures to recreate the antihelical fold.
    - Severe constriction may require complete auricular reconstruction.
- *Stahl's Ear—"Spock ear".*
  - Deformity—A third accessory crus extends from the antihelix in a transverse orientation, disrupting the helical rim and scapha contour; the concha is intact.
  - Management—wedge excision of the third crus with helical advancement.

- *Cryptotia.*
  - *Deformity.*
    - Superior parts of the ear appear "buried" beneath the skin.
    - Absence of the superior auriculocephalic sulcus.
  - *Management.*
    - Creation of a new superior auriculocephalic sulcus.
    - The superior aspect of the auricular cartilage is advanced from under the scalp such that the edge of the helical rim is clearly visible. An incision is placed along this line, freeing the cartilage framework, and the resulting medial deficiency from cartilage advancement is grafted or covered with a scalp advancement flap.
- *Ear Molding.*
  - Must distinguish between malformation (part of ear skin or cartilage is *absent*) vs deformation (all parts present but abnormal).
  - Molding can be used to restore normal contour in the above ear deformations (malformations require reconstruction).
  - High plasticity of auricular cartilage early in life (due to circulating maternal estrogens) permits the use of ear molding to correct prominent ear and other deformities:
    - Maternal estrogens peak at day 3 and return to normal by week 6.
    - Many infants will have spontaneous resolution of ear deformities within the first week of life—wait till 1 week of age to begin molding therapy.
- Acquired.
  - *Epidemiology.*

Malignancy

- Squamous cell carcinoma (SCC).
  - *Most common malignancy of the ear.*
- *Chondrodermatitis nodularis chronica helicis.*
  - Painful inflammatory papule on the helix.
  - High recurrence rate—Treat with excisional biopsy and avoid sleeping on the affected side.
- *Trauma.*
  - *Hematoma—requires immediate evacuation* and *bolster* (fluid accumulation between the perichondrium and skin disrupts skin vascular supply and causes skin necrosis and can calcify/fibrose causing *cauliflower ear deformity*).

- *Lacerations.*
  - *Simple lacerations*—repair in a single layer.
  - *Complex/large lacerations*—reapproximate the cartilage in addition to the skin.
- *Avulsions.*
  - Replantation determined by multiple factors including mechanism of injury, presence of donor/recipient vessels and location/level of amputation/avulsion.
- *Specific Acquired Deformities and Management.*
  - *Acquired.*
    - *Partial Thickness.*
      - *Perichondrium present:*
        - Small defects—will heal by secondary intention/wound care.
        - Large defects—require full-thickness skin graft.
      - *No perichondrium present:*
        - Helical rim: Advancement flaps, if <1.5 cm, can convert to full thickness and perform wedge excision of the helical rim.
        - Conchal bowel: trapdoor flap, postauricular island "revolving door" flap.
    - *Full-Thickness Defects of the Upper Third.*
      - *Primary closure.*
        - Defects <1.5 cm (otherwise ☐ size discrepancy with contralateral ear).
        - Star pattern excision limits buckling.
      - *Local skin flaps*—preauricular flap or retroauricular flap.
        - Can be transposition (preauricular) or advancement flaps (retroauricular).
        - Defects >25% of helical rim require cartilage support.
      - *Helical advancement (Antia-Buch flap, Fig. 21.4).*
        - *Defects up to 3 cm.*
        - Incision made in helical sulcus along entire length from the scapha to lobule through the anterior skin and cartilage—the posterior skin is preserved.
        - Posterior skin elevated in supraperichondreal plane to create chondrocutaneous composite flap based on posterior skin and advanced to close defect.
        - V-Y advancement of the helical root provides additional length.

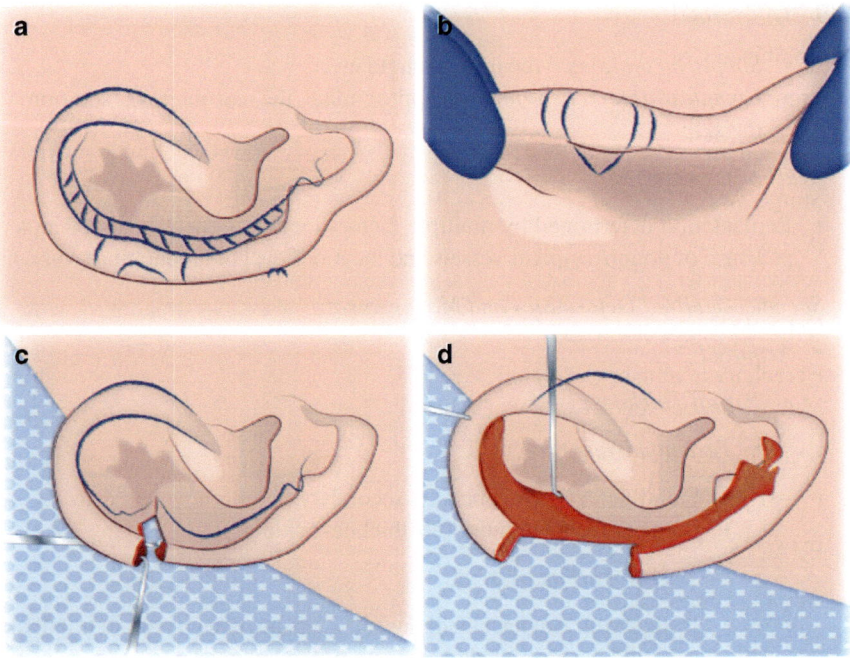

Fig. 21.4 (*note the title should read Anti*a*-Buch helical advancement flap (the current title is missing an "a"). Schematic of Antia-Buch helical advancement flap. The incisions and area to be undermined are outlined (**a**). The planned helical rim defect margins are shown (**b**). After creation of wedge-shaped, full-thickness, helical rim defect (**c**). Full-thickness incisions through the skin and cartilage (but not posterior auricular skin) are made along the internal margin of the helical rim. The retroauricular skin is then undermined and prepared for advancement and closure of the defect. (https://link.springer.com/chapter/10.1007/978-3-030-66865-5_25. Stavrakas, M., Trigkatzis, P. (2021). Common Local Flaps. In: Stavrakas, M., Khalil, H.S. (eds) Rhinology and Anterior Skull Base Surgery. Springer, Cham. https://doi.org/10.1007/978-3-030-66865-5_25. Permissions: 5331530033103)

- *Conchal cartilage graft* (contralateral ear) covered with retroauricular flap:
  - Defects <1.5 cm.
  - Composite grafts will have predictable pattern of color changes during process of graft take: white (ischemia, up to 24 hrs), blue (venous congestion, 24–72 hrs), and pink (neovascularization, 3–7 days).
- *Tubed retroauricular graft* (for isolated defects of the helical rim).
- *Full-Thickness Defects of the Middle Third.*
  - Primary closure + excision of accessory triangles.
  - Helical advancement (Antia-Buch).
  - Conchal cartilage graft and retroauricular flap.

- *Conchal Defects.*
    - Revolving door flap.
        - Can replace the entire concha with this flap.
        - A circular skin paddle involving the posterior ear and mastoid is raised posteriorly and anteriorly, keeping vascular attachments at a midline axis that becomes a pivot point to rotate the flap anteriorly into the conchal defect.
        - Posterior defect is closed primarily.
- *Lobe.*
    - Various techniques described:
        - All involve folding a local flap over itself with or without cartilage graft for support.
- *Microtia/Anotia.*

Background

- *Epidemiology*: 1:6000 births; male/female, 2:1; R/L/bilateral, 5:3:1.
- *Etiology*: typically sporadic/isolated but can also be related to ischemia (in utero tissue ischemia due to obliteration of the stapedial artery or hemorrhage into the developing ear—degree of hemorrhage dictates degree of deformity), teratogens (thalidomide), or infection (rubella).
- *Associated syndromes*: hemifacial microsomia, Goldenhar, Treacher Collins.
- *Presentation*
    - Due to different embryologic origins of inner and outer ears—inner ear is often spared while defects of outer and middle ear are common.
        - Usually leads to *conductive (80%)* > *sensorineural* hearing loss due to EAC atresia or stenosis.
            - Most hearing loss in microtia/anotia is treated with conductive hearing aids—anchoring these in the bone with osseo-integrated or bone-anchored "BAHA" hearing aids improves coaptation/effectiveness.
    - Classification
        - Grade I—small auricle but normal surface topographic anatomy.
        - Grade II—small auricle + malformed surface topographic anatomy.
        - Grade III—small remnant of "peanut-shaped" external cartilage and skin + atresia of the EAC.
        - Grade IV—complete absence of the auricle (anotia) + EAC atresia.

- *Preop Workup*
  - Family history and genetics evaluation.
  - Audiometric evaluation (determine conductive vs sensorineural hearing loss).
  - Temporal bone imaging (CT of middle ear ossicles for planning otologic surgery + MRI to determine course of facial nerve—can be displaced).
- *Timing*
  - Audiogram + bone conduction hearing aid ASAP after diagnosis.
  - Ear reconstruction at age 6–8.
    - Timing depends on the availability of donor rib cartilage, psychosocial factors, and need for acoustic surgery (perform reconstruction prior to canaloplasty).
    - Recommended to wait until *patient* not parent's requests reconstruction as this indicates willingness to comply with postoperative care.
  - Canaloplasty (at time of second stage ear reconstruction or later).
- *Techniques*
  - *Brent* [1].
    - Can be performed as early as age 6 (requires less initial cartilage harvest).
    - Four stages.
      - *Stage I*: Cartilage framework fabricated from contralateral costochondral rib cartilage of the synchondrosis of sixth to eighth ribs, placed in subcutaneous pocket.
      - *Stage II*: Lobule transposition.
      - *Stage III*: Elevation of construct and skin grafting of retroauricular sulcus.
      - *Stage IV*: Conchal graft from contralateral ear to create tragus.
  - *Nagata* [2].
    - Delayed till age 10 or chest circumference of 60 cm (requires significant initial cartilage harvest).
    - Two stages.
      - *Stage I*: *Ipsilateral* rib cartilage harvest from ribs 6–9, perichondrium left intact to minimize deformity and permit regrowth. Framework—including tragal component—constructed and placed in subcutaneous pocket. Lobule also transposed in this stage.
      - *Stage II*: Framework re-elevated, retorauricular sulcus created with wedge of cartilage from the fifth rib, posterior aspect of reconstructed ear is covered with a tunneled temporoparietal fascial flap and split-thickness skin graft.

- *MEDPOR* (porous polyethylene) [3].
  - Custom fabricated porous polyethylene implant is placed in a subcutaneous pocket and covered with a temporoparietal fascial flap.
  - Higher rates of infection and implant extrusion, however, no donor site morbidity.
- *Complications*
  - *Skin necrosis.*
    - *Prevention is key.*
      - Requires meticulous dissection to preserve subdermal plexus, avoiding injury to superficial temporal vessels and maintaining integrity of temporoparietal fascia flap during elevation.
      - Avoid pressure dressings—closed suction drains instead of bolsters decreased rate of skin necrosis.
    - Exposure requires early intervention to salvage the framework.
      - Small (< 1 cm) exposure: treat with local wound care.
      - Large (>1 cm) exposure: requires debridement and coverage with local flap.
  - *Infection.*
    - *Early detection is key.*
      - Superficial infections—may be managed with antibiotics alone.
      - Deep infections (gross purulence/suppurative chondritis)—require removal of ear framework.
  - *Hematoma.*
    - Requires immediate clot evacuation.
  - *Pneumothorax.*
    - May require intraoperative catheter or red rubber to evacuate air.
    - Evaluate with chest radiograph in recovery and POD 1.
  - *Chest wall deformity.*
    - Harvest with intact perichondrium decreases risk of deformity.
    - Higher risk in younger donors.
  - *Resorption of cartilage graft.*
    - Usually due to infection or an excessively tight skin envelope.

References

1. Brent B. Auricular repair with autogenous rib cartilage grafts: two decades of experience with 600 cases. Plast Reconstr Surg. 1992;90(3):355–74. discussion 375–376
2. Nagata S. A new method of total reconstruction of the auricle for microtia. Plast Reconstr Surg. 1993;92(02):187–201.
3. Reinisch J, Tahiri Y. Polyethylene Ear Reconstruction: A State-of-the-Art Surgical Journey. Plast Reconstr Surg. 2018 Feb;141(2):461–70. https://doi.org/10.1097/PRS.0000000000004088.
4. Thorne CH, Wilkes G. Ear deformities, otoplasty, and ear reconstruction. Plast Reconstr Surg. 2012;129(4):701e–16e. https://doi.org/10.1097/PRS.0b013e3182450d9f.

Chapter 22
Nasal Reconstruction

Sumun Khetpal and Nirbhay S. Jain

Anatomy

- Regions of the nose [1]
    - Proximal third: nasal bones, bony septum
    - Middle third: upper lateral cartilages, cartilaginous septum
    - Distal third: nasal tip, lower lateral cartilages, nasal alae
- Nasal subunits [2]
    - The nose has nine subunits: dorsum, two side walls, tip, two soft triangles, columella, and two alae
        - If >50% of subunit is involved/damaged, often best to excise whole subunit and reconstruct (Fig. 22.1)
- Layers of the nose
    - Skin
    - Subcutaneous fat
    - SMAS/muscles
    - Deep fat
    - Perichondrium/periosteum
    - Mucosa
    - *In order to have a successful reconstruction, need to take into account "all" layers*

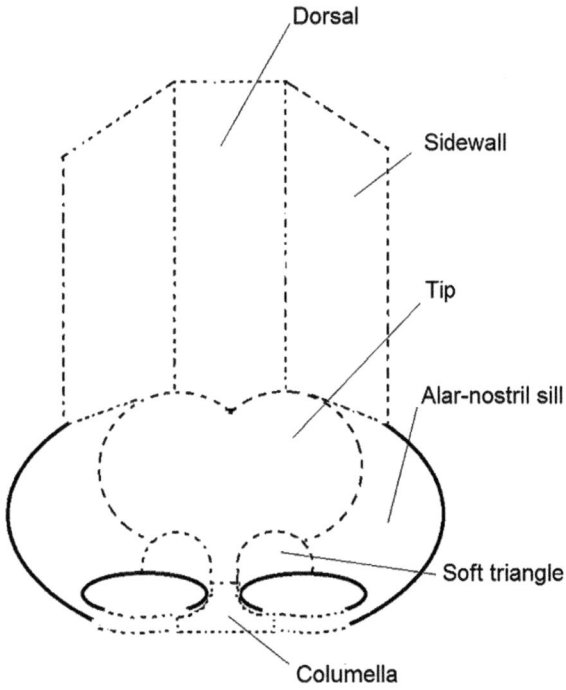

Fig. 22.1 Subunits of the nose

- Vasculature of the nose [1–4]
  - ECA - > facial - > angular - > lateral nasal
  - ECA - > facial - > superior labial - > columellar
  - ECA - > internal maxillary - > infraorbital
  - ICA - > ophthalmic - > dorsal nasal, supratrochlear, supraorbital
  - Specific areas of anastomosis
    - Septum (Kiesselbach triangle): anterior ethmoid, posterior ethmoid, sphenopalatine, superior labial, greater palatine
    - Lateral nasal wall: anterior ethmoid, posterior ethmoid, sphenopalatine
- Nerves to the nose [1–4]
  - Sensation: divided between branches of V1 (supratrochlear, infratrochlear, external nasal) and V2 (infraorbital)
    - The septum has anterior ethmoidal (V1) and nasopalatine (V2)
    - The lateral nasal wall has anterior ethmoidal and pterygopalatine
  - Motor: branches of VII, mainly zygomatic and buccal
- Cartilage structure
  - Septal cartilage midline
  - Flanked by the upper lateral cartilage (underneath nasal bone) and lower lateral cartilage (on top of the upper lateral cartilage)

Preoperative Evaluation for Nasal Reconstruction [3–4]

- Need to understand the who/what/where/when/why of the defect before determining the how
    - Who: Characteristics of the patient (comorbidities, psychiatric, patient goals)
    - What: What layers are involved (skin only, mucosa, cartilage) and how big (less than 2 sq. cm could get away with local flap)? Is there appropriate imaging?
    - Where: Where on the nose is it (proximal, middle, or distal $\frac{1}{3}$, which subunits are involved)?
    - When: Can this be done immediately, or does it have to be delayed? Are margins clear? Is further workup needed? Is radiation or adjunctive treatment needed?
    - Why: What is the etiology? Is it cancer, trauma? Has there been other surgeries done to attempt this?

Surgical Approaches to Nasal Reconstruction

- Objectives of surgery
    - Restore anatomic structure, including all layers of the nose involved.
        - Failure in reconstruction often comes from a lack of accounting for all layers of the nose (mucosa, cartilage, and cover).
        - Break the nose down into structural components and build outward.
    - Maintain functional airway.
    - Optimize aesthetic result.
- Restoring the bone/cartilage of the nose
    - The goal is to restore the "tetrapod" M of the nose, which provides the underlying support.
        - Involves the L-shaped septal framework and alar struts (Fig. 22.2).
- Can be done with the cartilage (rib, ear, cadaveric, septal)
- Can be done with cantilevered cranial graft
- Can be done with septal pivot flap
- Allows for support and redraping of the mucosa and skin
- Allows for airway patency
- Restoring the nasal lining [2]
    - Failure to do so appropriately can lead to gross nasal deformity from wound contraction
    - Need to restore epithelial surface, can be the mucosa or skin

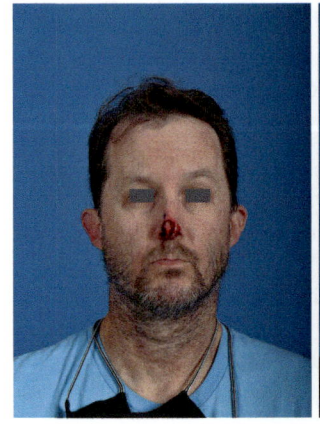 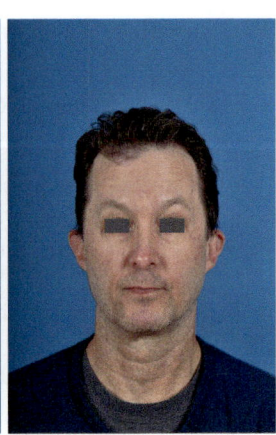

Fig. 22.2 Pre- and post-operative (1 year) frontal view photograph of patient who underwent Mohs reconstruction of his nasal tip with forehead flap, septorhinoplasty with alar grafts and composite ear cartilage graftn

- Basal options include lining advancement and skin grafts
    - Skin grafts have to be on vascular bed and cannot be placed onto the cartilage
- Local flaps
    - External skin turnover flap
    - Septal composite flap (ipsilateral or contralateral)
    - Mucoperichondrial flaps
    - Facial artery musculomucosal flap (better for midvault)
    - Nasolabial flap
    - Forehead flap
- Free flap
    - Radial forearm
    - TPF flap
- Restoring the skin
    - Areas of concavity (radix) can be treated well with secondary healing.
    - Areas of convexity (tip) do poorly with secondary healing.
    - Composite grafts can be done from the ear with the helical cartilage and skin for the ala, often fail if >1.5 cm, high risk of congestion.
    - Small defects are often treated with local flaps.
        - Dorsal nasal flap: good for proximal and middle thirds
        - Nasolabial flap: sidewall and alar defects.
        - Bilobed flaps: sidewall and alar defects, not good for tip. Usually limited to 1.5 cm
        - Forehead flap: best for tip and larger defects
            - Requires two stages: inset and division

- Large defects may need free flaps
    - Most commonly radial forearm free flap, though ulnar forearm fibula (if the maxilla is involved) and even rectus abdominis have been used

Complications [2]

- Infection
- Flap necrosis, especially at distal tip
- Risk factors
    - Narrow pedicle base.
    - Pivot point too high, resulting in vascular compromise from excess tension.
    - Radiation.

References

1. Janis JE, Ahmad J, Rohrich RJ. Rhinoplasty. In: Thorne CH, editor. *Grabb and Smith's Plastic Surgery*. Lippincott Williams & Wilkins; 2014. p. 512–29.
2. Menick FJ. Nasal reconstruction. Plast Reconstr Surg. 2010;125:138e–50e.
3. Lee MR. Rhinoplasty. In: Janis JE, editor. Essentials of plastic surgery. Thieme Medical Publishers; 2017. p. 1203–27.
4. Pessa JE, Rohrich RJ. Nasal analysis and anatomy. In: Neligan PC, editor. Plastic surgery. Elsevier; 2018. p. 373–86.

Chapter 23
Scalp Reconstruction

Jack D. Sudduth and Jessica L. Marquez

Introduction

- Scalp trauma is a relatively common injury ranging from small defects to total scalp avulsion. Because of the robust blood supply to the scalp, reconstruction can typically be achieved through local flaps. However, in cases of partial or total scalp avulsion, replantation is considered the gold standard approach.

Anatomy

Layers (Fig. 23.1)

- The scalp consists of five layers, often remembered by the mnemonic: SCALP.
- S (skin)—thick layer of the skin (3–8 mm)
- C (connective tissue)—also known as the *subcutaneous layer*
  - Location of nerves, vessels, and lymphatics
- A (aponeurotic layer)—also known as the *galea aponeurotica* or "galea"
  - This layer is a dense fibrous tissue that serves as the central tendinous junction of the frontalis anteriorly and occipitalis posteriorly.

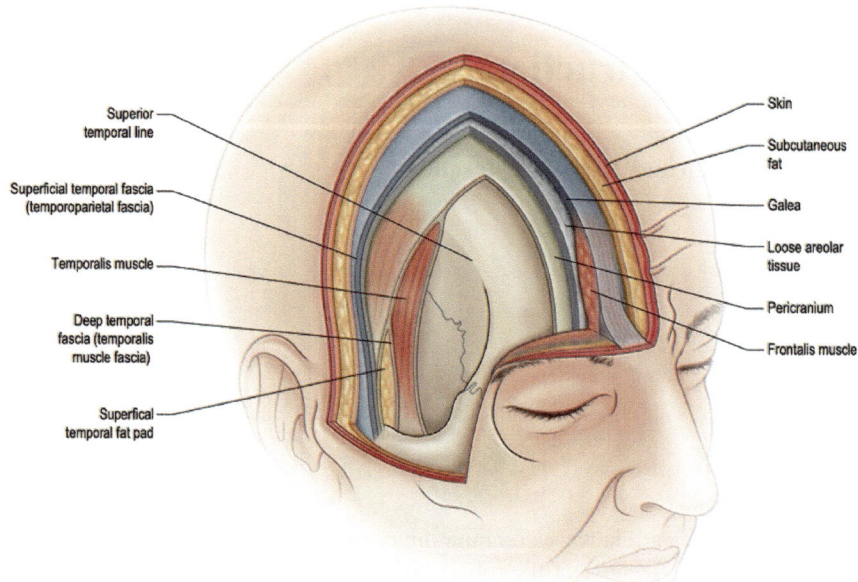

Fig. 23.1 Layers of the scalp

- L (loose areolar tissue)—also known as *subgalea fascia* or *innominate fascia*
  - This layer provides mobility to the outer layers of the scalp.
  - This is the most common plane for scalp avulsion injuries to occur.
- P (pericranium)—This is the periosteum of the calvarium.
  - Firmly attached to the skull
  - Laterally continuous with the deep temporal fascia

Vascular

- Consists of four territories: anterior, lateral, posterior, posterolateral
- Internal carotid (anterior territory)—supplies the anterior scalp and forehead
  - Supraorbital artery
  - Supratrochlear artery
- External carotid
  - Superficial temporal artery (lateral territory)
    - Supplies the temporal and central scalp

- Postauricular artery (posterolateral territory)
  - Supplies the mastoid region
  - Smallest of main vessels of the scalp
  - Not enough to support the entire scalp in replantation
- Occipital artery (posterior territory)
  - Supplies the posterior scalp above the nuchal line
- Because of extensive collateral flow between these vessels, replantation can be possible with a singular vascular anastomosis [1]

Neurological (Fig. 23.2)

- Motor
  - Frontal branch of the facial nerve (CN VII)—also known as *temporal branch*
    - Innervates the frontalis muscle
  - Posterior auricular branch of the facial nerve (CN VII)
    - Innervates the anterior and posterior auricular muscles and occipitalis muscle
  - Deep temporal nerve of the trigeminal nerve (CN V)
    - Innervates the temporalis muscle

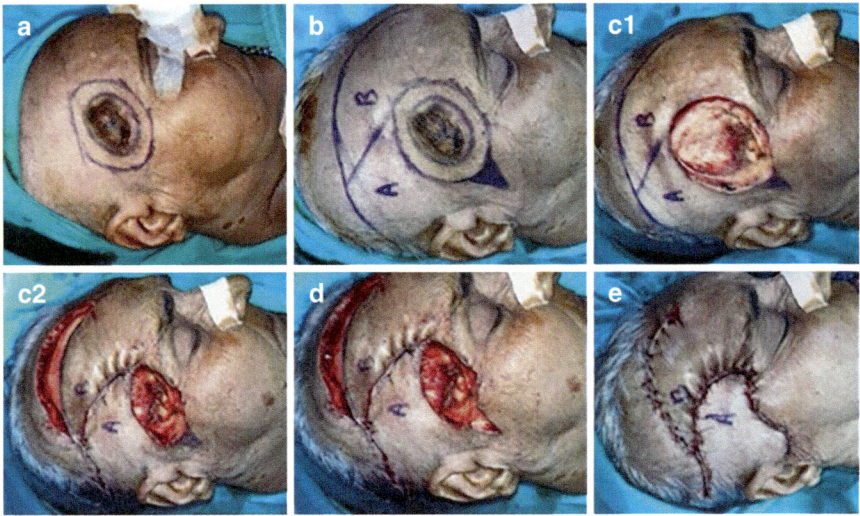

Fig. 23.2 Orticochea flaps

- Sensory
  - Supraorbital nerve
    - Superficial division—supplies sensation to the forehead and anterior hairline
    - Deep division—supplies sensation to the frontoparietal scalp
  - Supratrochlear nerve
    - Supplies sensation to the forehead along with supraorbital nerve
  - Zygomaticotemporal nerve—V2 branch of CN V
    - Supplies sensation to the anterior temporal area
  - Auriculotemporal nerve—V3 branch of CN V
    - Supplies sensation to the posterior temporal area
  - Greater and lesser occipital nerves—C2/C3 spinal nerves
    - Supplies sensation to the posterior scalp

Principles

Trauma

- Open wounds need irrigation and debridement of devitalized edges prior to closure.
- Excessive bleeding of the scalp is expected since the scalp has robust vascularity.
- Quick closure and hemostasis can be achieved with full-thickness sutures or staples.
- Microvascular anastomosis is the gold standard for major scalp avulsions.
  - Replantation must occur within 30 hours of accident.

Hair and Hairline

- Defects in hair-bearing areas should be covered with hair-bearing scalp.
- The hairline can be distorted with excessive undermining so minimal undermining is recommended in these areas.

Galea

- Defects of the galea require closure since it is the layer that confers strength in the scalp.

Oncologic Reconstruction

- Clear margins of malignancy are necessary before undergoing reconstruction.
- Temporary reconstruction using dermal regeneration templates with skin grafts in combination with wound care can be used to temporize when clear margins are unable to be confirmed.

Reconstructive Options

Primary Closure

- Acceptable for defects up to 3 cm in diameter.
- Undermining in the subgaleal plane can increase mobility of the scalp.

Secondary Closure

- Always an option, but not recommended.
- The scar will produce no hair and can negatively affect cosmesis of the scalp.
- Exposed bone with compromised pericranium is at risk for osteomyelitis.

Split-Thickness Skin Grafts (STSG)

- Able to be placed directly on the subcutaneous tissue, galea, or pericranium.
- Provides coverage of a primary defect, donor area of local flap, or coverage for skinless flap:
  - Expect alopecia and skin color mismatch
  - Low shear force tolerance
  - Usually not meshed for better cosmetic outcomes

- Can be used as a temporary reconstruction before definitive coverage is placed.
- Intact pericranium is needed for optimal uptake when grafting over the calvarium.
- With exposed calvaria, all devitalized bone needs to be debrided before placing coverage to prevent graft failure.

Dermal Regeneration Templates

- Integra (Integra LifeSciences, Plainsboro, NJ) is a synthetic bilaminate bovine collagen construct that can be placed directly on wounds to promote formation of a robustly vascular wound bed [2]:
    - Helpful to use when vascular supply is compromised or when increased thickness of the wound bed is needed to help prevent a contour deformity
    - Can be placed on most surfaces, including the bone, but there needs to an underlying blood supply (i.e., punctate bleeding on the calvarium) in order to promote angiogenesis
- A few weeks after Integra placement, the sheet is removed, and the STSG is placed on the wound bed.
- Can also be combined with negative pressure wound therapy for optimal neovascularization.
- Can be cost-prohibitive in some cases.

Local Flaps

- Designed as partial or full-thickness flaps:
    - Full-thickness scalp flaps (FTSF)—preferred as they provide superior functional and aesthetic results
        - Covers most defects from 3 to 6 cm in diameter:
            - Donor sites closed primarily
        - For defects 6–9 cm in diameter, one scalp flap with a major pedicle can be used:
            - Secondary defect will require skin grafting.
        - Created as axial flaps based on a major vessel
        - Long, wide flaps preferred to small flaps.
        - Steps to increase mobilization of the flaps:
            - Wide undermining
            - Galeal scoring

- Performed perpendicular to the axis of advancement.
- Incisions are made 1–2 cm apart:
  - Each incision score line allows 1–2 mm of advancement.
- Back cutting of the flap
- Partial flaps (pericranial and galea flaps)—create a vascularized wound bed that can receive a skin graft
  - Pericranial flap—includes pericranium and loose areolar tissue
  - Galea flap—includes the galea
  - Can be skin grafted immediately
  - Preferred when FTSFs are unavailable
- Incorporate at least one named scalp vessel into flaps.
- Scars from previous oncologic reconstruction, previous radiation therapy, and burns limit the utility of local flaps.
- Infections need to be controlled prior to creating a flap.
- Dog ears are typically acceptable in the scalp and do not require resection or revision as they usually flatten out over time.

Tissue Expansion

- Able to replace hair-bearing skin with hair-bearing skin.
- Indicated when hair-bearing skin is needed and there is inadequate tissue for primary closure or local flap arrangement.
- Placed in the subgaleal plane at the flap margin, typically between the skin and skin graft junction:
  - Must have separate incision for remote filling port
- Fluid added to the expander sequentially over time to allow skin to expand:
  - Typically filled every week starting 4–6 weeks after the index surgery.
  - Larger wounds may require more rounds of expansion than smaller wounds.
- Alopecia not concerning for tissue expansion unless reconstruction exceeds 50% of the scalp.
- Avoid expansion in irradiated or infected scalps.

Regional Flaps

- Most useful for mastoid, temporal, and occipital regions.
- Options include trapezius musculocutaneous flap, latissimus dorsi musculocutaneous flap, and pectoralis major flap.

- Orticochea flap [3]—three-flap technique with two lateral flaps based on the superficial temporal vessels and one large, posterior flap based on the occipital arteries (Fig. 23.2)
  - Can result in poor aesthetic outcomes

Free Flaps

- Covers scalp defects greater than 9 cm in diameter.
- Options include musculocutaneous and fasciocutaneous flaps:
  - Latissimus dorsi or anterolateral thigh flaps are traditionally used [4].
  - Muscle and omental flaps can also be used in combination with STSGs.

Replantation

- Considered the gold standard for partial or total avulsion injuries to the scalp.
- Can achieve the best aesthetic and functional result compared to other options.
- Traditionally, scalps must be replanted within 30 hours of avulsion.
- Can have successful replant with only one artery and vein, but additional anastomoses are preferred:
  - Temporal vessels preferred, followed by occipital vessels [5]

General Guidelines

- Small defects can be closed primarily, with small rotation advancement flaps or with V-Y flaps.
- Moderate defects can be closed with rotation advancement flaps, V-Y flaps, or pedicled subcutaneous flaps.
- Large defects can be closed with large rotation advancement flaps, Orticochea flaps, tissue expansion, or free tissue transfer.
- Avulsions can be treated with replantation or free tissue transfer.
- Parietal region allows the most advancement of scalp tissue:
  - Most amenable to undermining and primary closure
  - Can provide full advancement coverage of other areas of the scalp

References

1. Christiano JGB, Nicholas; Langstein, Howard N. Reconstruction of the scalp, calvarium, and forehead. In: Thorne CH, editor. Grabb and Smith's plastic surgery. 7: Wolters Kluwer; 2015. p. 342–51.
2. Iorio ML, Shuck J, Attinger CE. Wound healing in the upper and lower extremities: a systematic review on the use of acellular dermal matrices. Plast Reconstr Surg. 2012;130(5 Suppl 2):232S–41S.
3. Arnold PG, Rangarathnam CS. Multiple-flap scalp reconstruction: Orticochea revisited. Plast Reconstr Surg. 1982;69(4):605–13.
4. Song P, Pu LLQ. Microsurgical scalp reconstruction: an overview of the contemporary approach. J Reconstr Microsurg. 2022;38(7):530–8.
5. Lin SJ, Hanasono MM, Skoracki RJ. Scalp and calvarial reconstruction. Semin Plast Surg. 2008;22(4):281–93.

Chapter 24
Eyelid Reconstruction

Zachary Dezeeuw

Summary

A. Purpose of eyelid reconstruction

  (i) Provide coverage and protection for the globe
  (ii) Proper functioning of the nasolacrimal system
  (iii) Unobstructed visual field
  (iv) Aesthetics [1]

Anatomy (Figs. 24.1 and 24.2)

A. Dimensions

  (i) Horizontal fissure: 28–30 mm
  (ii) Vertical fissure: 10–11 mm [2]
  (iii) Tarsal plate [3]

   1. *Superior: 10-mm height*
   2. *Inferior: 3.5–4-mm height* [3]
   3. *Length: 29 mm*

  (iv) Lamellae

Z. Dezeeuw (✉)
Department of Ophthalmology and Visual Sciences, University of Texas Medical Branch, Galveston, TX, USA
e-mail: zadezeeu@UTMB.EDU

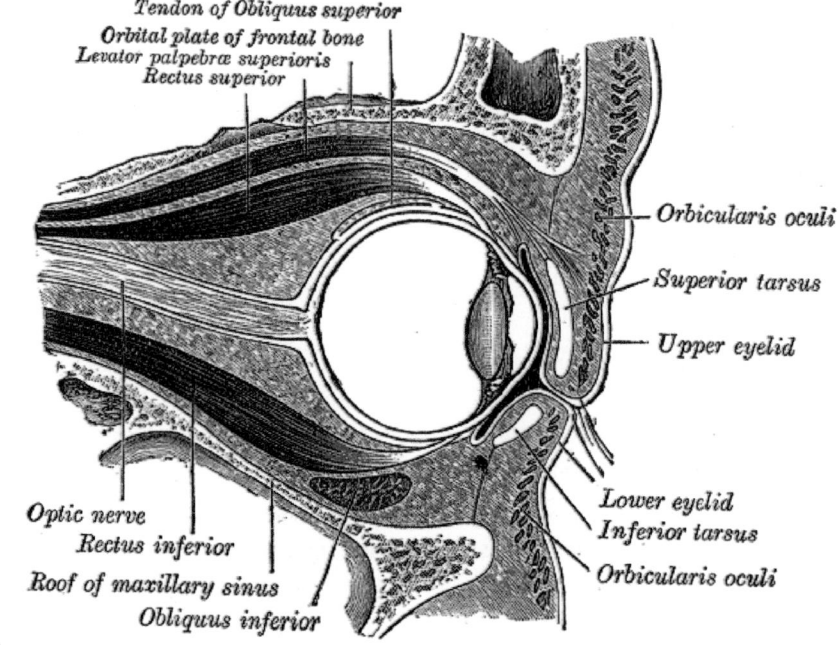

Fig. 24.1 Cross section of the eye

1. Anterior—skin + orbicularis oculi
2. Posterior—tarsal plate + conjunctiva
3. Middle—septum

B. Muscle and connective tissue T

(i) **Orbicularis oculi**

1. *Type of muscle: sphincter*
2. *Location: periocular*

    (a) *Two sections*

    (i) **Orbital**—insertions of anterior medial canthal tendon and lateral palpebral raphe
    (ii) **Palpebral**—further divided into preseptal and pretarsal

3. *Primary function: closes the eye*
4. *Secondary function: activation of lacrimal pump system* [4]

    (a) *Causes compression of meibomian gland and secretion of lipids for tear film*

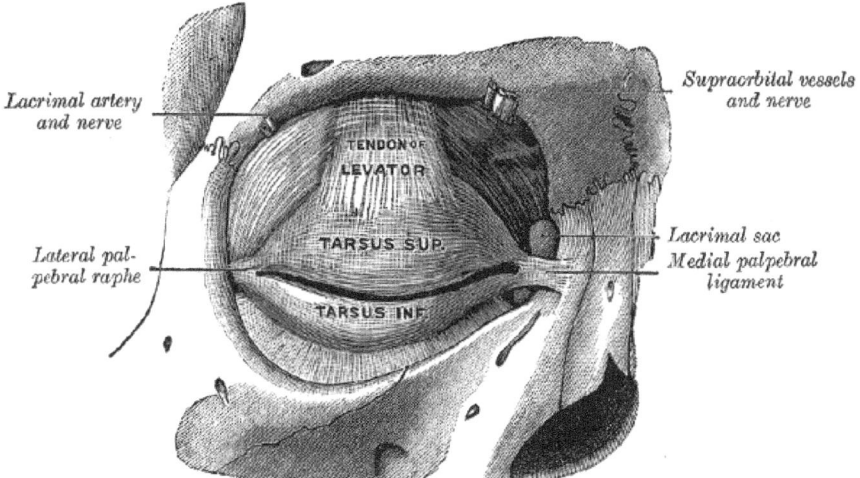

Fig. 24.2 Anatomy of the eyelids

- (ii) **Levator palpebrae superioris**
    1. *Type of muscle: triangular skeletal muscle*
    2. *Location: origin on the lesser wing of the sphenoid, traverses anteriorly to become the levator aponeurosis*
    3. *Primary function: elevation and retraction of the superior eyelid* [5]
    4. *Related: superior tarsal (muller) muscle*
- (iii) **Inferior tarsal muscle**
    1. *Type: smooth muscle*
    2. *Function: lower eyelid retraction*
    3. *Analogous to the levator palpebrae of the upper eyelid*
- (iv) **Tarsal plate**
    1. *Connective tissue*
    2. *Location: posterior lamellae of upper and lower eyelids*
    3. *Primary function: provide structural support for the eyelids*
- (v) **Canthal tendons**
    1. *Medial canthal tendon*
    2. *Lateral canthal tendon*

C. Blood supply [4–6]

- (i) **Internal carotid branches**
    1. *Ophthalmic artery -> Medial palpebral artery*

    2. *Lacrimal artery -> Lateral palpebral artery*
    3. *Supratrochlear artery*
    4. *Supraorbital artery*
  (ii) **External carotid branches**
    1. *Facial artery*
    2. *Superficial temporal artery*
      D. Lacrimal system [7]
        (i) Gland located superotemporally in the lateral orbit
          1. *Two lobes bisected by the tendon of the levator palpebrae superioris*
            (a) *Orbital lobe*
            (b) *Palpebral lobe*
        (ii) Function: production and distribution of tear film
          1. *Meibomian glands in the tarsus produce lipids that help stabilize the tear film.*
        (iii) Drainage: through the superior and inferior punctum located near the medial canthus -> into the nasolacrimal duct system

Indications

A. Any defects in the eyelid that could be contributing a deficit in eyelid function
   (i) Trauma/burns
   (ii) Neoplasms
   (iii) Congenital malformations

Evaluation

A. Thickness of involvement
   (i) Full thickness vs posterior lamellae vs anterior lamellae
B. Location
   (i) Upper vs lower eyelid
   (ii) Medial, lateral, central
   (iii) Pre-tarsal, preseptal, eyelid-cheek
   (iv) Canthal involvement?

(v) Lacrimal system involvement?
C. Patient factors
- (i) Age
- (ii) Laxity of tissue
- (iii) Anatomical variation

Techniques

A. Lower lid

  (i) Pretarsal

    1. *Full thickness*

      (a) *Small <25%*

        (i) Primary closure

      (b) *Medium 25–75%*

        (i) Myocutaneous flap, lesion 25–50%

          1. Tenzel semicircular flap (perform lateral canthotomy and rotate lateral tissue)

        (ii) Tarsoconjunctival flap for lesion >50%

          1. Hughes flap

      (c) *Large >75%*

        (i) Hughes tarsoconjunctival flap (Fig. 24.3)

        (ii) Mustarde cheek rotation flap [8]—brings in cheek tissue to replace large defects of the lower eyelid

  (ii) Preseptal [1, 9, 10]

    1. *Full-thickness skin grafts*
    2. *V-Y flaps*
    3. *Hatchet flaps*

B. Upper lid

  (i) Pre-Tarsal

    1. *Small to medium <25–75%*

      (a) *Can be handled in much the same way as lower lid lesions*

        (i) Myocutaneous flap

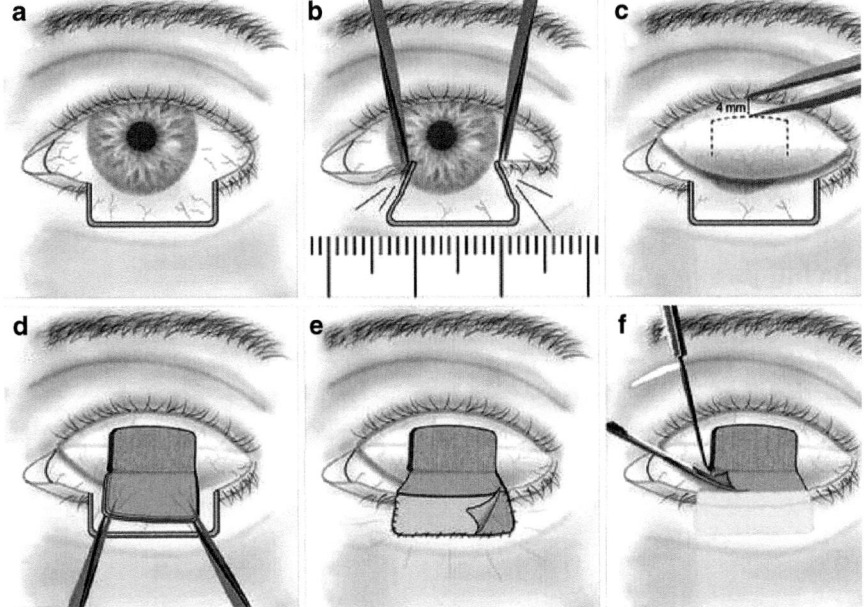

Fig. 24.3 Hughes tarsoconjunctival flap

      (b) *Lesions >50%*

          (i) Tarsoconjunctival flap

   2. *Large >75%*

      (i) Cutaneoconjuctival flap

          1. Cutler-Beard flap [11]—two-stage procedure to (Fig. 24.4)

      (ii) Orbicularis sandwich flap [12]
      (iii) Mustarde's lid switch flap [13]—Perform Mustarde cheek flap on the lower lid, and transpose the lower lid to the upper lid.

  (ii) Preseptal

      1. *Local skin graft*
      2. *Blepharoplasty*

C. Canthal involvement

  (i) Medial canthus

      1. *Suspect injury to the lacrimal duct system or medial canthal tendon (MCT) given anatomic proximity.*

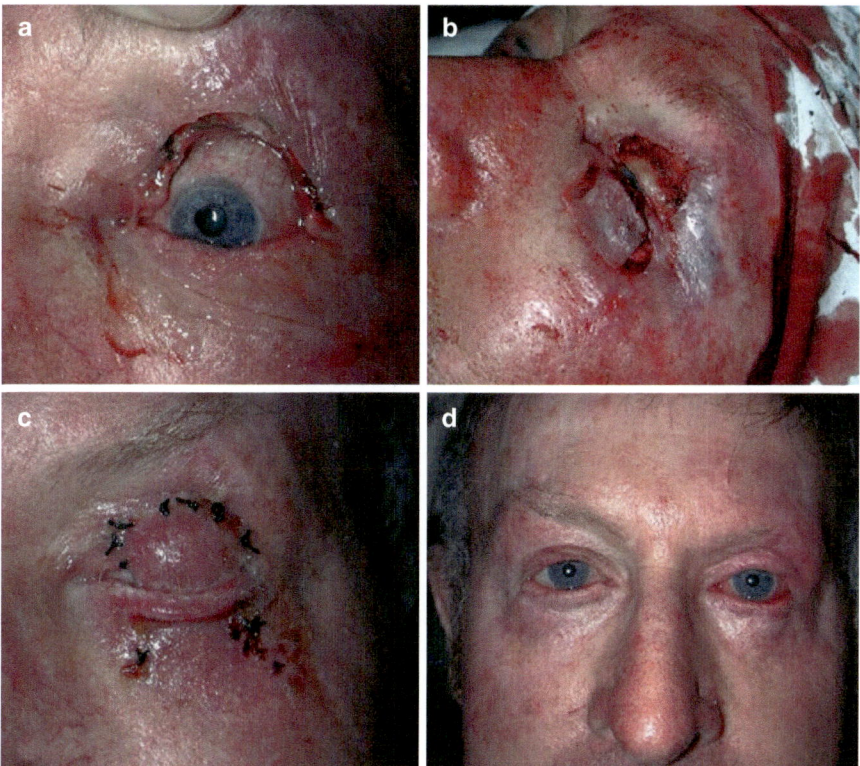

Fig. 24.4 Cutler beard flap

   (a) *Lacrimal duct system*

      (i) Stent placement with potential canaliculostomy and canthoplasty [1]

   (b) *Medial canthal tendon*

      (i) If traumatic, repair immediately.
      (ii) If secondary to malignancy, immediate repair is not warranted [8]

2. *"Laissez-faire" method*

   (a) *Small defect*
   (b) *Spontaneous healing*

3. *Full-thickness skin graft*
4. *Glabellar flap*

   (a) *Transposition flap from forehead region*

(b) *Used in lesion with exposed bone*

(ii) Lateral canthus

1. *Skin graft if non-lid involving*
2. *Large defect*

    (a) *Transposition flap*
    (b) *Island flap*

3. *Reconstruction*

    (a) *Anchoring of the eyelid tarsal plate with a periosteal flap from the lateral orbit [8] in a canthopexy or canthoplasty*

Common Complications [1, 14]

A. Retrobulbar hematoma
B. Globe perforation
C. Infection
D. Corneal abrasion
E. Lagophthalmos
F. Dry eye and chemosis
G. Graft/flap failure
H. Wound dehiscence

References

1. Alghoul MS, Kearney AM, Pacella SJ, Purnell CA. Eyelid reconstruction. Plast Reconstr Surg Glob Open. 2019;7(11):e2520. https://doi.org/10.1097/GOX.0000000000002520. PMID: 31942310; PMCID: PMC6908339
2. Blomquist PH, et al. Practical ophthalmology: a manual for beginning residents. San Francisco: American Academy of Ophthalmology; 2021.
3. Cochran ML, Lopez MJ, Czyz CN. Anatomy, head and neck, eyelid. [Updated 2021 Aug 11]. In: StatPearls [Internet]. Treasure Island: StatPearls Publishing. p. 2022. Available from https://www.ncbi.nlm.nih.gov/books/NBK482304/.
4. Tong J, Lopez MJ, Patel BC. Anatomy, head and neck, eye orbicularis oculi muscle. [Updated 2021 Jul 26]. In: StatPearls [Internet]. Treasure Island: StatPearls Publishing; 2022. Available from https://www.ncbi.nlm.nih.gov/books/NBK441907/.
5. Knight B, Lopez MJ, Patel BC. Anatomy, head and neck, eye levator palpebrae superioris muscles. [Updated 2021 Aug 11]. In: StatPearls [Internet]. Treasure Island: StatPearls Publishing; 2022. Available from https://www.ncbi.nlm.nih.gov/books/NBK536921/.
6. Djordjević B, Novaković M, Milisavljević M, Milićević S, Maliković A. Surgical anatomy and histology of the levator palpebrae superioris muscle for blepharoptosis correction. Vojnosanit Pregl. 2013;70(12):1124–31.

7. Machiele R, Lopez MJ, Czyz CN. Anatomy, head and neck, eye lacrimal gland. [Updated 2021 Jul 26]. In: StatPearls [Internet]. Treasure Island: StatPearls Publishing; 2022. Available from https://www.ncbi.nlm.nih.gov/books/NBK532914/m.
8. Cies WA, Bartlett RE. Modification of the Mustardé and Hughes methods of reconstructing the lower lid. Ann Ophthalmol. 1975;7(11):1497–502. PMID: 1200561
9. Gurunluoglu R, Williams SA, Olsen A. Reconstructive outcomes analysis of lower eyelid and infraorbital skin defects using 2 hatchet flaps: a 6-year experience. Ann Plast Surg. 2014;72:657–62.
10. Marchac D, de Lange A, Bine-bine H. A horizontal V-Y advancement lower eyelid flap. Plast Reconstr Surg. 2009;124:1133–41.
11. Fischer T, Noever G, Langer M, Kammer E. Experience in upper eyelid reconstruction with the cutler-beard technique. Ann Plast Surg. 2001;47(3):338–42.
12. Morley AM, deSousa JL, Selva D, Malhotra R. Techniques of upper eyelid reconstruction. Surv Ophthalmol. 2010;55(3):256–71. https://doi.org/10.1016/j.survophthal.2009.10.004. Epub 2010 Jan 18. PMID: 20083289
13. Subramanian N. Reconstructions of eyelid defects. Indian J Plast Surg. 2011;44(1):5–13. https://doi.org/10.4103/0970-0358.81437. PMID: 21713158; PMCID: PMC3111123
14. Omari A, Shaheen KW. Upper eyelid reconstruction. [Updated 2022 Apr 30]. In: StatPearls [Internet]. Treasure Island: StatPearls Publishing; 2022. Available from: https://www.ncbi.nlm.nih.gov/books/NBK551694/.

Chapter 25
Lip Reconstruction

Emily L. Geisler

Introduction

The lips are an essential component to human physiology, communication, and expression. As the dynamic center of the lower third of the face, lip reconstruction poses a particular challenge to the plastic surgeon. Reconstructive goals include functional outcomes such as oral competence, sensation, and speech, as well as aesthetic restoration for proportion and symmetry. The focus in this chapter will be based on acquired lip defects, such as from cancer excision or traumatic injury.

Anatomy

Layers and Landmarks

A. Superficial (Fig. 25.1)
   - Skin
   - Commissure
   - Cupid's bow
   - Philtral columns
   - Tubercle
   - White roll: vermillion-cutaneous junction

E. L. Geisler (✉)
Division of Plastic Surgery, The University of Texas Medical Branch, Galveston, TX, USA
e-mail: elgeisle@UTMB.EDU

© The Author(s), under exclusive license to Springer Nature Switzerland AG 2025
J. Roostaeian et al. (eds.), *Plastic Surgery Clerkship*, Contemporary Surgical Clerkships, https://doi.org/10.1007/978-3-031-99098-4_25

Anatomy Of The Human Lip

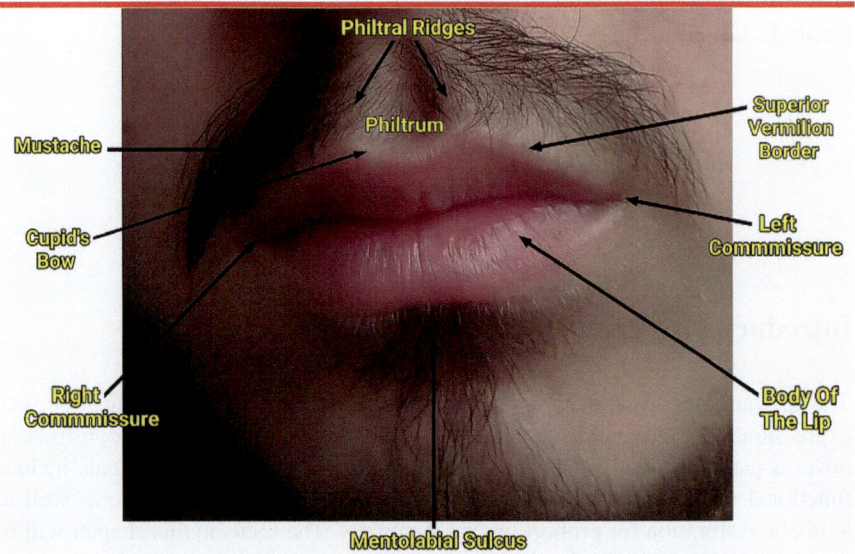

Fig. 25.1 Anatomy of the human lip

- Vermillion
- Red line: junction between dry keratinized squamous epithelium and wet non-keratinized squamous epithelium (oral mucosa).

B. Deep
  - Subcutaneous fat
  - Orbicularis oris muscle

Aesthetic Subunits

A. Upper lip
  - Lateral
  - Medial/philtral

B. Lower lip (one unit)
C. Chin subunit

Innervation

A. Sensory:
   - Upper lip: V2 (infraorbital nerve)
   - Lower lip: V3 (mental nerve)

B. Motor: buccal branch of VII (facial nerve) for zygomaticus major (smile muscle), marginal mandibular for the mentalis, and depressor anguli oris (pouting muscle)

Blood Supply

- Superior and inferior labial arteries, which are branches of the facial artery

Classification

Classification of lip defects is based on size (length and % of total lip), depth, and commissure involvement:

A. Vermillion only
B. Partial thickness
C. Full thickness

   - Up to 1/3 of the lip
   - One third to two thirds
   - Greater than two thirds

Etiology

A. Trauma
B. Cancer

   - Squamous cell carcinoma most common in general
   - Basal cell carcinoma most common on the upper lip

Treatment

Vermillion Realigning the vermillion is essential since small defects (>1 mm) are noticeable from a short distance.

A. Small, volume-only defects:
- Primary repair: Sutures should avoid crossing white roll.
- Healing by secondary intention.
- V-Y advancement: good for notches.
- Fat grafting: volume replacement.

B. Subtotal defects (<50%)
- Myovermillion advancement flap
- Myomucosal V-Y advancement flap
- Lip switch: where ipsilateral tissue isn't available for reconstruction, replaces wet and/or dry vermillion with identical tissue (avoiding chronically dry lips if dry vermillion is replaced with wet vermillion)

C. Large defects (>50%)
- Tongue flap: tissue from lateral or ventral tongue should be used to avoid papillae. Typically performed as a two-stage procedure

D. Total vermillion deficiency
- Buccal mucosal advancement flap: Wet mucosa replaces deficient vermillion (prone to chronic desiccation).

Partial-Thickness Defects

A. Superficial defects can be reconstructed in a variety and combination of ways. Local flaps are usually advancement or transposition flaps using cheek and/or lip tissue, which frequently require removal of redundancy. Patient gender should be considered in order to maintain the boundaries of hair-bearing areas.

Full-Thickness Defects Require attention to obtain three-layer closure of the mucosa, muscle, and skin. It is important to obtain a watertight seal of the mucosa, to realign the muscle fibers allowing for tension-free coaptation, and alignment of any vermillion defects to avoid aesthetically distracting scarring. A general algorithm for suggested reconstructive methods is below; however, each defect and patient must be carefully evaluated to determine appropriateness of any particular method.

Small FT Defects (<40%)

A. Layered closure, with attention to reestablishing landmarks
B. Full-thickness excisions, lying at anatomical boundaries, to facilitate symmetric anatomic closure

Large FT Defects Involve recruiting tissue from the opposite lip or adjacent cheek. Recruiting lip tissue, although aesthetically superior, is limited by the amount of redundant lip tissue and risks microstomia. When there is insufficient lip tissue for recruitment, cheek advancement can be utilized for better functional outcome.

A. Central upper or lower lip:
   - Abbe flap, +/− lateral cheek advancement w/ excision of perialar crescents; two-stage procedure requiring division at 2–3 weeks postop (Fig. 25.2)
B. Central lower lip
   - Bernard-Burow: laterally based horizontal advancement flap, adynamic, requires tension setting to maintain oral competence
   - Karapandzic flap: musculocutaneous rotation advancement flap; dynamic because it preserves facial nerve function; critical microstomia is the limit of flap design. Can be used for upper or lower lips one third to two thirds defects
C. Lateral upper or lower lip: with involvement of commissure
   - Estlander flap: medially based rotation advancement flap from the opposite lip, may require secondary commissuroplasty

Total Lip Recon (>80%)

A. Regional tissue transfer:
   - Submental flap: Island flap based on submental branch of the facial artery, superior cosmetic results due to similarity of local tissues.
   - Facial artery myomucosal (FAMM) flap: Axial, intraoral flap including facial artery and buccinator, tendency to desiccate.
B. Free tissue transfer: Total lip defects are often accompanied by resections of surrounding tissue, which may require multi-flap reconstructions.
   - Radial free forearm flap: Involves composite harvest of the palmaris longus tendon for weaving into the remaining orbicularis oris; adynamic, poor color match; useful for irradiated tissues.
   - Partial face transplantation: Considered for soft tissue defects of both lips, +/− underlying bony defects.

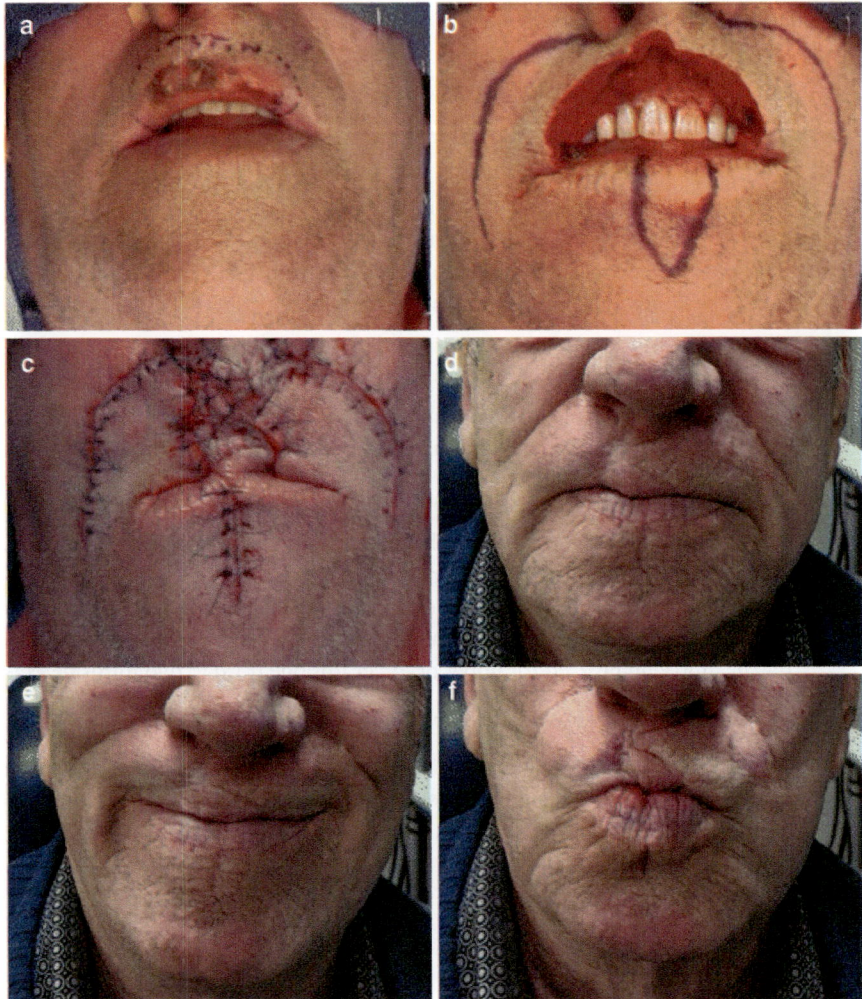

Fig. 25.2 a) preoperative markings of resection, **b)** near complete resection of upper lip and markings for Abbe and Karapandzic flaps, **c)** immediate postop of inset flaps, **d)** postop after Abbe flap division and healing, at rest, **e)** functional assessment of smile, and **f)** of pursing

C. Lip replantation:

- When traumatic amputation occurs, all possible efforts should be made for replantation to restore native tissue since it is superior to any reconstruction.

Of note, many lip reconstructions require secondary revisions after interim healing. Consideration of the appearance, symmetry, anatomic integrity, and function of the lip, as well as the patient's goals, are of utmost importance.

Conclusion

Lip reconstruction poses a complex challenge to the plastic surgeon, requiring meticulous attention to restoration of function and form. A wide variety of reconstructive options exist for creative application to each unique patient and defect.

Suggested Reading

1. Janis JE. Essentials of plastic surgery. 2nd ed. Boca Raton: CRC Press; 2014.
2. Thorne C, Chung KC, Gosain A, Guntner GC, Mehrara BJ. Grabb and Smith's plastic surgery. 7th ed. Philadelphia: Wolters Kluwer/Lippincott Williams & Wilkins Health; 2014.
3. Baumann D, Robb G. Lip reconstruction. Semin Plast Surg. 2008;22(4):269–80.
4. David L. Brown, Gregory H. Borschel, Benjamin L. Michigan manual of plastic surgery. 2nd ed. Beaverton: Ringgold, Inc; 2015.

Chapter 26
Facial Fractures

Brendan J. Cronin

Anatomy

- *Facial skeleton/bones*
  - Figure 26.1: *Buttresses of the facial skeleton*
  - Bony buttresses are thick columns or beams of bone that provide structural support to the facial skeleton—restoring these buttresses is key to restoring functional stability in the setting of facial fractures.
  - The face has both vertical and horizontal buttresses:
    - *Vertical*: nasomaxillary, zygomaticomaxillary, pterygomaxillary, vertical mandibular
    - *Horizontal*: Frontal bar (supraorbital rim), upper (infraorbital rim) and lower transverse (hard palate) maxillary, upper and lower transverse mandibular
- See Chap. 12 for a detailed explanation of head and neck anatomy including innervation and vascular supply of the face.

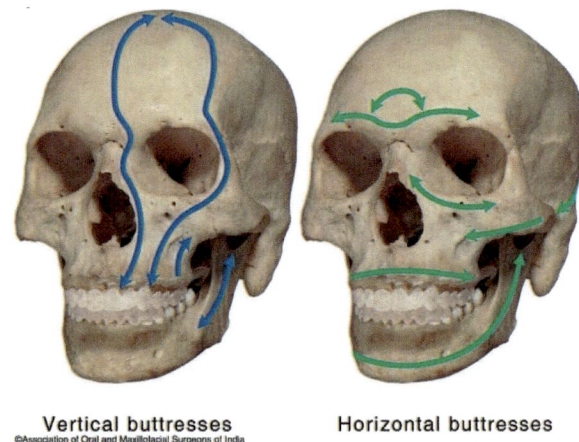

Fig. 26.1 Buttresses of the facial skeleton. Vertical buttresses (from medial to lateral above) include the nasomaxillary, zygomaticomaxillary, pterygomaxillary, and mandibular. Horizontal buttresses (from superior to inferior above, right) include the frontal bar, the upper (infraorbital rim) and lower (hard palate) transverse maxillary, and the mandibular. (https://link.springer.com/chapter/10.1007/978-981-15-1346-6_55 (Fig. 55.2). Jacob and Prathap [6]. Permissions: CC BY open source article)

Emergency Department Evaluation

- *ABCs—Perform primary and secondary survey.*
    - CF trauma is not often life-threatening, but fractures of certain facial structures (frontal bone, maxilla, mandible) indicate high-velocity injuries that are often associated with life-threatening injuries of other organ systems (C-spine).
        - 10% of patients with facial fractures have concomitant C-spine injury.
- *History*
    - *Mechanism of injury* (blunt vs penetrating vs avulsive)—informs likelihood of tissue loss and degree of injury.
    - *Time of injury.*
    - *Loss of consciousness.*
    - *Subjective complaints*—diplopia, malocclusion, loss of vision/color vision, altered sense of hearing, rhinorrhea
        - *Note preexisting malocclusion or enophthalmos which can otherwise cause significant distraction and misallocation of resources
    - *Catalog of injuries*—other associated traumas (intracranial, thoracic, abdominal, dysvascular extremities).
    - *Assess impedances to surgical management of facial fractures:*

- Stable airway established? Hemodynamically stable? C/T/L spine injuries and stabilization? Planned operations by other teams (i.e., craniotomy by neurosurgery)?
- *Focused CF Exam*
  - *Equipment*: tongue blades, light source, visual chart, nasal speculum
  - *Inspection*
    - *Scalp*—Evaluate for lacerations, abrasions, and hematomas.
    - *Eyes*—Evaluate visual acuity, direct and indirect pupillary reflex, extraocular movements (*rule out entrapment, may require forced duction test in unconscious or sedated patients*), globe injury/rupture, conjunctival hemorrhage, enophthalmos (indicate massive orbital floor fractures), exophthalmos (may indicate retrobulbar hematoma), hyphema (blood in the anterior chamber, risk for acute elevation intraocular pressures), and telecanthus (possible NOE fractures).
    - *Ears*—Lacerations, perichondral hematoma (requires drainage and application of bolster), tympanic rupture or hemotympanum, and postauricular bruising (Battle's sign) concerning for basilar skull fracture.
    - *Nose*:
      - *External exam*—lacerations, abrasions, deviation (nasal fracture is a *clinical diagnosis;* ask the patient: "Does your nose look different?")
      - *Intranasal exam*—septal deviation, turbinate hypertrophy, septal hematoma (hematoma disrupts mucoperiosteal blood supply to underlying septum—requires emergent drainage to prevent septal necrosis)
    - *Midface/cheeks*—Note any malar depression, downward-slanting canthal tilt, ecchymoses, or any lacerations in proximity to Stenson's duct (runs in the middle third region of a line from tragus to lateral commissure).
    - *Mouth/lips*:
      - *Intraoral*—loose/missing teeth, occlusion, wear facets, floor of mouth ecchymoses (pathognomonic for mandibular fracture).
      - Palpate TMJ directly and in external auditory canal with mouth opening/closing.
      - Evaluate for anterior/posterior open bite and cross bites.
  - *Palpation*
    - Palpate frontal bone, orbital rims, and zygomatic arches for tenderness or step-offs.
    - Perform bimanual exam to assess for maxillary mobility (mobility indicates possible pterygomaxillary disjunction also known as Le Fort I fracture pattern).
    - "Gruss sign" (apply downward pressure to bony dorsum of the nose) to evaluate nasal support—may indicate NOE and need for cantilever bone graft.

- *CN Exam*
  - Evaluate CN's II–XII.
- *Diagnostic Imaging*
  - Gold standard = CT maxillofacial with 1-mm thickness cuts.
  - Panorex may be useful for mandibular fractures (though may miss symphyseal fractures!).
  - Historically, various plain radiographs were used to evaluate facial trauma but have fallen out of fashion given the accessibility of CT

Facial Fractures

Frontal Bone

Anatomy/Epidemiology

- Frontal bone has a thick anterior table, thin floor (orbital roof), and thinner posterior table.
  - Requires greatest force to break of any facial bone (800–1600 lbs of force) [Janis]
- Nasofrontal duct is posterior and medial and runs through the anterior ethmoid bone to drain into the *middle meatus*.
- Sinus not present at birth, begins forming at 2 years and fully formed by age 12.

Presentation

- Palpable deformity, supraorbital/supratrochlear paresthesias, inferior globe displacement by orbital roof:
  - CSF rhinorrhea (test for beta-transferrin, less accurate but more rapid/available tricks include using a urine dipstick to test for glucose or look for the "halo sign" on gauze)
- Often associated with NOE or globe fractures.
- Evaluating nasofrontal duct obstruction: instill methylene blue into sinus, and place cotton tip applicator endonasally for confirmation of flow.

Management

- Key variables to assess include the location of fracture (anterior vs posterior table), presence of displacement, and presence of nasofrontal outflow tract obstruction:
  - In *posterior* table fractures, the presence of CSF leak is another important consideration.
- General guidelines:
  - Displaced fractures require operative reduction and fixation; non-displaced fractures can be treated with antibiotics (the sinus is "dirty" and colonized with bacteria) and observation.
  - Nasofrontal outflow tract obstruction requires removal ("exenteration") of sinus mucosa and nasofrontal duct/sinus obliteration to prevent the formation of a mucocele.
  - Disruption of the posterior table risks exposing the brain to sinus/nasal microbiota—this requires isolating the cranial cavity from the upper airway (duct obliteration).
  - The presence of a CSF leak merits longer durations of antibiotics (14 vs 7 days) given the risk of meningitis.
- *Displaced anterior table*: ORIF with low-profile miniplates, may need intraosseous wiring if fracture is comminuted.
- *Displaced anterior table + nasofrontal duct obstruction*: ORIF + obliteration of sinus/duct + exenteration of the sinus mucosa.
- *Posterior table fracture without CSF leak*: ORIF + obliteration of sinus/duct + exenteration of the sinus mucosa.
- *Posterior table fracture with CSF leak*: Cranialization + exenteration of sinus mucosa + obliteration of duct.
  - Cranialization involves removing posterior table and allowing brain to fill the space of the sinus after removal of sinus mucosa.

Orbital Fractures

Anatomy/Epidemiology

- Orbit comprised of seven bones—maxilla, lacrimal bone, ethmoid, sphenoid (greater + lesser wings), frontal bone, zygoma, palatine bone (Fig. 26.2):
  - The orbital floor is weakest and most prone to fracture medially in the region of the ethmoid, lacrimal, and medial maxilla.
- Fissures and foramen allow passage of critical structures through and adjacent to the greater and lesser wings of the sphenoid:

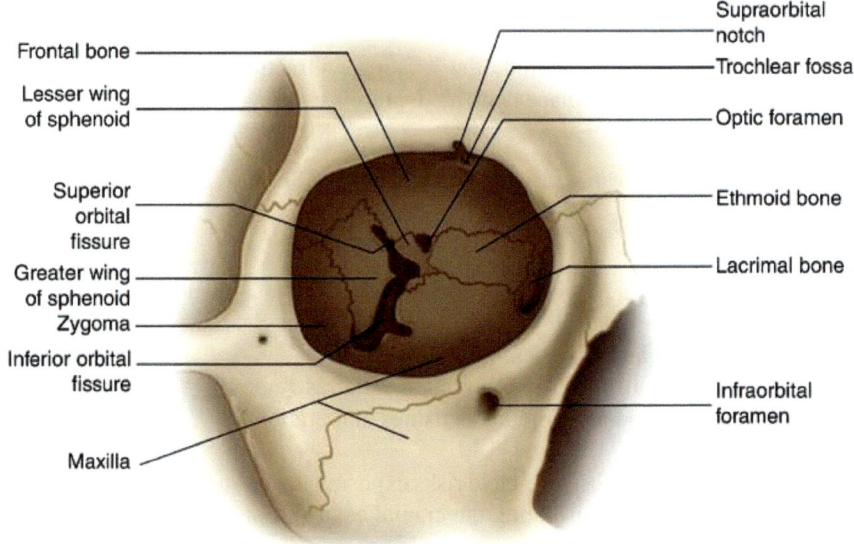

Fig. 26.2 Orbital anatomy. The orbit is comprised of seven bones as shown above. The medial wall ("lamina papyracea") and the floor, especially medial to the infraorbital foramen, are most prone to fracture. The orbit assumes a "cone" shape with the posterior aspect of the maxilla slanting upward to meet the ethmoid. Restoring this geometry is key during orbital reconstruction to prevent excess orbital volume and enophthalmos. (https://link.springer.com/chapter/10.1007/978-3-030-28841-9_2. Schulz et al. [7]. Permissions license number: 5333700730704)

- *Superior orbital fissure*—divided into two parts by the origin of the lateral rectus muscle:
  - *Superolateral portion*: trochlear nerve (IV), sensory branches of V1 (lacrimal, frontal)
  - *Inferomedial portion*: CN's 3 (oculomotor), V (nasociliary), VI (abducens)
- *Optic canal/foramen*—optic nerve + ophthalmic artery
- *Infraorbital groove*—along the middle aspect of the inferior orbital fissure; the infraorbital nerve passes in a bony tunnel beneath the orbital floor

Presentation

- Periorbital edema and ecchymoses, diplopia, V2 paresthesia +/− enophthalmos (*posterior* globe displacement), and dystopia (*vertical* globe displacement):
  - Enophthalmos is usually seen in a delayed fashion following orbital fat atrophy but can be seen in large blowout fractures.
- Evaluate for globe injury, globe rupture, elevated intraocular pressure, *entrapment* (accompanied by nausea, vomiting, and bradycardia due to oculocardiac reflex), diplopia, altered vision/color vision, hyphema, and V2 paresthesias.

Associated Syndromes

Superior Orbital Fissure Syndrome

- Fracture that affects the oculomotor, trochlear, abducens, and trigeminal nerves
- Findings: ptosis, proptosis, ophthalmalgia, V1 numbness, fixed/dilated ipsilateral pupil

Orbital Apex Syndrome

- Superior orbital fissure syndrome + *loss of vision* due to optic nerve injury

Management

- Prevent further injury to the globe (nose blowing precautions); minimize periorbital edema (elevate HOB, cold compresses).
- No good evidence to suggest the use of prophylactic or postop antibiotics (intraop recommended).
- Determine if *urgent surgical intervention is required* (Table 26.1).

Technique—orbital reconstruction with autogenous graft (particularly in pediatric patients) or allograft (titanium mesh vs MEDPOR implant) via transconjunctival approach

NOE (Naso-Orbital-Ethmoidal) Fractures

Anatomy/Epidemiology

- Involves fracture of the nasal bones, frontal processes, lacrimal bone, and ethmoid bone

Table 26.1 Indications for ORIF

Timing	Indication
Emergent	Entrapment +/− Enophthalmos (*Acute enophthalmos indicates massive fracture and significantly increased orbital volume*)
Delayed (within 2 weeks)	Persistent diplopia Enophthalmos >2 mm >50% orbital floor defect or >1 cm^2 defect

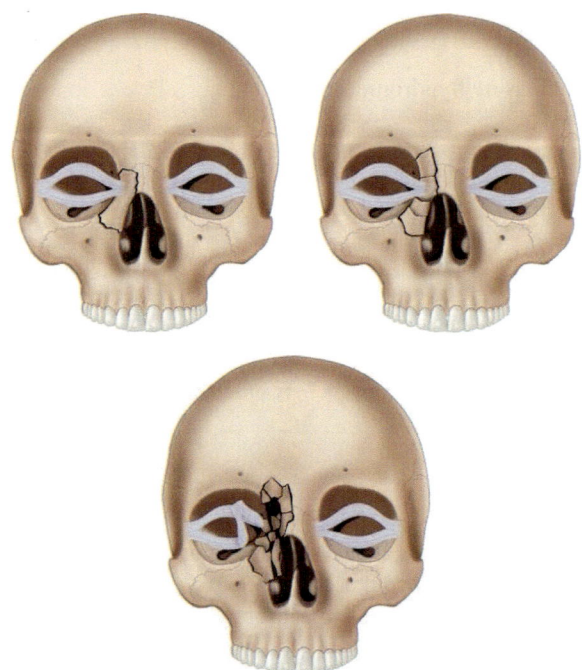

Fig. 26.3 Markowitz classification of NOE fractures. Type I (top left) fractures are characterized by a large, non-comminuted central fragment with an intact medial canthal tendon origin. Type II (top right) fractures have comminution of the bony fragments but nonetheless have an intact canthal insertion. Type III fractures are severely comminuted with disruption of the medial canthal tendon insertion. (https://link.springer.com/chapter/10.1007/978-1-4614-8341-0_18. Bruckman et al. [8]. Permissions license number: 5333700882128)

- *Markowitz classification* (Fig. 26.3)—categorizes the fracture based on the state of the central fragment and the bony attachment of the medial canthal tendon
- Classically caused by facial trauma from steering wheel in unrestrained drivers, less common with the advent of the seatbelt (Table 26.2)

Presentation

- Telecanthus
  - Normal intercanthal distance = 30–34 mm
  - Due to displacement of bony segment with medial canthal tendon origin
- Short and depressed nose without dorsal support (Gruss sign)
- Epiphora (disruption of nasolacrimal duct)
- CSF rhinorrhea
- Mobile medial canthal tendon on exam ("bowstring test")

Table 26.2 Markowitz classification of NOE fractures

Type	Fracture pattern	Medial canthal tendon
I	Single noncomminuted fracture fragment	Intact
II	Comminuted fragment	Intact
III	Comminuted	Avulsed

Management

- *Goals*: Restore medial canthal position, reconstruct the orbit, and restore nasal projection.
- *Exposure*: *Wide exposure* obtained through coronal incision, existing lacerations, transconjunctival incision with lateral canthotomy, occasionally upper buccal sulcus incision required for complete reduction.
- *Reconstruction*:
  - Cantilever bone graft from split calvarial bone or rib is utilized to restore nasal projection.
  - Transnasal wiring is used to restore the anatomic position of the medial canthal tendon:
    - If avulsed, the vector of resuspension is posterior and superior to recreate the appropriate tension of the canthal sling and prevent ectropion.
  - Miniplates are used to secure bony fragments when possible.
  - Orbital reconstruction performed with bone graft or implant.

Nasal Bone

Anatomy/Epidemiology

- Most common type of facial bone fracture
- Paired "wedge-shaped" nasal bones:
  - Superior portion is thicker and well supported by articulations with the frontal bone and maxilla—less likely to fracture.
  - Lower portion is broad and thin, more liable to injury.
- Often accompanied by fractures of the bony and cartilaginous septum

Presentation

- Periorbital ecchymoses
- Nasal deviation/deformity and swelling

- Epistaxis
- Difficulty with nasal breathing
- Septal hematoma (must rule out otherwise risk septal necrosis)
- Clinical diagnosis! Ask the patient: "Does your nose look different?" CT is unnecessary.

Management

- Closed vs open reduction
  - Closed
    - Indicated for minimally to mildly displaced fractures within 2 weeks of injury
    - Needs to be performed either shortly after injury (prior to obfuscating effects of swelling) or after swelling subsides (3–5 days) but prior to 2 weeks (after which manipulation of bony fragments becomes challenging)
  - Open
    - Indicated in patients with persistent deformity after closed reduction or those with significant displacement/deformity or septal fracture/dislocation
- After acute period
  - If bones not reduced within first 2 weeks or residual deformity after close reduction, wait for ~6 months, and perform formal rhinoplasty.

ZMC

Anatomy/Epidemiology

- *Zygoma has a "quadrilateral" shape with four key articulations*—(1) frontal, (2) maxillary, (3) sphenoid, and (4) temporal:
  - Exposing these four sutures is key for assessing anatomic reduction of the fracture fragment—the zygomaticosphenoid suture is the most important for assessing accurate reduction.
- *Four muscle insertions*—masseter, temporalis, zygomaticus major and minor:
  - Masseter = key displacing force on ZMC fractures
- *High-energy* vs *low-energy fractures*:
  - High-energy fractures often have comminuted fracture fragments at suture articulations—requires wider exposure for appropriate reduction.
  - Low-energy fractures often have less comminution and require less aggressive exposure.

Presentation

- Malar flattening with down-slanting palpebral fissure (lateral canthal tendon is attached to Whitnall's tubercle of the zygoma)
- Trismus (inferior displacement of zygomatic arch entraps coronoid process of the mandible)
- Infraorbital paresthesias
- Enophthalmos

Management

- *Goals*: Restore malar projection and facial width; correct orbital dystopia.
- *Exposure*:
    - Upper blepharoplasty incision (ZF suture access)
    - Upper buccal sulcus incision (ZM buttress access)
    - Coronal (for wide exposure to arch and lateral orbit)—not typically necessary
    - Transconjunctival (orbital floor + zygomaticomaxillary suture access)
- ORIF
    - Secure the ZF suture with a 1.0–1.5-mm miniplate (sets the vertical height of the fragment while still allowing manipulation in the other planes) or wire fixation.
    - Perform ZM buttress fixation (typically 1.5–2-mm L-plate) via buccal sulcus incision.
    - Carroll-Girard screw allows 3D manipulation of the arch to establish reduction.

Zygomatic Arch

Anatomy/Epidemiology

- Isolated fractures of the zygomatic arch are purely aesthetic in nature aside from those that cause trismus.

Presentation

- Palpable/visible deformity
- Trismus

Management

- Reduce via Gillies approach (dissect deep to the deep temporal fascia within the temporal fat pad to access the zygomatic arch and "pop out" the fragment to obtain reduction) or Keen approach (intraoral).
- Fixation rarely needed. If unstable in reduced position can use percutaneous sutures to hold in place.

Mandible

Anatomy/Epidemiology (Table 26.3)

- *Mandible biomechanics play a key role in fracture patterns and management*:
    - Forces across mandible create zones of *tension* (superior mandibular border) and *compression* (inferior mandibular border).
    - Muscular insertions on mandible exert displacing or stabilizing forces on fractures depending on their orientation:
        - "unfavorable fracture:" fracture parallel to vector of muscle pull leads to displacing force which causes fracture displacement at "rest"
        - "favorable fracture:" fracture perpendicular to vector of muscle pull acts as a stabilizing force resulting in no displacement at "rest"
- *Innervation*
    - V3 distribution of trigeminal nerve □ inferior alveolar nerve □ mental nerve
        - Inferior alveolar nerve enters lingula and travels within the cancellous bone of the mandible and is prone to injury during osteotomies or plating. Exits as the mental nerve to provide sensation to the lip at the second bicuspid.
- *Blood supply*
    - Mandible has different types of blood supply in different regions which is key to understand for surgical exposures to various fracture locations:

Table 26.3 Regions of the mandible and incidence of fracture per region

Region	Boundaries	Fracture incidence (%)
Symphysis	Canine to canine	14
Body	First premolar to third molar	21
Angle	Third molar to gonial angle	20
Ramus	Gonial angle to sigmoid notch	3
Condyle	Superior to the sigmoid notch (can be condylar neck or condylar head)	36

- *Symphysis/body*—periosteal blood supply (more stripping/exposure ☐ greater devascularization of fragments)
- *Ramus/angle*—mix
- *Condyle*—*predominantly* endosteal via branch of inferior alveolar artery in the neck of condylar process, capsular blood supply from TMJ capsule, supply via muscular attachments of lateral pterygoid

Presentation

- Malocclusion
- Anterior open bite (bilateral condylar fracture)
- Crossbite
- Floor of mouth ecchymoses
- Mental nerve paresthesias
- Chin deviation or mandible deviation with opening (condylar fracture)

Management

- *Antibiotics*
  - Prophylactic abx (anaerobic coverage) until reduction of fracture shown to decrease infection risk
  - No evidence for postoperative abx administration
  - Peridex for open fractures
- *Teeth in the line of fracture*
  - Teeth within line of fx considered "open" fractures
  - *Remove if* grossly mobile, periodontal compromise, root fracture, exposed apices
- *Fixation*
  - *Maxillomandibular fixation*
    - Re-establish occlusion using inter-dental wiring, arch bars (secured with interdental wiring) or hybrid arch bars (secured with screws)
  - ORIF
    - *Principles of Fixation*
      - *Rigid fixation*—School of thought that both tensile *and* compressive forces are detrimental for fracture healing. Aims to achieve complete fixation of fracture fragments:
        - Indicated for comminuted fractures or multiple mandibular fractures
        - Achieve using large recon plate or tension band + stabilization plate

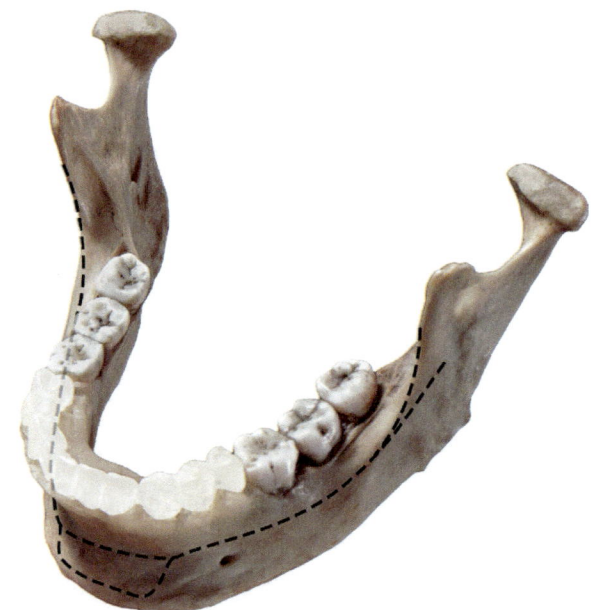

Fig. 26.4 Champy's ideal lines of osteosynthesis. Champy defined "ideal" lines of osteosynthesis where placement of a single monocortical miniplate (posterior to the canine) or two miniplates (symphysis) would neutralize tensile forces. Plates are monocortical to limit damage to tooth roots. Anteriorly, a thicker bicortical plate can be used on the inferior line of osteosynthesis given the lack of tooth roots or nerves in this region. (https://link.springer.com/chapter/10.1007/978-981-15-1346-6_51. Yadav [9]. Permissions: CC BY license Fig. 51.9)

- *Functional stabilization*—proposes that *only* tensile forces are detrimental for fracture healing. Fixation that neutralizes only tensile forces:
    - Indicated in uncomplicated isolated mandibular fractures
    - Achieve using miniplates along Champy's lines of ideal osteosynthesis (Fig. 26.4 and Table 26.4)

Maxilla

Anatomy/Classification

- The maxilla comprises majority of midfacial skeleton and contains maxillary sinus and dentition.
- Four processes: alveolar, zygomatic, palatine, and frontal.
- Three key buttresses provide strength (Fig. 26.4):

Table 26.4 Management by fracture type/region

Fracture	Management
Symphysis	Lag screws, box plate, superior monocortical 1-mm miniplate with inferior bicortical 2-mm stabilization plate, arch bar, and inferior border plate
Parasymphysis/body	Superior monocortical 1-mm miniplate with inferior bicortical 2-mm stabilization plate
Angle	Angle has highest complication rate of all mandible fractures Third molar within fracture line = risk of infection *Functionally stable fixation*: Single Champy plate (external oblique ridge) Easiest with lowest complication rate *Rigidly stable fixation*: Champy plate +2-mm lower border miniplate (below inferior alveolar nerve)
Ramus	*Non-displaced + normal occlusion*: MMF 6–8 weeks *Displaced or malocclusion*: ORIF (rigid or functionally stable fixation)

Condyle	Considerations include location of fracture (intracapsular vs extracapsular vs condylar neck), open vs closed approach and duration of MMF
	Intracapsular—MMF ×2–3 weeks followed by guiding elastics
	    Higher risk of TMJ ankylosis, challenging to access for ORIF or fixate due fragment size
	Extracapsular/condylar neck—MMF ×4–6 weeks vs ORIF
	    Lower risk of TMJ ankylosis permits longer duration MMF and better rates of fracture union
	    Surgical access is challenging and risks facial nerve injury and scarring

Bilateral fractures	May require ORIF with rigid fixation given inherent instability of disrupted mandibular arch
Comminuted fractures	ORIF with recon plate + miniplates to stabilize fracture fragments
Pediatric fractures	Typically treated with closed reduction because fractures are typically greenstick + minimally displaced Limited opportunities for fixation (missing/partially erupted teeth ☐ challenging MMF application, risk of disrupting tooth growth with plating/screws) Peds have thicker periosteal envelope and higher capacity for remodeling
Edentulous mandible	8% of US population Risk of fibrous nonunion inversely related to mandibular height Necessitates ORIF in this population Consider load-bearing recon plate via extraoral approach (challenging to obtain adequate exposure for large plates via intraoral approach)

- Zygomaticomaxillary
- Nasomaxillary
- Pterygomaxillary
- *Alternating thin segments of bone and thick buttresses create predictable fracture patterns (below).

Classification (Fig. 26.5)

- *Dentoalveolar*—involves teeth and supporting osseous structure
- *Le Fort I—Transverse*
  - Separates tooth-bearing maxilla from the midface
  - Fracture at the level of tooth apices above the palate and alveolus that extends from pyriform aperture posteriorly through the nasal septum, anterior maxillary wall, lateral nasal wall, and pterygoid plates
  - *All Le Fort pattern fractures involves *fractures* of the pterygoid plates.
- *Le Fort II—Pyramidal*
  - Fracture line extends through frontonasal junction along the medial orbital wall, through the orbital rim at the zygomaticomaxillary suture; continues posteriorly through pterygoid plates.
  - Nasal bones and maxilla are freely mobile as a single unit.
- *Le Fort III—Craniofacial Disjunction*
  - The entire midface is mobile and detached from the cranial base.
  - Fracture extends from nasofrontal junction through the medial orbital wall, along the inferior orbital fissure and out the lateral orbital wall:
    - Can be subtle! May present only as occlusion problems.
    - Maxilla/nasofrontal and zygomaticofrontal regions will be jointly mobile.
    - High level fracture through pterygoid plates

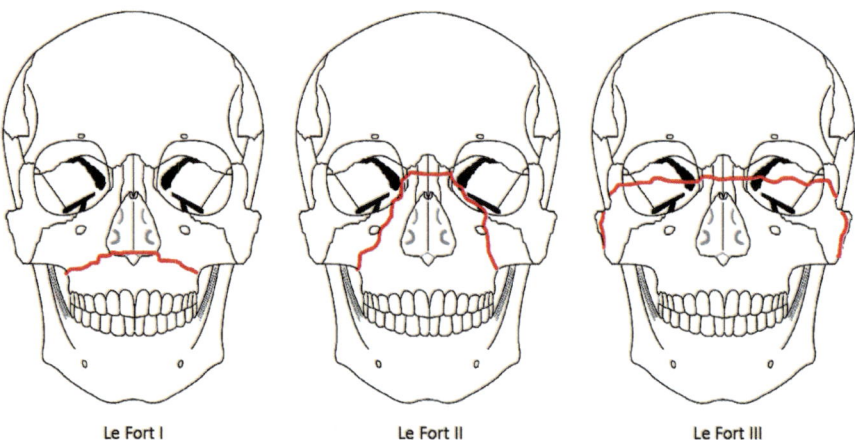

Fig. 26.5 Classification of Le Fort-type fractures. Le Fort fracture patterns are distinct patterns created by the juxtaposition of strong facial buttresses next to segments of thinner weaker bone. All Le Fort-type fractures involve fracture of the pterygoid plates. (CC BY-SA 3.0. Modified from "Le Fort 3 Fracture", Own Work, June 2007, RosarioVanTulpe. https://commons.wikimedia.org/wiki/File:LeFort3b.png)

Management

- ABCs
- Rigid fixation +/− bone grafts
    - IMF ×4–6 weeks.
    - Ensure proper reduction of nasomaxillary and zygomaxillary buttresses.

Pan-Facial Fractures

- Challenging due to the lack of stable reference from which to reconstruct the facial skeleton.
- Fixation should proceed from a bottom-to-top, back-to-front, and then top-down manner:
    - Begin with reconstructing the mandibular arch and re-establishing posterior facial height (need to reconstruct condyle in bicondylar fractures).
    - Once mandibular height is re-established, reconstruction proceeds from the frontal process inferiorly to the maxilla.
    - The zygoma is reconstructed to re-establish facial projection.
    - The maxilla/Le Fort I level is the last area to be stabilized and re-establishes occlusion.
- The goal is to re-establish the *major determinants of the facial form*:
    - Mandibular height
    - Anteroposterior projection (zygoma)
    - Vertical facial height (condyles, maxilla, NOE region)
    - *If these are established, then small malreductions *above* the area of maxillary dentition are tolerable.

References

1. Yavuzer R, Sari A, Kelly CP, Tuncer S, Latifoglu O, Celebi MC, Jackson IT. Management of frontal sinus fractures. Plast Reconstr Surg. 2005;115(6):79e–93e; discussion 94e–95e. https://doi.org/10.1097/01.prs.0000161988.06847.6a. PMID: 15861045.
2. Gart MS, Gosain AK. Evidence-based medicine: orbital floor fractures. Plast Reconstr Surg. 2014;134(6):1345–55.
3. Morrow BT, Samson TD, Schubert W, Mackay DR. Evidence-based medicine: mandible fractures. Plast Reconstr Surg. 2014;134(6):1381–90.
4. Marcowitz BL, Manson PN, Sargent L, et al. Management of the medial canthal tendon in nasoethmoid orbital fractures: the importance of the central fragment in classification and treatment. Plast Reconstr Surg. 1991;87:843–53.
5. Evans BGA, Evans GRD. MOC-PS(SM) CME article: zygomatic fractures. Plast Reconstr Surg. 2008;121(1 Suppl):1–11.

6. Jacob OA, Prathap A. Maxillary fractures. In: Bonanthaya K, Panneerselvam E, Manuel S, Kumar VV, Rai A, editors. Oral and maxillofacial surgery for the clinician. Singapore: Springer; 2021. https://doi.org/10.1007/978-981-15-1346-6_55.
7. Schulz C, Meredith P, Shinton A. Anatomy of the eye, orbit and visual pathway. In: Liu C, Lee H, editors. Fundamentals in ophthalmic practice. Cham: Springer; 2020. https://doi.org/10.1007/978-3-030-28841-9_2.
8. Bruckman KC, Boucree TS, Garri JI, Wolfe SA. Nasoorbitoethmoid (NOE) fractures. In: Taub P, Patel P, Buchman S, Cohen M, editors. Ferraro's fundamentals of maxillofacial surgery. New York: Springer; 2015.
9. Yadav A. Principles of internal fixation in maxillofacial surgery. In: Bonanthaya K, Panneerselvam E, Manuel S, Kumar VV, Rai A, editors. Oral and maxillofacial surgery for the clinician. Singapore: Springer; 2021. https://doi.org/10.1007/978-981-15-1346-6_51.

Chapter 27
Head and Neck Tumors

Kshipra Hemal, Allyson R. Alfonso, and Jasmine Lee

Demographics, Incidence, and Epidemiology

- HNC accounts for 3% of all malignancies, with an estimated 54,000 Americans developing HNC annually and about 11,230 dying from the disease [1].
- Tobacco use is associated with a fivefold increase in incidence of HNC, alcohol with a ninefold increase, and concomitant use of tobacco and alcohol with a 35-fold increase [2].
- In recent years, HPV-mediated oropharyngeal squamous cell carcinomas have risen in incidence; the HPV-16 strain is associated with a 15- to 230-fold increased risk of oropharyngeal squamous cell carcinoma [3, 4].
- It is important to distinguish HPV-associated and tobacco-associated HNCs:
  - The 5-year survival is 28% for HPV-negative cancers versus 65% for HPV-positive cancers [5].
  - HNCs related to smoking and alcohol exposure are more often associated with mutations in tumor suppressor genes such as TP53, which makes them less sensitive to chemoradiation [6].
  - HPV-positive cancers have unique gene expression and DNA methylation profiles, which make them possible to treat with targeted therapies [6].

Classification of Head and Neck Cancers [7]

- Tumors of the head and neck arise from one of five major subunits:

- Oral cavity
  - The lip is the most common site of HNC—the lower lip is involved more frequently than the upper lip.
  - Tumors of the tongue typically present on the lateral border of the middle third of the tongue.
  - Tumors of the buccal mucosa comprise <10% of all oral cavity cancers.
- Oropharynx
  - 60% of oropharyngeal tumors arise from the tonsils.
  - Cancer at the base of the tongue is considered to be part of the oropharynx and is more often caused by HPV infection, as opposed to oral tongue cancers which are most commonly related to tobacco use.
- Hypopharynx
  - Hypopharyngeal tumors are the least common HNCs and have high rates of metastatic spread on initial presentation: 80% present with nodal disease while 25% with distant metastases.
- Larynx
  - The larynx consists of the supraglottis, glottis, and subglottis; the supraglottis has rich lymphatic drainage network, as such supraglottic tumors typically present at higher stages than glottic tumors.
- Salivary glands
  - The majority of salivary gland tumors arise from the parotid gland, while the sublingual gland has the highest rate of malignancy relative to overall tumor occurrence.

Staging

- The American Joint Committee on Cancer (AJCC) divides head and neck cancers into location-based categories, each with its own staging criteria [8]. Staging varies between tumor types but generally depends on tumor size (T), lymph node involvement (N), and presence of metastasis (M).
- The National Comprehensive Cancer Network (NCCN) publishes treatment recommendations for head and neck cancers including that of the lip, oral cavity, pharynx, larynx, ethmoid and maxillary sinuses, and salivary glands [9].

Diagnosis

- History
  - The etiology of injury or presenting cancer-related symptoms such as facial pain or numbness, weight loss, signs of throat or nasal obstruction, and shortness of breath should be reviewed.
  - Past medical and surgical histories should be documented while paying close attention to predictors of reconstructive complications such as diabetes and malnutrition [10].
  - Family history and social history, particularly history of smoking, is important, and smoking cessation should be recommended [11].
- Physical Exam
  - Emphasis should be placed on evaluating all tissue layers with a focus on facial coverage, lining, and integrity of underlying structures such as bone and cartilage.
  - Notation should include aesthetic unit(s) involved, skin quality, scarring, position of hair-bearing skin, and skin texture or color mismatch.
  - A full head and neck exam should include testing cranial nerve function, inspecting oral cavity and mucosal lining, performing anterior rhinoscopy, and inspecting and palpating salivary glands, in addition to the neck for adenopathy or masses [12].
- Laboratory Tests
  - Laboratory studies are not required to make the diagnosis but may be obtained to rule and determine a patient's suitability to a variety of treatment options.
- Imaging
  - Computed tomography angiography (CTA) allows for preoperative planning of microvascular free tissue transfer by assessing both donor and recipient sites [13].
  - Computerized surgical planning (CSP) converts high-resolution CT scan to three-dimensional reconstructions of the facial skeleton and donor site in order to interactively plan surgical reconstruction. Comparison can be made postoperatively to evaluate reconstruction [14].

Head and Neck Surgical Anatomy

- Bony Skeleton: The bony skeleton of the face includes the frontal bone, mandible, and midface [15].

- The midface consists of the maxilla, zygomatic bones, nasal bone, temporal bones, sphenoid, palatine bones, lacrimal bones, ethmoid bones, and vomer.
- Soft Tissue: Upon dissecting through the epidermis and dermis of the face, surgeons can appreciate a layer of superficial fat that is partitioned into separate anatomical compartments, which give volume and youthful appearance [16].
  - The superficial musculoaponeurotic system (SMAS) is a fibrofatty superficial fascia that connects the underlying muscle layer to overlying dermis [17].
  - The SMAS plane spans the entire head and neck, as it is continuous with the platysma, superficial temporal fascia, and galea aponeurotica [18].
  - Careful dissection in the SMAS is necessary to minimizing facial palsies, as the facial nerve runs directly underneath the SMAS in the lower face and runs in the superficial temporal fascia above the zygomatic arch [19].
- Muscles
  - The muscles of the face can be divided into muscles of facial expression and muscles of mastication.
    - The muscles of facial expression derive from the second pharyngeal arch, are innervated by the facial nerve (CN 7), and consist of three groups: periorbital, perioral, and nasal.
    - The muscles of mastication derive from the first pharyngeal arch, are innervated by the trigeminal nerve (CN 5), and include the temporalis, masseter, and medial and lateral pterygoid muscles.
    - Muscles of the neck include the platysma, which is continuous with the SMAS and is offset from deeper neck muscles by the superficial cervical fascia.
- Neck
  - The neck can be anatomically divided in several ways:
    - In oncologic terms, nodes are classified by triangles and levels [20]. There are two large triangles, anterior and posterior, which are separated by the sternocleidomastoid muscle.
      - The anterior triangle can be divided into submandibular, submental, muscular, and carotid triangles (Levels I through IV).
      - The posterior is comprised of the supraclavicular and occipital triangles (Level V).
    - The neck may also be divided into three axially divided zones, with implications for trauma surgery.
- Neurovasculature
  - The muscles of the face are innervated as described above and are perfused by branches of the external carotid artery and drained by the internal jugular vein.
  - Facial sensation is innervated by the trigeminal nerve (CN 5).

References

1. Siegel RL, Miller KD, Jemal A. Cancer statistics, 2016. CA Cancer J Clin. 2016;66(1):7–30.
2. Blot WJ, McLaughlin JK, Winn DM, Austin DF, Greenberg RS, Preston-Martin S, et al. Smoking and drinking in relation to oral and pharyngeal cancer. Cancer Res. 1988;48(11):3282–7.
3. Gillison ML, D'Souza G, Westra W, Sugar E, Xiao W, Begum S, et al. Distinct risk factor profiles for human papillomavirus type 16–positive and human papillomavirus type 16–negative head and neck cancers. J Natl Cancer Inst. 2008;100(6):407–20.
4. D'Souza G, Gross ND, Pai SI, Haddad R, Anderson KS, Rajan S, et al. Oral human papillomavirus (HPV) infection in HPV-positive patients with oropharyngeal cancer and their partners. J Clin Oncol. 2014;32(23):2408.
5. Goodman MT, Saraiya M, Thompson TD, Steinau M, Hernandez BY, Lynch CF, et al. Human papillomavirus genotype and oropharynx cancer survival in the United States of America. Eur J Cancer. 2015;51(18):2759–67.
6. Canning M, Guo G, Yu M, Myint C, Groves MW, Byrd JK, et al. Heterogeneity of the head and neck squamous cell carcinoma immune landscape and its impact on immunotherapy. Front Cell Dev Biol. 2019;7:52.
7. Brockstein BE, Stenson KM, Song S, Fried MP, Brizel DM. Overview of treatment for head and neck cancer. In: Ross ME, editor. UptoDate. Waltham: UpToDate, Inc; 2015.
8. Huang SH, O'Sullivan B. Overview of the 8th edition TNM classification for head and neck cancer. Curr Treat Options in Oncol. 2017;18(7):40.
9. Colevas AD, Yom SS, Pfister DG, Spencer S, Adelstein D, Adkins D, et al. NCCN guidelines insights: head and neck cancers, Version 1.2018. J Natl Compr Cancer Netw: JNCCN. 2018;16(5):479–90.
10. Eskander A, Kang S, Tweel B, Sitapara J, Old M, Ozer E, et al. Predictors of complications in patients receiving head and neck free flap reconstructive procedures. Otolaryngol Head Neck Surg. 2018;158(5):839–47.
11. Crippen MM, Patel N, Filimonov A, Brady JS, Merchant AM, Baredes S, et al. Association of smoking tobacco with complications in head and neck microvascular reconstructive surgery. JAMA Facial Plast Surg. 2019;21(1):20–6.
12. 1.0 Approach to the otolaryngology–head and neck surgery patient. In: Handbook of otolaryngology [Internet]. Stuttgart: Georg Thieme Verlag; 2011.
13. Chang EI, Chu CK, Chang EI. Advancements in imaging technology for microvascular free tissue transfer. J Surg Oncol. 2018;118(5):729–35.
14. Levine JP, Patel A, Saadeh PB, Hirsch DL. Computer-aided design and manufacturing in craniomaxillofacial surgery: the new state of the art. J Craniofac Surg. 2012;23(1):288–93.
15. Ferneini EM, Goupil MT, McNulty MA, Niekrash CE. Applied head and neck anatomy for the facial cosmetic surgeon. Springer; 2021.
16. Rohrich RJ, Pessa JE. The fat compartments of the face: anatomy and clinical implications for cosmetic surgery. Found Pap Oculoplast. 2007;119:13.
17. Mitz V, Peyronie M. The superficial musculo-aponeurotic system (SMAS) in the parotid and cheek area. Plast Reconstr Surg. 1976;58(1):80–8.
18. Broughton M, Fyfe GM. The superficial musculoaponeurotic system of the face: a model explored. Anat Res Int. 2013;2013:794682.
19. Agarwal CA, Mendenhall SD 3rd, Foreman KB, Owsley JQ. The course of the frontal branch of the facial nerve in relation to fascial planes: an anatomic study. Plast Reconstr Surg. 2010;125(2):532–7.
20. Robbins KT, Shaha AR, Medina JE, Califano JA, Wolf GT, Ferlito A, et al. Consensus statement on the classification and terminology of neck dissection. Arch Otolaryngol Head Neck Surg. 2008;134(5):536–8.

Chapter 28
Complex Head and Neck Reconstruction

Alexandre J. Bourcier and Edward H. Nahabet

Introduction

Trauma and neoplasms of the head and neck can lead to significant functional and cosmetic deformities. Reconstruction of such deformities is highly dependent on etiology, extent of the defect, overall patient disease status, and prognosis. Depending on the size and defect, free flaps are often considered the preferred option for head and neck reconstruction due to the paucity of local tissue and difficulty recruiting regional tissue from below the neck.

Cancer Treatment

- General knowledge of head and neck cancer treatments is important as they can impact decision-making with regard to the type of reconstruction necessary.

Lymph Node Dissections

- Advanced cancer treatment often involves lymph node dissections (LND) [1, 2].

- Previously explored necks with prior neck dissections may contain fewer options with regard to usable recipient vessels.
- The types of neck dissection are as follows:
  - Selective Neck Dissection/Modified Radical Neck Dissection
    - Targeted removal of appropriate nodal regions and preservation of non-lymphoid structures.
    - Deemed the standard of care for primary treatment.
    - All other structures are left in place.
  - Radical Neck Dissection
    - Considered in advanced or metastatic cancers
    - Removal of all nonvital structures of the neck
    - Structures sacrificed include
      - Internal jugular vein (IJV)
      - Sternocleidomastoid
      - CN XI
    - Only considered in salvage setting

Radiotherapy

- Adjuvant radiation therapy is commonplace in head and neck cancer after resection and reconstruction.
- In the setting of prior radiation or anticipated radiation therapy, the importance of bringing healthy, non-radiated, vascularized tissue cannot be overstated.
- Radiation of the head and neck can also result in osteoradionecrosis, most commonly of the mandible, which requires complex head and neck reconstruction.
- Additionally, radiated recipient vessels can be diminutive in size, friable, and backup options should be considered.

Patient Evaluation

- Head and neck patients that will require reconstruction should undergo complete evaluation of any comorbidities that may impact outcomes including but not limited to hypertension, diabetes, and smoking [3].
- History of past radiotherapy and prior procedures at the location of interest and donor site should be documented as these can impact decision-making with regard to treatment [4].

Physical Exam

- Examination involves evaluation of the disease process with focus on the expected size and volume of the defect [5, 6].
- Identification of involved tissue components, i.e., the skin, mucosa, and bone, is a crucial component in determining the reconstructive options.
- Assess available recipient vessel options with focus on length and reach for free flap reconstruction.
- Routine head and neck examination should also be performed including a complete cranial nerve exam, lymph node examination, and examination of potential donor sites.

Preoperative Planning

- Routine neoplastic workup can include chest X-ray and PET scan to evaluate for metastatic disease [5, 6].
- Additional imaging performed by the reconstructive team can include CT or CTA to further evaluate the defect and regional vasculature.
- Due to disease etiology, many head and neck patients suffer from malnutrition, and preoperative optimization can be integral in preventing postoperative wound issues—consider a nutritional consultation.
- If operating near or around the airway, patients will require a tracheostomy to allow protected ventilation during the postoperative recovery—this can be performed prior to the day of the ablative procedure and reconstruction.
- Similarly, patients that will undergo reconstruction involving the oral cavity or hypopharynx should receive a gastric tube or Dobhoff to allow feeding in the postoperative period and prevent malnutrition.
- Ultimately, the exact size and extent of a cancer ablative defect may not be known until the resection is completed.
- A multidisciplinary approach and frequent communication with the ablative surgeons helps plan as best as possible for the expected defect; however, planning should involve considering scenarios where the defect is larger than anticipated.

Recipient Vessels

- The quality of the recipient vessels is central to the success of head and neck reconstruction [7].
- Consider what vessels may be available to you in the setting of a prior or concurrent neck dissection.

- Additionally, consider the length of flap pedicle and reach to the recipient vessels, especially in scalp vertex reconstruction.

Arteries (Fig. 28.1)

- Facial artery
    - Branches off the external carotid artery (ECA)
    - Crosses the inferior border of the mandible anterior to the mandibular angle

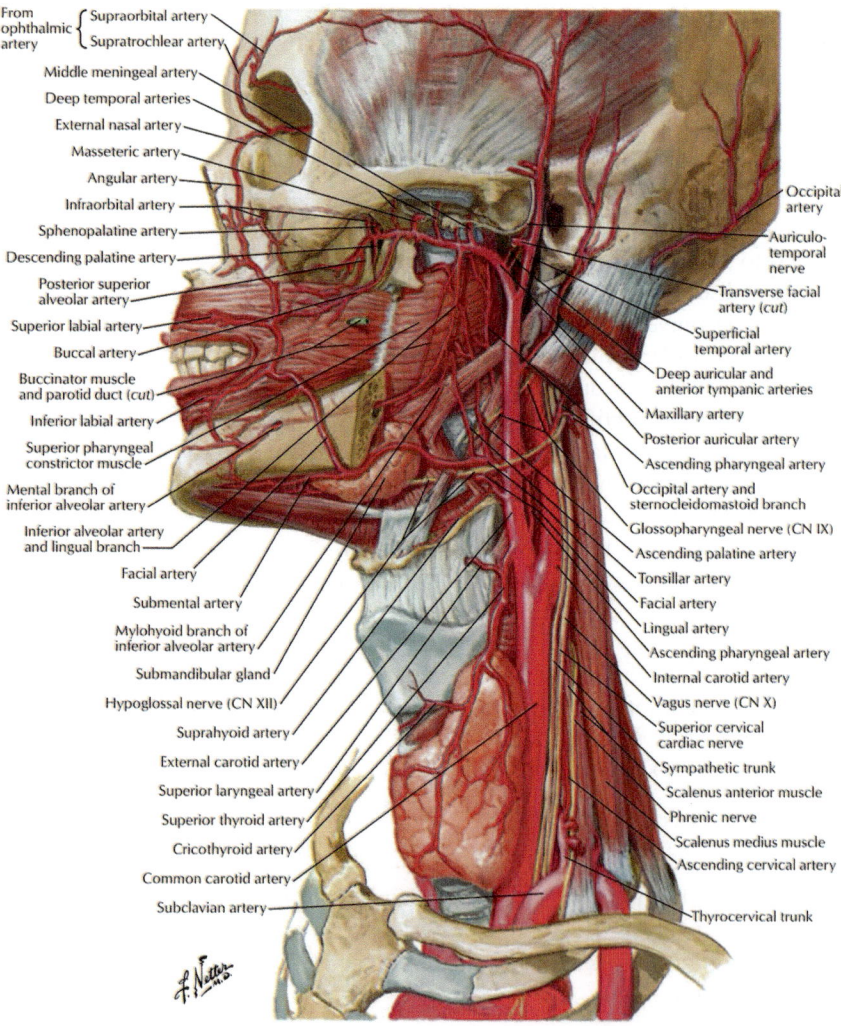

Fig. 28.1 Arteries of the head and neck. (Obtained from Neligan et al. [6])

- Superior thyroid artery
  - Branches off the ECA
  - Excellent flow and good proximity to IJV
- Superficial temporal artery
  - Branches off the ECA
  - Easy access
  - Ideal for scalp and midface reconstruction
- Transverse cervical artery
  - Branches off the thyrocervical trunk
  - Often spared in neck dissection
  - Travels within the posterior triangle of the neck

Veins (Fig. 28.2)

- Common facial vein
  - Good caliber and in close proximity to the facial artery
  - May not be available if the patient had a prior neck dissection
- Jugular veins
  - Most commonly used jugular vein is the external jugular.
  - Extra pedicle length may be necessary to reach scalp defects.

Interpositional Vein Grafts

- In the event that additional pedicle length is needed, an interpositional vein graft can be utilized.
- The lesser saphenous vein from the lower extremity is a commonly used option.

Arteriovenous (AV) Loop

- AV loops are an alternate method of gaining length to reach your recipient vessels.
- This technique connects the recipient artery to the recipient vein with a vein graft harvested from elsewhere, thus creating an AV loop.

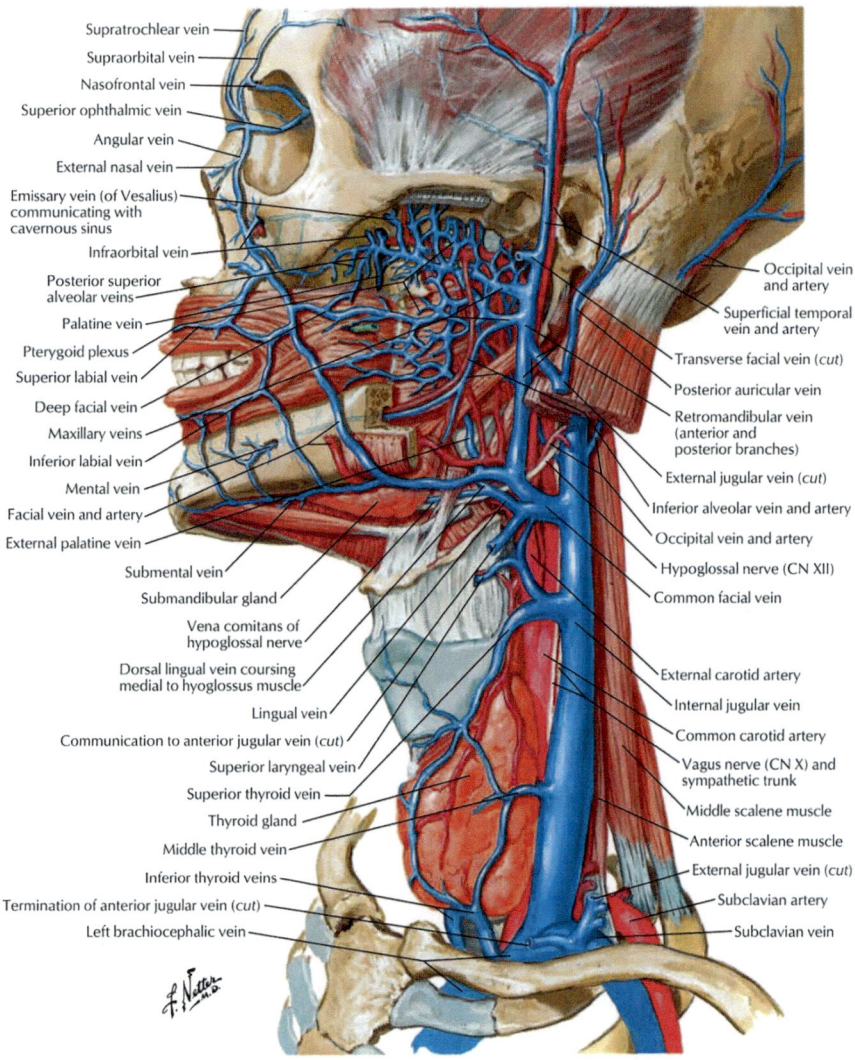

Fig. 28.2 Veins of the head and neck. (Obtained from Neligan et al. [6])

- The AV loop is left in place to allow the vessel to dilate and subsequently divided in half, thereby extending the reach of the recipient vessels to the flap vessels for anastomosis.

Scalp Reconstruction

- In the setting of scalp reconstruction, evaluation requires determination of the soft tissues involved and the presence of bony involvement [8].

Cranioplasty

- In the setting of bony involvement, a cranioplasty may be required to reconstruct the calvarial defect.
- This procedure is typically performed in conjunction with neurosurgery and is performed most commonly by means of alloplastic materials or autologous reconstruction.
- Alloplastic materials:
  - The most commonly used alloplastic material for calvarial reconstruction remains the titanium mesh plate.
  - Benefits of alloplastic reconstruction include unlimited supply, lack of donor site morbidity, and ease of use; disadvantages include risk for extrusion or infection.
  - Alternative alloplastic materials for complex head and neck reconstruction include custom-fashioned polyetheretherketone (PEEK) implants and polymethyl methacrylate—these materials are not typically used in the setting of primary defects.
- Autologous reconstruction:
  - Autologous calvarial reconstruction such as split calvarial bone grafts are an alternative option.
  - Benefits include the lack of foreign material and lower risk for infection; disadvantages include donor site morbidity and increased operative time.
  - Split thickness calvarial graft involves separating the inner and outer cortices of healthy calvarial bone and using a single cortex to reconstruct the bony defect.

Soft Tissue Reconstruction

- Locoregional scalp flaps are capable of covering large defects, although may be limited in patients with multiple prior surgeries or radiation.
- Free flaps offer a reliable solution for coverage of complex scalp defects following cranioplasty or if there is no bony involvement [9].
- The most commonly used free flaps for scalp reconstruction include the latissimus dorsi and anterolateral thigh flaps as they are both large flaps with long vascular pedicles to reach recipient vessels in the head and neck.
- The latissimus dorsi flap can be taken as a musculocutaneous flap or a muscle flap in conjunction with skin grafting and has a long vascular pedicle that allows reach to the recipient vessels in the neck.
- The anterolateral thigh (ALT) flap is a large fasciocutaneous flap capable of covering large scalp defects and has a good length vascular pedicle to reach recipient vessels with good source vessel diameter for anastomosis.

Tongue Reconstruction

- The goal of tongue reconstruction is to restore mobility and bulk for articulation, deglutition, and airway protection [10, 11].
- Treatment of tongue malignancies can be surgical resection, neck dissection, and adjuvant radiotherapy.

Tongue Defects Classification (Fig. 28.3)

- Mucosectomy—Resection of the mucosa
- Partial glossectomy—Resection of the mucosa, submucosa, and intrinsic muscles
- Hemiglossectomy—Resection of the mucosa, submucosa, and intrinsic and extrinsic muscles ipsilateral to the lesion
- Subtotal glossectomy—Resection of the anterior tongue with preservation of part or whole base of the tongue
- Total glossectomy—Complete resection of the tongue at the level of the vallecula

Reconstructive Algorithm

- Tongue lesions <4 cm of the anterior and middle 1/3
    - Can be closed primarily

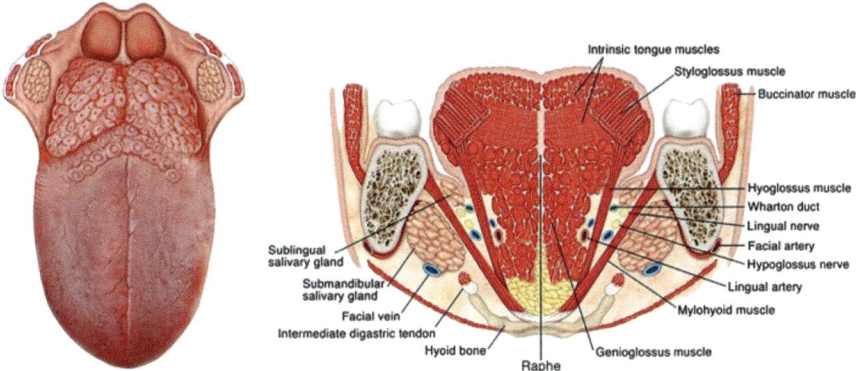

Fig. 28.3 Tongue anatomy. (Obtained from Ansarin et al. [11])

- Larger lesions involving >1/3 of the base of the tongue
  - Reconstruction via fasciocutaneous free flaps (radial forearm, ALT, medial sural artery perforator)
- Subtotal and total tongue resection
  - Reconstruction with free ALT flap, which provides both mobility and bulk

Mandibular Reconstruction

- The goal of mandibular reconstruction is to restore shape and integrity of the mandible for mechanical functions [12, 13].
- Defects can generally be thought of as those requiring soft tissue reconstruction, bony reconstruction, or both [14].

Soft Tissue Reconstruction

- Pedicled pectoralis major
  - Used when neck coverage is needed
  - Reliable and easy to harvest
- Radial forearm flap
  - Fasciocutaneous flap useful for intraoral reconstruction
- ALT
  - Utilized for larger soft tissue reconstructions

Bone Reconstruction

- Nonvascularized bone grafts
  - Used for traumatic or benign tumor defects <6 cm long
  - Should not be subjected to radiotherapy due to the risk of osteoradionecrosis
- Vascularized bone free flaps, i.e., fibula flap, deep circumflex iliac artery (DCIA), scapular flap, and osteocutaneous radial forearm flap
  - Treatment of choice when nonvascularized bone grafts are contraindicated
  - Provide greater strength and functional outcomes than nonvascularized flaps

Virtual Surgical Planning

- Creation of 3D computer images of the mandible and fibula [15] (Fig. 28.4)
- Particularly useful for mandibular reconstruction, especially when planning dental rehabilitation
- Provides significant benefits including
  - Improved accuracy of reconstruction
  - Reduction in operative time
  - Shorter hospital admission

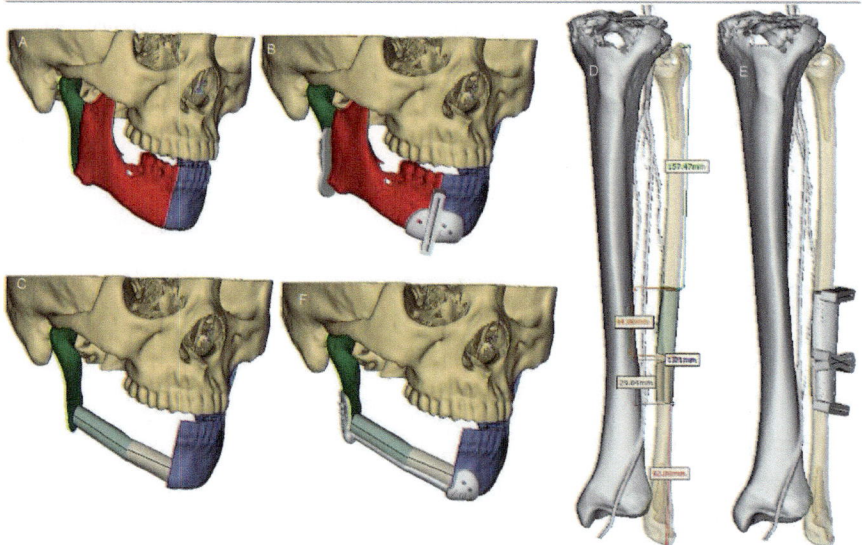

Fig. 28.4 Virtual surgical planning of mandibular reconstruction [20]

Pharyngeal Reconstruction

- The goal of pharyngeal reconstruction is to protect the airway and restore speech and swallow functions [16].

Anatomy (Fig. 28.5)

- Nasopharynx
    - Space and structures surrounding the nasal cavity and above the soft palate
- Oropharynx
    - Space between the soft palate and the aryepiglottic folds
- Hypopharynx
    - Space from the aryepiglottic folds at the level of the hyoid bone to the esophageal inlet

Primary Closure

- If there is adequate mucosa and/or velopharyngeal function is preserved, then primary closure is indicated.
- In the setting of prior or anticipated radiotherapy, it is crucial to transfer healthy well-vascularized tissues.

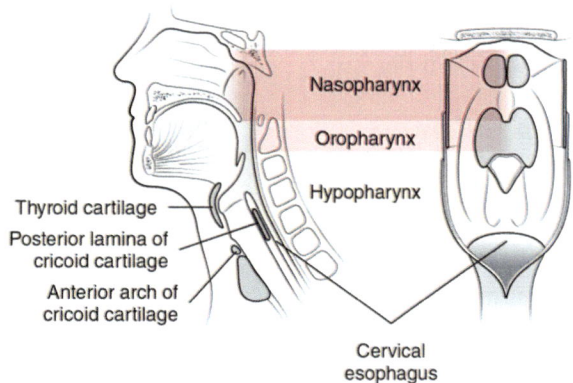

Fig. 28.5 Subdivisions of the pharynx [5]

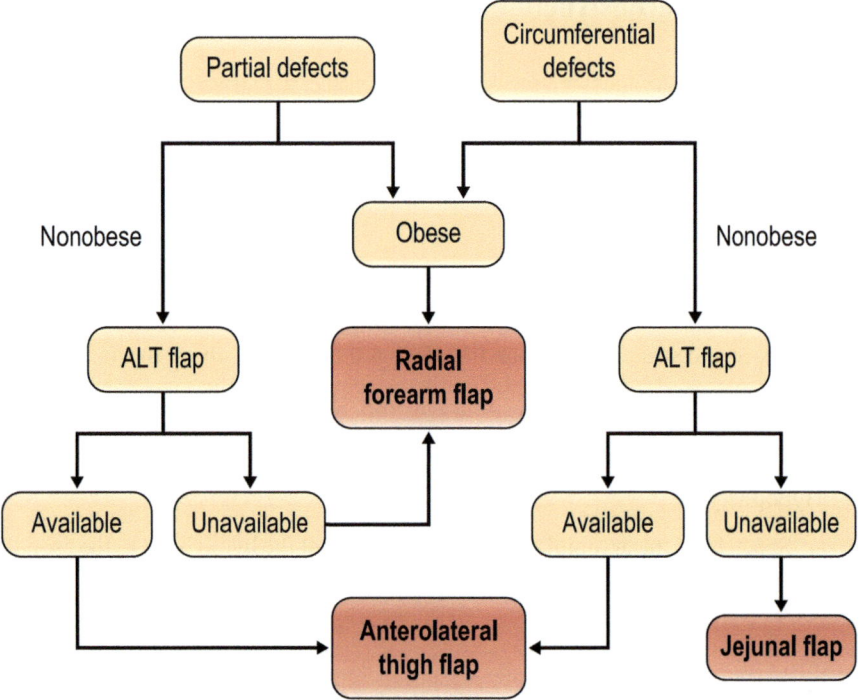

Fig. 28.6 An algorithm of flap selection for pharyngoesophageal reconstruction [6]

Free Flap

- Free flap options are dependent on the type of defect, comorbidities, and donor site availabilities (Fig. 28.6)
- Commonly used options include the ALT flap, the radial forearm flap, and the free jejunal flap.

Complications

Flap Failure

- Common causes include arterial or venous thrombosis, systemic coagulative disorders, and technical errors [17–19].
- Flap compromise should be addressed with urgent re-exploration and attempted salvage.
- Flap loss should only be addressed after etiology of initial failure is determined and addressed and should consider the use of virgin recipient vessels.

Vessel Blowout

- Sudden bleeding in a previously irradiated neck, typically at the site of anastomoses to the carotid system [17–19].
- This is a surgical emergency and requires immediate operative exploration and repair.

Hardware Exposure

- Exposure of implants such as titanium mesh in the scalp reconstruction or mandibular plates in mandibula reconstruction [17–19]
- Can be treated conservatively in the acute setting and with hardware removal and reconstruction if necessary in the prolonged postop period

Fistula

- Salivary leaks can present as orocutaneous fistulas in head and neck reconstruction [17–19].
- Treatment involves parenteral feeding, nutritional optimization, and if necessary debridement and reconstruction.

Cancer Recurrence

- A possibility for any cancer patient undergoing reconstruction [18, 19].
- Postoperative monitoring, adjuvant treatment, and surveillance are important.

References

1. Cotter CS, Stringer SP, Landau S, Mancuso AA, Cassisi NJ. Patency of the internal jugular vein following modified radical neck dissection. Laryngoscope. 1994;104:841–5.
2. Medina JE. A rational classification of neck dissections. Otolaryngol Head Neck Surg. 1989;100:169–76.
3. Kademani D, Mardini S, Moran SL. Reconstruction of head and neck defects: a systematic approach to treatment. Semin Plast Surg. 2008;22:141–55.
4. Wehage IC, Fansa H. Complex reconstructions in head and neck cancer surgery: decision making. Head Neck Oncol. 2011;3:14.
5. Janis J. Essentials of plastic surgery. Thieme; 2014.
6. Neligan PC. Plastic surgery: 6-volume set. Elsevier; 2017.

7. Wei F-C, Mardini S. Flaps and reconstructive surgery. Elsevier; 2016.
8. Leedy JE, Janis JE, Rohrich RJ. Reconstruction of acquired scalp defects: an algorithmic approach. Plast Reconstr Surg. 2005;116:54e–72e.
9. Labow BI, Rosen H, Pap SA, Upton J. Microsurgical reconstruction: a more conservative method of managing large scalp defects? J Reconstr Microsurg. 2009;25:465–74.
10. Haughey BH. Tongue reconstruction: concepts and practice. Laryngoscope. 1993;103:1132–41.
11. Ansarin M, et al. Classification of GLOSSECTOMIES: proposal for tongue cancer resections. Head Neck. 2019;41:821–7.
12. Hanasono MM, Zevallos JP, Skoracki RJ, Yu P. A prospective analysis of bony versus soft-tissue reconstruction for posterior mandibular defects. Plast Reconstr Surg. 2010;125:1413–21.
13. Momoh AO, et al. A prospective cohort study of fibula free flap donor-site morbidity in 157 consecutive patients. Plast Reconstr Surg. 2011;128:714–20.
14. Schultz BD, et al. Classification of mandible defects and algorithm for microvascular reconstruction. Plast Reconstr Surg. 2015;135:743e.
15. Barr ML, et al. Virtual surgical planning for mandibular reconstruction with the fibula free flap: a systematic review and meta-analysis. Ann Plast Surg. 2020;84:117–22.
16. Sokoya M, et al. Pharyngeal reconstruction with microvascular free tissue transfer. Semin Plast Surg. 2019;33:78–80.
17. Razdan SN, Albornoz CR, Matros E, Paty PB, Cordeiro PG. Free jejunal flap for pharyngoesophageal reconstruction in head and neck cancer patients: an evaluation of donor site complications. J Reconstr Microsurg. 2015;31:643–6.
18. Salgado CJ, Chim H, Schoenoff S, Mardini S. Postoperative care and monitoring of the reconstructed head and neck patient. Semin Plast Surg. 2010;24:281–7.
19. Wu C-C, Lin P-Y, Chew K-Y, Kuo Y-R. Free tissue transfers in head and neck reconstruction: complications, outcomes and strategies for management of flap failure: analysis of 2019 flaps in single institute. Microsurgery. 2014;34:339–44.
20. Wang YY, Zhang HQ, Fan S, Zhang DM, Huang ZQ, Chen WL, Ye JT, Li JS. Mandibular reconstruction with the vascularized fibula flap: comparison of virtual planning surgery and conventional surgery. Int J Oral Maxillofac Surg. 2016;45:1400–5.

Chapter 29
Facial Paralysis

Shervin Etemad

Facial Nerve Anatomy

- Intracranial: Upper motor neurons originate in the primary motor cortex, descend contralaterally, and reach the facial nucleus in the pons.
- Intratemporal: Facial nerve passes through the internal auditory meatus of the temporal bone and enters the facial canal in the petrous temporal bone.
- Extratemporal: Facial nerve exits the stylomastoid foramen. Five branches of the facial nerve innervate the muscles of facial expression: temporal branch, zygomatic branch, buccal branch, mandibular branch, and cervical branch.
  - Nerves split in between the lobes of the parotid gland.
    - Temporal travels over zygomatic arch, area of injury.
    - Marginal mandibular travels along border of mandible posterior to facial vessels before crossing over.
  - Temporal and marginal mandibular are most prone to injury because of lack of redundant fibers.
- All muscles are innervated on deep surface except for buccinator, levator anguli oris, and mentalis.

S. Etemad (✉)
Plastic and Reconstructive Surgery, Keck Medicine of USC, Los Angeles, CA, USA
e-mail: shervin.etemad@med.usc.edu

© The Author(s), under exclusive license to Springer Nature Switzerland AG 2025
J. Roostaeian et al. (eds.), *Plastic Surgery Clerkship*, Contemporary Surgical Clerkships, https://doi.org/10.1007/978-3-031-99098-4_29

History of Facial Paralysis

- Need to know progression, duration, associated conditions/exposures/surgeries/diseases
- Isolate concerns anatomically:
  - Eye: dry eye, tearing, vision changes
  - Nose: breathing difficulty
  - Mouth: drooling, smile, speaking

Examination

- Examine at rest and in motion
  - Rest: loss of wrinkles, presence of brow ptosis, ectropion, effacement of nasolabial fold, oral commissure drooping (Fig. 29.1)
  - Activity: break up for each branch of the nerve

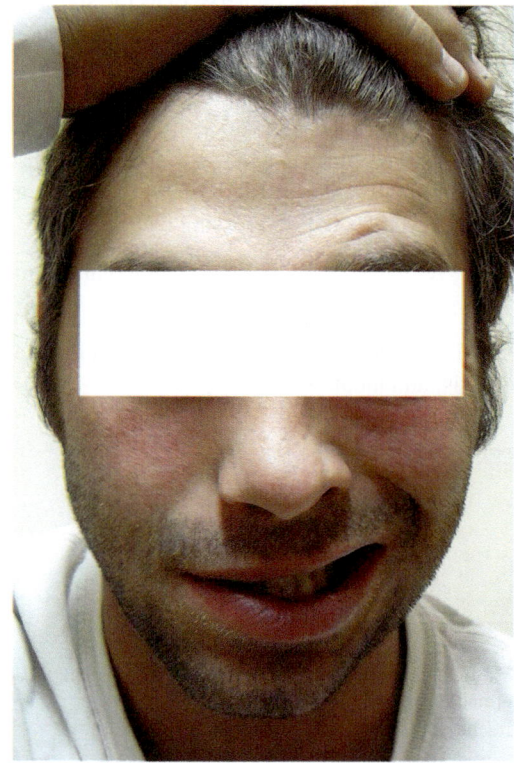

Fig. 29.1 Right-sided Bell's palsy facial paralysis

- Temporal: brow elevation (frontalis)
- Zygomatic: eye closure (orbicularis oculi)
- Buccal: smile (zygomaticus major)
- Marginal mandibular: pursing lips (mentalis)
- Full dental smile: marginal mandibular and cervical (depressor anguli oris, mentalis, platysma):
  - Isolating the marginal mandibular and cervical can be challenging.
  - The side with more depression of the lower lip has normal function.
  - If full dentured, smile is present without lip pursing, then cervical is intact, and marginal is out.
  - The reverse can be difficult to assess.
- Isolating upper motor v lower motor neuron injury
  - There are redundancies in brow elevation in an upper motor neuron injury (if an upper motor neuron is injured, then contralateral *lower* facial paralysis is seen only).
  - There are no redundancies in lower motor neuron injury (if a lower motor neuron is injured, then ipsilateral *total* facial paralysis is seen).
- Other associated issues
  - Hyperacusis due to loss of nerve to the stapedius
  - Dysgeusia due to loss of the chorda tympani
- Synkinesis
  - Sign of reinnervation of the facial nerve in poor form
  - Includes hyperlacrimation and gustatory sweating
- Classify by House-Brackmann scale (Table 29.1)

Table 29.1 House-Brackmann scale of facial paralysis

	Forehead	Eye	Mouth
I (normal)	Normal	Normal	Normal
II (mild)	Slightly weak	Can close completely easily	Slightly weak
III (moderate)	Moderate movement	Hard to close but can close	Moderate movement, not disfiguring
IV (moderate severe)	Disfiguring	Incomplete closure	Asymmetric at rest
V (severe)	Barely perceptible	Barely perceptible	Barely perceptible
VI (total loss)	No movement	No movement	No movement

Adjunctive Studies

- Electrodiagnostics can be used to determine if regeneration is occurring (done multiple weeks after injury).
- Audiogram is used to assess hearing.
- MRI/CT can be used in setting of trauma or suspected tumor.

Etiologies of Paralysis

Bell's Palsy [1]

- Most common cause of unilateral facial nerve paralysis
- Associated with reactivation of latent herpes infection
- Acute presentation with 3–7-day progression
- Treatment consists of early steroids and antiviral therapy
- Most often self-limited, but some patients may have incomplete recovery

Infection

- Herpes zoster oticus (Ramsay Hunt syndrome): varicella-zoster reactivation resulting in facial paralysis, otalgia, auricular vesicle eruption
    - Treat with valacyclovir
- Lyme disease (*Borrelia burgdorferi*)
    - Treat with doxycycline
- Ear infections [2]

Neoplasm

- Facial nerve tumors (neuroma, hemangioma)
- Nerve adjacent tumors (parotid tumors, cutaneous tumors, posterior fossa tumors, acoustic neuroma—associated with tinnitus)
- Metastatic tumors

Trauma

- Temporal bone fracture
- Zygomatic arch fracture (temporal branch)

- Lacerations
- Iatrogenic injuries (obstetrical use of forceps)

Developmental

- Hemifacial microsomia (unilateral)
- Moebius syndrome (bilateral CN6 and CN7 palsies, along with CN12)

Nonsurgical Treatment

- Depends on etiology and goals
- Early steroids and antivirals in suspected Bell's palsy or Ramsay Hunt syndrome
- Doxycycline for suspected Lyme disease
- Intervention for corneal protection
  - Artificial tears
  - Eye taping
  - Eye patch
- Botulinum toxin
  - Used to promote dynamic symmetry by weakening the contralateral side (in the case of brow) or static symmetry by weakening the contralateral side (in the case of lip elevation from loss of the marginal mandibular)
- Facial therapy for facial functionality and mime therapy for biofeedback and movement training

Surgical Management

Principles of Surgical Management

- Direct nerve repair may be indicated in traumatic lacerations:
  - Exploration must occur within 72 hours of injury so distal targets can be stimulated; otherwise, neurotransmitters depleted.
  - Nerve repair or reconstruction can be performed up to 12 months after injury before target muscles and neuromuscular junction atrophy.
- Static procedures rely on soft tissue suspension for improved symmetry.
- Dynamic procedures rely on innervated muscle for reanimation.

Static Reconstruction

- The goal is to restore symmetry at rest and prevent exposure-related injury.
- Depends on anatomic unit:
  - Brow: brow lift
  - Upper lid: gold weight, tarsorrhaphy
  - Lower lid: tendon sling, canthoplasty
  - Lower lip: neuromodulators to unaffected side, tensor fascia lata graft for oral commissure elevation (static sling), or depressor anguli oris resection (unaffected side)

Dynamic Reconstruction [3, 4]

- Direct nerve repair or reconstruction with nerve graft
  - More synkinesis in nerve grafting
- Secondary repair
  - Need to bring in healthy functioning nerve to either reinnervate injured muscle (if <12 months from injury) or innervate a transferred muscle
- Cross-facial nerve graft with free muscle transfer
  - Stage 1: Sural nerve graft used to connect donor nerve from unaffected side to the affected side.
    - Typically target buccal branch to restore zygomaticus major
  - Stage 2: free muscle transfer with accompanying nerve, artery, and vein. Most often the gracilis is used for the second stage.
  - Can be done in single stage with babysitter procedure with transfer of hypoglossal nerve into muscle to prevent denervation while cross-facial nerve graft grows.
  - Best option for restoration of spontaneous smile
- Free muscle transfer can be done for other donor nerves, again lacking spontaneous smiling.
- Ipsilateral nerve transfers:
  - Ipsilateral hypoglossal and masseter nerves may be used in the acute phase of paralysis.
  - Does not provide spontaneous smile.
  - Unwanted smile animation can occur with mastication.
- Local muscle transfers:
  - Resting symmetry and non-spontaneous voluntary smile.
  - Masseter, temporalis, and temporalis tendon are commonly used (Fig. 29.2).

Fig. 29.2 Cross-facial nerve grafting

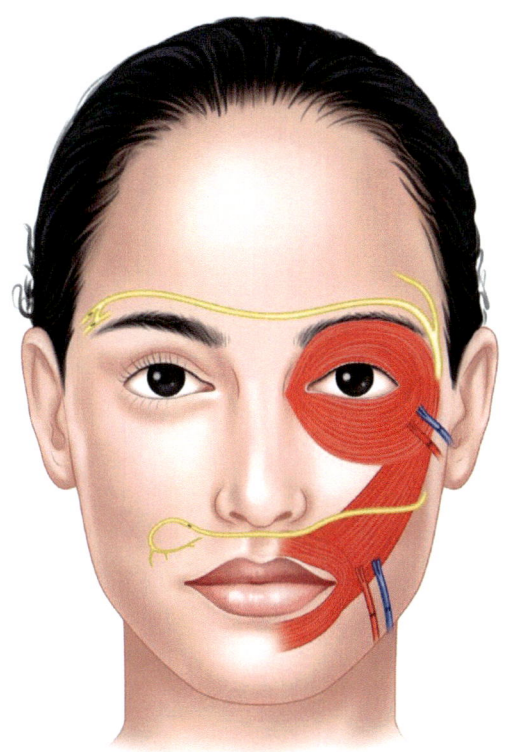

References

1. Eviston TJ, Croxson GR, Kennedy PG, Hadlock T, Krishnan AV. Bell's palsy: aetiology, clinical features and multidisciplinary care. J Neurol Neurosurg Psychiatry. 2015;86(12):1356–61. https://doi.org/10.1136/jnnp-2014-309563. Epub 2015 Apr 9. PMID: 25857657.
2. Makeham TP, Croxson GR, Coulson S. Infective causes of facial nerve paralysis. Otol Neurotol. 2007;28(1):100–3. https://doi.org/10.1097/01.mao.0000232009.01116.3f. PMID: 17031324.
3. Pinkiewicz M, Dorobisz K, Zatoński T. A comprehensive approach to facial reanimation: a systematic review. J Clin Med. 2022;11(10):2890. https://doi.org/10.3390/jcm11102890. PMID: 35629016; PMCID: PMC9143601.
4. Owusu JA, Stewart CM, Boahene K. Facial nerve paralysis. Med Clin North Am. 2018;102(6):1135–43. https://doi.org/10.1016/j.mcna.2018.06.011. Epub 2018 Sep 20. PMID: 30342614.

Chapter 30
Breast Anatomy

Shamit Prabhu

- Structure [1]

  - The borders of the breast are the second rib superiorly, sternal border medially, inframammary fold inferiorly, and latissimus/axilla laterally.
  - The upper medial portion of the breast overlies the pectoralis major.
  - The breast consists of groups of 15–20 lobes divided by fibrous bands of connective tissue termed the suspensory ligaments of the breast (Cooper's ligaments). These ligaments extend from the clavipectoral fascia to the dermis, providing structure and shape to the breast. These ligaments weaken with time, resulting in breast ptosis (Fig. 30.1).
  - Lobes are comprised of lobules containing tubuloalveolar glands that are stimulated by prolactin to produce milk.
  - Lactiferous ducts carry milk and converge at the nipple.
  - Nipple position is typically centered on the breast mound but can shift downward with breastfeeding and age.
  - The nipple is surrounded by a pigmented, circular area of the skin termed the areola. The areola surface has small, raised areas which are areolar glands, also known as glands of Montgomery. Together, with the nipple, it is termed the nipple-areolar complex (NAC).

- Arterial supply [1]

  - Arterial supply can be subdivided into the arterial supply to the skin and to the underlying parenchyma.
  - Skin

S. Prabhu (✉)
UCLA Division of Plastic Surgery, Los Angeles, CA, USA
e-mail: sprabhu@mednet.ucla.edu

Fig. 30.1 Basic breast anatomy

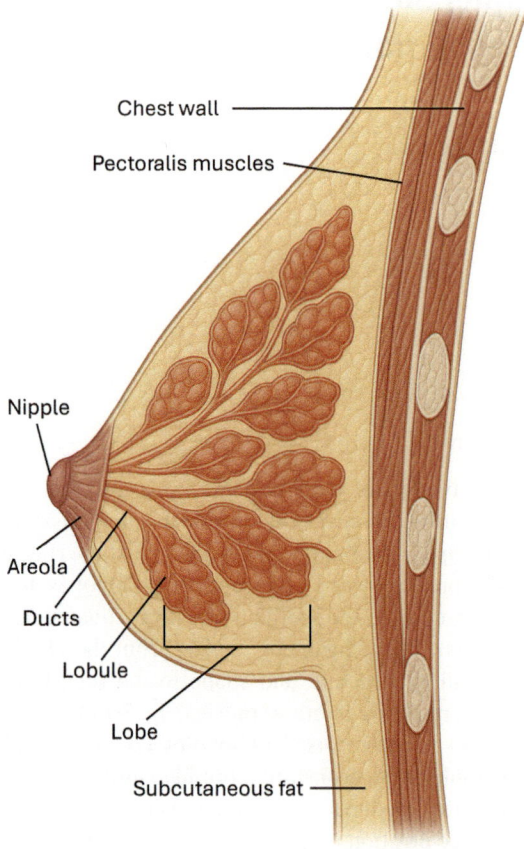

- Supplied by a network of small vessels traversing the subdermal plane called the subdermal plexus.
- The NAC is reliant on the subdermal plexus after a nipple-sparing mastectomy.

– Parenchyma

- Internal thoracic artery perforators
- Lateral thoracic artery
- Second, third, and fourth intercostal artery perforators
- Thoracodorsal artery
- Thoracoacromial artery

– NAC

- Dominant supply by internal thoracic perforators with secondary supply from anterior intercostal arteries and lateral thoracic artery [2]

- Venous drainage [1]
    - Veins typically travel alongside arteries and drain into the axillary vein with smaller tributaries to the internal thoracic vein and second, third, and fourth intercostal veins.
- Innervation [1, 3, 4]
    - The breast is innervated by the anterior and lateral cutaneous nerve branches of the second to sixth intercostal nerves.
    - The nipple is innervated by the third through fifth intercostal nerves.
        - Primary innervation is the most consistent by the lateral cutaneous branch (LCB) of the fourth intercostal nerve.
        - Secondary innervation by the anterior cutaneous branch (ACB) of the third and fourth intercostal nerves.
        - Würinger's septum—septum that originates along the pectoral fascia at the level of the fifth rib and travels anteriorly to the nipple. Carries the main supplying nerve for the nipple (LCB of the fourth intercostal). The septum lies between a vascular network comprised of the thoracoacromial artery and branch of the lateral thoracic artery cranially and perforating intercostal arteries caudally.
- Lymphatics [1]
    - Multiple lymph nodes drain the breast with the majority draining into the axillary lymph nodes.
    - Some drainage occurs via the parasternal lymph nodes and intercostal/internal mammary lymph nodes.
    - With the majority of breast drainage occurring via the axillary lymph nodes, these are the nodes dissected and tested during sentinel lymph node biopsies and axillary node dissections.
    - The location of axillary nodes relative to the pectoralis minor is clinically relevant during axillary node dissections and are categorized as follows:
        - Level I: lateral to the pectoralis minor
        - Level II: deep to the pectoralis minor
        - Level III: medial to the pectoralis minor
    - Lymph nodes between the pectoralis major and minor are termed Rotter's nodes

References

1. Netter F. Mammary gland. In: Atlas of human anatomy. 7th ed. Elsevier; 2019. p. 188–91.
2. van Deventer PV. The blood supply to the nipple-areola complex of the human mammary gland. Aesth Plast Surg. 2004;28(6):393–8.

3. Smeele HP, Bijkerk E, van Kuijk SMJ, Lataster A, van der Hulst RRWJ, Tuinder SMH. Innervation of the female breast and nipple: a systematic review and meta-analysis of anatomical dissection studies. Plast Reconstr Surg. 2022;150(2):243–55.
4. Würinger E, Mader N, Posch E, Holle J. Nerve and vessel supplying ligamentous suspension of the mammary gland. Plast Reconstr Surg. 1998;101(6):1486–93.

Chapter 31
Gynecomastia

Laurel D. Ormiston and Kaylee B. Scott

Introduction

Gynecomastia is the benign proliferation of breast tissue in a male and can be attributed to many different causes. It can be unilateral or bilateral and is usually asymptomatic. Most cases resolve spontaneously. Persistent gynecomastia that occurs for greater than 1 year may be addressed surgically if the patient desires treatment.

Definitions

- Gynecomastia is a benign proliferation of mammary glandular tissue in males [1].
- In contrast, pseudogynecomastia is characterized by proliferation of only the fatty tissue in the breast region in males [2].

L. D. Ormiston (✉) · K. B. Scott
University of Utah, School of Medicine, Division of Plastic Surgery, Salt Lake City, UT, USA
e-mail: laurel.ormiston@hsc.utah.edu; kaylee.scott@hsc.utah.edu

Etiology

Physiologic Causes

- Gynecomastia is often due to an imbalance in the ratio of free estrogen to free androgen, which commonly occurs at periods of hormonal changes [1]. Therefore, there is a trimodal age distribution, occurring in infancy, puberty, and older age [2].
- Within these age groups, gynecomastia is common, occurring in 60–90% of male infants, 48–64% of pubertal males and greater than 50% of older males aged 50 years or older. Typically, physiologic gynecomastia will resolve spontaneously, although it can persist.
- Higher BMI is also associated with gynecomastia [1].

Pharmacologic Causes

- Various drug classes are associated with gynecomastia, including estrogens, gonadotropins, androgens, anti-androgens, calcium channel blockers, chemotherapy agents, ACE inhibitors, antihypertensives, dopamine antagonists, drugs of abuse (alcohol, heroin, and marijuana), and highly active antiviral therapy for HIV [1, 3, 4]. Common etiologies include cimetidine, spironolactone, and ketoconazole. This list is not exhaustive, and many different drugs can lead to development of gynecomastia.

Pathologic Causes

- Gynecomastia may be due to testicular tumors, including Leydig tumors, Sertoli tumors, and germ-cell tumors. Adrenocortical tumors and hCG-producing tumors can also cause gynecomastia [3].
- Gynecomastia can also be caused by metabolic and endocrine dysfunction, including primary or secondary hypogonadism, hyperthyroidism, liver disease, renal disease, androgen insensitivity, and familial or sporadic aromatase excess syndrome [2, 3].
- Klinefelter syndrome is a genetic condition in which a male has an extra X chromosome (XXY). Approximately 80% of patients with Klinefelter syndrome will exhibit gynecomastia. Among Klinefelter patients, gynecomastia carries an increased risk of breast cancer [2]. There are reports of 10–20 times greater risk, and as high as 66% increased incidence of breast cancer in Klinefelter patients compared to non-Klinefelter patients with gynecomastia [5, 6]. Gynecomastia due to other causes (non-Klinefelter) has a cancer risk equal to that in the general male population [7].

Idiopathic Gynecomastia

- The most common cause of gynecomastia is idiopathic or unknown [7].

Clinical Evaluation

- Evaluate for use of gynecomastia-inducing drugs. Physical exam should include exam of the testes, breast exam for masses, thyroid exam, abdominal exam for hepatomegaly or adrenal mass, and observation for physical signs of virilization [2]. Screening labs should be tailored to the patient based on the history and physical but may include serum hCG, LH, growth hormone, testosterone, estradiol, dehydroepiandrosterone (DHEA), liver enzymes, and thyroid function. Further workup may also include testicular ultrasound [3]. If Klinefelter syndrome is suspected, karyotype analysis can confirm.
- Consider mammography if there is concern for cancer [7]. Consultation and further management with endocrinology, urology, or general medicine is appropriate if the workup is suggestive of a pathological or pharmacological etiology.
- If the history and physical are negative, or further workup is normal, persistent gynecomastia <12 months may simply be observed. Persistent gynecomastia for greater than 12 months can be managed surgically [4, 7].

Classification of Gynecomastia

Simon, Hoffman, and Kahn [8]

- Grade 1: Small, visible breast enlargement. No skin redundancy
- Grade 2A: Moderate breast enlargement without skin redundancy
- Grade 2B: Moderate breast enlargement with skin redundancy
- Grade 3: Marked breast enlargement with marked skin redundancy, i.e., pendulous female breasts

American Society of Plastic Surgery Practice Parameters

- ASPS has since put forth a modified classification system which was adapted from the McKinney and Simon, Hoffman, and Kahn scales. This scale is commonly referenced by insurance companies in guiding coverage for treatment in the United States [9].

- Grade I: Small breast enlargement with localized button of tissue that is concentrated around the areola.
- Grade II: Moderate breast enlargement exceeding areola boundaries with edges that are indistinct from the chest.
- Grade III: Moderate breast enlargement exceeding areola boundaries with edges that are distinct from the chest with skin redundancy present.
- Grade IV: Marked breast enlargement with skin redundancy and feminization of the breast.

Rohrich et al.

- Another classification system was put forth by Rohrich et al. [4], which describes a classification system as well as guidance for treatment including the utility of ultrasound-assisted liposuction (Table 31.1):

Table 31.1 Gynecomastia classification

Classification	Treatment
Grade I—Minimal hypertrophy (<250 g of breast tissue) without ptosis IA. Primarily glandular IB. Primarily fibrous	IA. Ultrasound-assisted liposuction or suction-assisted lipectomy IB. Ultrasound-assisted liposuction
Grade II—Moderate hypertrophy (250–500 g of breast tissue) without ptosis IIA. Primarily glandular IIB. Primarily fibrous	IIA. Ultrasound-assisted liposuction or suction-assisted lipectomy IIB. Ultrasound-assisted liposuction
Grade III—Severe hypertrophy (>500 g of breast tissue) with grade I ptosis—Glandular or fibrous	III. Ultrasound-assisted liposuction with or without staged excision
Grade IV—Severe hypertrophy with grade II or III ptosis: glandular or fibrous	IV. Ultrasound-assisted liposuction with or without staged excision

Adapted from Rohrich et al. [4]

Treatment

Nonsurgical

- Nonsurgical treatment typically involves withdrawal of the offending agent or treatment of the underlying cause. However, in patients with a lengthy duration of gynecomastia, the gynecomastia may persist despite treatment of the underlying etiology [4, 7].
- Treatments can include anti-estrogens, selective estrogen blockers, synthetic testosterone, and aromatase inhibitors, as well as radiation, although efficacy is variable and side effects must be considered [1].

Surgical

- Suction-assisted lipectomy or ultrasound-assisted liposuction may be used alone or as an adjunct to surgical excision.
- Surgical excision usually involves a periareolar incision, leaving a 1–1.5 cm thick cuff of tissue deep to the nipple-areolar complex to prevent depression of the nipple postoperatively. The fibrous or glandular subareolar tissue is then excised, and any skin redundancy may be addressed at the time of initial surgery or after a period of delay to allow for maximal skin retraction [4, 7, 10].
- If significant excess skin requires excision, then elliptical excision with grafting of the nipple may be required. This is typically avoided, if possible, given greater scarring.
- Due to increased risk of breast cancer in patients with Klinefelter syndrome, en bloc excision is recommended in this population and the tissue should be sent for pathological analysis [4].
- Hematoma is the most common early complication, while under-resection of tissue is the most common long-term complication of surgery [7].

Financial Disclosure Statement None.

References

1. Ladizinski B, Lee KC, Nutan FN, Higgins HW 2nd, Federman DG. Gynecomastia: etiologies, clinical presentations, diagnosis, and management. South Med J. 2014;107(1):44–9.
2. Bembo SA, Carlson HE. Gynecomastia: its features, and when and how to treat it. Cleve Clin J Med. 2004;71(6):511–7.
3. Braunstein GD. Clinical practice. Gynecomastia. N Engl J Med. 2007;357(12):1229–37.
4. Rohrich RJ, Ha RY, Kenkel JM, Adams WP Jr. Classification and management of gynecomastia: defining the role of ultrasound-assisted liposuction. Plast Reconstr Surg. 2003;111(2):909–23; discussion 24–5.
5. Jackson AW, Muldal S, Ockey CH, O'Connor PJ. Carcinoma of male breast in association with the Klinefelter syndrome. Br Med J. 1965;1(5429):223–5.
6. Korenman SG. The endocrinology of the abnormal male breast. Ann N Y Acad Sci. 1986;464:400–8.
7. Karp NS. Gynecomastia. In: Thorne CH, Chung KC, Gosain AK, Gurtner GC, Mehrara BJ, Rubin JP, et al., editors. Grabb and Smith's plastic surgery. Seventh ed. Philadelphia: Lippencott Williams & Wilkins; 2014.
8. Simon BE, Hoffman S, Kahn S. Classification and surgical correction of gynecomastia. Plast Reconstr Surg. 1973;51(1):48–52.
9. Surgeons ASoP. ASPS recommended insurance coverage criteria for third-party payers: gynecomastia. American Society of Plastic Surgeons; 2004. Available from: https://www.plasticsurgery.org/documents/members-only/health-policy/archives/practice-parameter-2004-gynecomastia.pdf?downloadId=20dddbfb-4867-4f09-b488-1d2720a53af6.
10. Hammond DC. Surgical correction of gynecomastia. Plast Reconstr Surg. 2009;124(1 Suppl):61e–8e.

Chapter 32
Breast Reduction

Katherine J. Choi

Pathophysiology [1]

- Most patients have normal estrogen levels and receptors, suggesting that there is an excessive growth response to an unknown stimulus.
- Fibrous and fatty growth > glandular tissue growth.

Symptoms

- Back and neck pain, headaches.
- Shoulder grooving from bra strap.
- Intertrigo and skin maceration.
- Inability to find well-fitting clothing and undergarments.
- Difficulty exercising.
- Symptoms are more important than breast volume and size in predicting health/quality of life benefits after reduction surgery [2].

Preoperative Workup

- Discuss motivations for seeking reduction mammaplasty
- Focal breast examination

K. J. Choi (✉)
Division of Plastic Surgery, Department of Surgery, University of California, Los Angeles, Los Angeles, CA, USA
e-mail: kjchoi@mednet.ucla.edu

- Family history of breast cancer
- Mammography for ages 40 years and above
- Schnur Sliding Scale [3]
    - Uses patient height and weight to determine amount of resection required to have insurance coverage for procedure (Table 32.1)

Resection Options

- Liposuction
    - Can be used alone or with excisional techniques
    - Benefits
        - Smaller scars
        - Nipple areolar complex (NAC) and lactation ability preserved
    - Limitations
        - Does not address ptosis or skin excess
        - Difficulty removing dense glandular tissue
- Inferior Pedicle
    - Internal mammary and intercostal perforators
    - Benefits
        - Most patients preserve lactation ability
        - Safe for large resections
    - Limitations
        - Squares breast borders
        - May predispose for late pseudoptosis
- Central Mound [4]
    - Benefits

Table 32.1 Schnur scale

Body surface area (m²)	Grams to remove
1.4	218
1.5	260
1.6	310
1.7	370
1.8	441
1.9	527
2.0	628

- Modification of inferior pedicle—same vascular supply
- Relies on glandular (not dermal) blood supply, safe for re-reductions, especially if previous pedicle unknown
- Can precisely establish base width
  - Limitations
    - More extensive dissection required between subcutaneous tissue and breast capsule
- Superomedial Pedicle [5]
  - First to fourth internal mammary artery (second internal mammary is dominant)
  - Benefits
    - Safe for large volume (up to 2000 g) resections
    - Inferior tissue excision addresses ptosis
  - Limitations
    - May not be appropriate in re-reduction patients with unknown original pedicle
- Lateral Pedicle
  - Lateral thoracic artery
  - Benefits
    - Maintains continuity of Wuringer's septum, resulting in improved NAC sensation preservation
  - Limitations
    - Limited resection in the axilla and ability to address lateral fullness

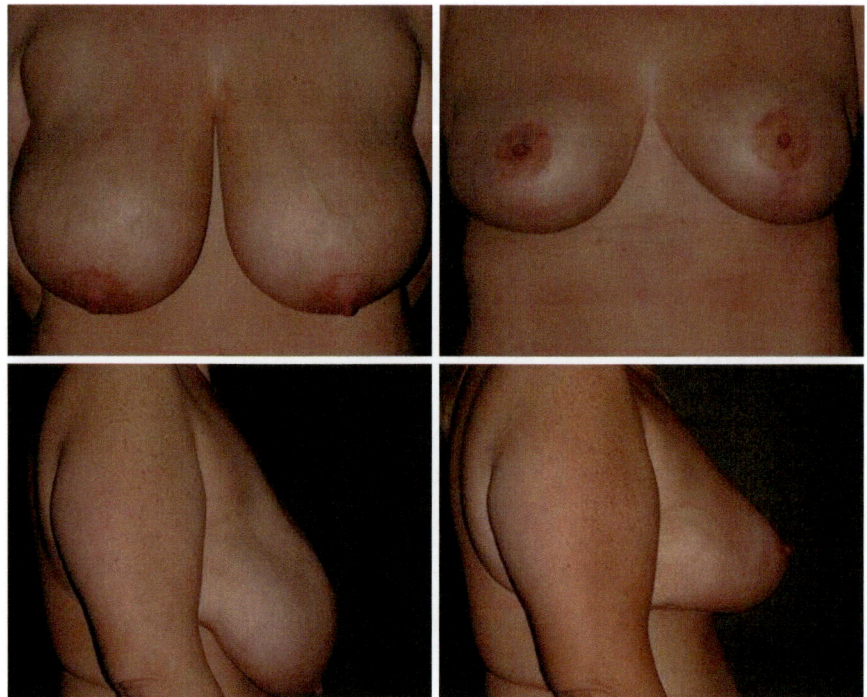

Fig. 32.1 Pre- and post-breast reduction with Wise pattern

Skin Resection Patterns

- Inverted T/Wise Pattern (Fig. 32.1)
  - Removes large areas of skin both vertically and horizontally
- Vertical
  - Relies on parenchyma to shape skin
  - Needs healthy skin
  - Higher incidence of dog ear revisions
- Circumareolar
  - Tends to widen NAC
  - Not recommended for ptotic breasts or large volume resections

Free Nipple Grafting

- For impaired blood flow to NAC due to length of pedicle in massive reductions, or systemic illnesses or previous radiation
- Disadvantages
    - Hypopigmentation
    - Loss of sensation and lactation
    - Loss of nipple projection

Post-Operative Care

- Front closing soft bra for 6–8 weeks.
    - Limit heavy lifting and upper body exercise to prevent wound breakdown and scar widening
- Bulb suction drains are commonly used.
- Complications are typically related to the amount of resection volume.
- Most patients maintain the ability to breastfeed and nipple sensation unless a free nipple graft is used.

Sources

1. Jabs AD. Mammary hypertrophy is not associated with increased estrogen receptors. Plast Reconstr Surg. 1990;86:64–6.
2. Miller AP, Zacher JB, Berggren RB, et al. Breast reduction for symptomatic macromastia: can objective predictors for operative success be identified? Plast Reconstr Surg. 1995;95:77–83.
3. Schnur PL, Hoehn JG, Ilstrup DM, et al. Reduction mammaplasty: cosmetic or reconstructive procedure? Ann Plast Surg. 1991;27(3):232–7.
4. DeLong MR, Chang I, Farajzadeh M, et al. The central mound pedicle: a safe and effective technique for reduction mammaplasty. Plast Reconstr Surg. 2020;146(4):725–33.
5. Nahai F, editor. The art of aesthetic surgery. 2nd ed. St Louis: Quality Medical Publishing; 2011.

Chapter 33
Breast Implants, Augmentation, and Mastopexy

Michael W. Wells and Irene A. Chang

Anatomy

- Vasculature: Branches of thoracoacromial artery, thoracodorsal artery, internal mammary artery, lateral thoracic artery, and intercostal perforators
- Innervation: Branches of third–sixth intercostal nerves and cervical plexus C3 and C4
- Musculature: Pectoralis major, pectoralis minor, serratus anterior, rectus abdominis, and external oblique
- Lymphatic drainage
  - Level 1 (lateral to pectoralis minor), Level 2 (posterior to pectoralis minor and inferior to axillary vein), Level 3 (medial to pectoralis minor), Rotter's nodes (between pectoralis major and minor)
- Structure
  - Lobules (functional unit of breast composed of acini).
  - Lactiferous duct forms sinuses that drain to the nipple.
  - Fat provides the majority of the shape and content of the breast.
  - Cooper's Ligaments.

Augmentation

Indications

- Reconstruction after mastectomy
- Developmental impairment
- Cosmetic enhancement
- One of the most commonly performed aesthetic surgery procedures in the United States at 300,000 augmentations a year

Contraindications

- Body dysmorphic disorder
- Medical comorbidities producing high anesthetic risk or poor wound healing
- Active smoking

Implants

- Two main categories of implants, based on what the implant is made of:
    - Saline implants: silicone shell filled with saline
    - Silicone implants: silicone shell with viscous silicone gel
- Saline versus silicone
    - Saline is able to adjust to body temperature faster than silicone.
    - Saline is more safely absorbed by the body and has less risk of inflammation.
    - Saline leaks are more easily detected.
    - Silicone has a more natural feel than saline.
    - Saline often feels heavier and ripples more.
    - Silicone implants for augmentation are indicated only for patients 22 and older.
    - BII: breast implant illness.
        - Poorly understood rheumatologic symptoms occurring in patients with breast implants.
        - FDA has included language about BII in the black box warning (Table 33.1).
- Implants can also be described as smooth versus textured based on the feel of the shell of the implant.
    - Textured implants are favored by some surgeons, and texturing is required for anatomic implants to prevent malrotation.

Table 33.1 Comparison of saline and silicone-filled implants [1]

Saline	Silicone
Harder, less natural	Soft, gummy
More rippling	Less rippling
Heavier	Lighter
No need for imaging	Routine ultrasound recommended
Easy to detect leak	Hard to detect leak

- Textured implants have been associated with a risk of breast implant-associated anaplastic large cell lymphoma (BIA-ALCL).
  - Thought that texturing process causes inflammation in the breast pocket resulting in development of a lymphoma.
  - Diagnosed via a late seroma with CD30+ and ALK- on flow cytometry.
  - Management is typically removal of the implant +/− chemotherapy.
  - High-risk brand, BioCell, textured devices were recalled in 2019.
- Implants also categorized by shape.
  - Anatomic has a shape to it to match a breast, typically textured.
    - Gives a teardrop shape to the implant so the breast mound is better defined.
  - Round assumes teardrop when standing, round when lying down.
    - Most common.
    - Various profiles give more projection/volume per width.

Incisions

- Typically chosen to optimize implant placement and aesthetic appearance while minimizing scar visualization
- Inframammary fold (IMF)
  - Most common site of incision.
  - IMF location is often lateral to the nipple to decrease visibility.
  - Believed to minimize contact with breast ducts, decreasing risk of infection/inflammation leading to capsular contracture.
- Periareolar
  - Incision at the lower half of the areola with stair-step dissection.
  - Well-hidden scar and no decreased nipple sensation.
  - Scar visibility and size may change with time (i.e., pigmentation).
- Transaxillary
  - Incision located away from the breast at the highest point of the axilla

- Undetectable with arms down
- Silicone implants are harder to insert (typically only an option for saline implants, which are inserted deflated)
- Can be associated with malposition requiring a secondary procedure
- Transumbilical
    - Only with saline, blind dissection w/o control of implant position
    - Not frequently used

Plane of Implant Insertion

- Subglandular Plane
    - Anterior to pectoralis muscle
    - Prevents distortion of the muscle and maintains good shape
    - Associated with a higher capsular contracture rate, obtrusive implant
- Subpectoral Plane
    - Posterior to pectoralis major but anterior to pectoralis minor
    - Lower contracture rates with intact nipple sensation
    - Associated with animation deformity and displacement of implant over time
- Dual Plane
    - Subpectoral with release of pectoralis inferiorly
    - Level of pectoralis separation from breast parenchyma (subpectoral dissection, to level of inferior NAC, or level of superior NAC) depends on degree of ptosis (i.e., more release for more ptotic breasts).

Postoperative Management

- Surgical bra with early mobilization.
- Avoid submersion in water.
- Monitor for complications.

Complications

- Capsular contracture (2.8–20.4%) [2]
    - Potentially due to biofilm formation from contamination of the implant. Involves myofibroblasts

- Management and prevention are a controversial topic.
- Baker grading:
  - Grade 1: soft capsule
  - Grade 2: palpable capsule
  - Grade 3: visible deformity from the capsule
  - Grade 4: painful capsule

- Implant rupture
  - Increased risk over time.
  - Saline is typically detectable from absorption of saline; silicone can often be "silent," so recommended screening is ultrasound at 5 years and then every 2–3 years after.
- BIA-ALCL [3]
- Nipple and breast loss of sensation/pain
- Hematoma
- Seroma
- Infection
- Asymmetry
- Malposition
  - Double bubble—implant positioned too high or low
- Screening for breast cancer is more difficult with implants but follows the normal protocol.

Mastopexy

Indications

- Goal is to improve breast shape without changing volume, typically for ptosis.
- Insufficient skin retraction and support in the context of volume loss.
- Ptosis by Regnault classification: grading scheme based on location of nipple-areolar complex relative to inframammary fold.
  - Grade I is for NAC at the level of the IMF.
  - Grade II is 1–3 cm below IMF.
  - Grade III is NAC located at the most inferior portion of the breast [4].

Approaches

- Periareolar or Circumareolar Technique

- Incisions made and closed around the areola, camouflaging scar
- Used for patients with mild ptosis with reasonable skin quality and glandular parenchyma
- Simple de-epithelialization: removal and repositioning of fascia and nipple without changes to parenchyma
- Benelli technique: repositioning of parenchyma in cone-like formation for larger-degree ptosis
- Potential drawbacks: flattened breast, skin pleating, areolar widening

- Vertical Technique
  - Incision inferiorly from the inferior border of the areola, followed by resection of skin, fat, and gland, liposuction, and/or undermining of the nipple
  - Any degree of ptosis
  - Drawback: upper pole fullness, inferior skin redundancy

- Inverted T-Scar Technique
  - W-shaped (wise-pattern) incision with parenchymal resection with inferior parenchymal support for breast tissue [5]
  - Useful for patients with poor skin quality, fatty parenchyma, and severe ptosis
  - Disadvantage: larger scar

- Combined Augmentation Mastopexy
  - Higher risk procedure for the devascularization of tissues
  - Can have higher revision rates than staged procedures
  - For grade I ptosis, augmentation alone may be sufficient by increasing volume in same skin envelope and producing tightening effect

Mastopexy Complications

- Hematoma
- Infection
- Asymmetry
- Scarring
- Recurrent ptosis
- Nipple perfusion or sensation issues
- Wound breakdown

References

1. Coombs DM, Grover R, Prassinos A, Gurunluoglu R. Breast augmentation surgery: clinical considerations. Cleve Clin J Med. 2019;86(2):111–22. https://doi.org/10.3949/ccjm.86a.18017.

2. Headon H, Kasem A, Mokbel K. Capsular contracture after breast augmentation: an update for clinical practice. Arch Plast Surg. 2015;42(5):532–43. https://doi.org/10.5999/aps.2015.42.5.532.
3. Nelson JA, McCarthy C, Dabic S, et al. BIA-ALCL and textured breast implants: a systematic review of evidence supporting surgical risk management strategies. Plast Reconstr Surg. 2021;147(5s):7s–13s. https://doi.org/10.1097/prs.0000000000008040.
4. Regnault P. Breast ptosis. Definition and treatment. Clin Plast Surg. 1976;3(2):193–203.
5. Wong C, Vucovich M, Rohrich R. Mastopexy and reduction mammoplasty pedicles and skin resection patterns. Plast Reconstr Surg Glob Open. 2014;2(8):e202. https://doi.org/10.1097/gox.0000000000000125.

Chapter 34
Prosthetic-Based Breast Reconstruction

Harsh Patel

Introduction

Breast reconstruction via the use of prosthetic devices is one of the most common surgical procedures done by plastic surgeons today. The goal of the procedure is to recreate the silhouette and shape of the breast tissue that was removed. Since its advent, breast prosthetics have come a long way in design, shape, and fill, with surgical techniques keeping pace to provide improved reconstructive outcomes [1–3].

Anatomy

(a) Key landmarks of breast tissue:
- (i) Lateral border: latissimus dorsi muscle (axilla)
- (ii) Inferior border: inframammary ridge
- (iii) Superior border: second rib inferior to clavicle
- (iv) Medial border: sternum
- (v) Deep border: pectoralis muscle and serratus anterior (inferolaterally)

(b) Blood supply to breast tissue: thoracoacromial artery, internal mammary perforators, lateral thoracic artery, thoracodorsal artery, terminal branches of intercostal perforators
- (i) Blood supply to breast skin: subdermal plexus

H. Patel (✉)
UCLA Division of Plastic Surgery, Los Angeles, CA, USA
e-mail: harshpatel@mednet.ucla.edu

© The Author(s), under exclusive license to Springer Nature Switzerland AG 2025
J. Roostaeian et al. (eds.), *Plastic Surgery Clerkship*, Contemporary Surgical Clerkships, https://doi.org/10.1007/978-3-031-99098-4_34

(c) Prepectoral versus subpectoral refers to where the prosthetic is placed in relation to the pectoralis muscle

History and Physical

(a) Cancer and breast history

  (i) Aggressive, inflammatory cancers may not be able to tolerate reconstruction. Typically wait up to a year before reconstructing after mastectomy for inflammatory cancer.
  (ii) Need for radiation complicates plans.
  (iii) Need for prophylactic mastectomy.

(b) Medical history

  (i) Risk factors for surgery include BMI and smoking diabetes.

(c) Examination pearls

  (i) Other incisions on the breast
  (ii) Nipple retraction, ulceration, and discharge
  (iii) Degree of ptosis

Decisions on Reconstruction

(a) Timing

  (i) Can be immediate (day of mastectomy)
  (ii) Can be delayed (after treatment is complete), history of radiation limits options

(b) Type of reconstruction

  (i) Autologous (discussed separately)
  (ii) Alloplastic
  (iii) Defer to patient goals as primary, but also need to take into consideration reconstructive needs

    1. Radiated tissue needs adjunctive tissue

Options for Alloplastic Materials

(a) Breast implant versus expander [4]

(i) Breast implants are available as silicone-filled or saline-filled.
(ii) Breast tissue expanders are temporary devices that can progressively be filled with air or liquid to slowly expand tissue and create space for a permanent implant. Expanders have tabs that allow precise positioning of the device without use of mesh products.
(iii) Selected based on desired fill substance, fill volume, projection, and base width (measurement from cleavage area to the lateral aspect of the breast).

(b) Acellular dermal matrix [5]

(i) Form of surgical mesh developed from human or animal skin that is devoid of cells but contains the structural support elements.
(ii) Approved for use for hernia surgeries, but used off-label for breast reconstruction.
(iii) Used by some surgeons to create a pocket for an expander or implant or sling to place the prosthesis.
(iv) Alternatives include other surgical meshes such as Vicryl mesh.
(v) Benefit Unclear.

Methodology for Alloplastic Reconstruction

(a) Single-stage

- Also known as direct to implant (DTI).
- Permanent implants can be placed at the time of mastectomy in a subset of patients with appropriate mastectomy flaps and other surgeon-dependent factors.
- Good for small volume, nonptotic breasts with thick mastectomy flaps (often prophylactic). Nipple sparing mastectomy patients are better candidates for DTI.

(b) Two-stage

(i) Breast tissue expander is placed to hold the space and safely expand the tissue that will encompass the final implant.
(ii) Usually slowly filled with air or fluid percutaneously in a clinic in a progressive manner over the course of multiple weeks to achieve the desired size.
(iii) To expand, the needle is placed into the expansion port, and filling material is injected; the port is magnetic or RFID and identified with a manufacturer-provided device.
(iv) Allows patient to have a representation of what their final reconstruction size would look like, while allowing for modifications on the volume without requiring a trial of various implant sizes.
(v) Requires second procedure to remove the expander and replace with implant or autologous tissue (see autologous reconstruction chapter) [6–8].

(vi) Often, tissue expanders are placed in the pocket if radiation is anticipated to allow for maintenance of the breast pocket until final cancer treatment and reconstruction.

(c) Planes of reconstruction

  (i) Alloplastic material can be placed as prepectoral or subpectoral

    1. Prepectoral: ideal for patients with thicker flaps, with less risk of implant exposure, cosmetically equivalent, with less pain and animation deformity
    2. Subpectoral: ideal for patients with thinner flaps, more painful with increased dissection and risk of animation deformity

Nipple Reconstruction

(a) In certain patients, the nipple-areolar complex is removed for oncologic reasons.
(b) Reconstruction can be skin flap-based using tissue rearrangement with or without tattoo that allows for recreation of pigmented appearance.
(c) 3-D tattooing can also be done to give the appearance of projection without requiring surgical reconstruction (Fig. 34.1).

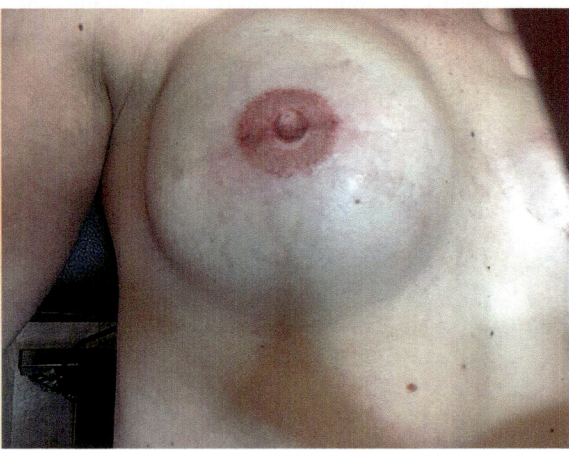

Fig. 34.1 Nipple reconstruction with skate technique and tattooing

Considerations

(a) A multitude of factors determine whether or not a patient is a candidate for prosthetic-based breast reconstruction, the primary of which are patient goals and anatomy.
(b) Other factors include, but are not limited to, surgeon-dependent, neoadjuvant and/or adjuvant therapy needs, previous surgical history (i.e., previous augmentation), and candidacy for autologous reconstruction.
(c) Radiated patients cannot undergo tissue expansion and have higher rates of all complications.
(d) Patients undergoing staged reconstruction usually will need to come multiple times for serial expansions.

Complications [9–11]

(a) Range from minor (i.e., seroma) to major (i.e., extrusion of prosthetic device)
(b) Capsular contracture—formation of scar tissue around the prosthesis that is firm, and can lead to prosthetic malposition, tightness, and pain
(c) Animation deformity—movement of the prosthetic device with movement of the pectoral musculature seen in submuscular reconstruction primarily (d) implant infection is much more common in reconstructive patients (compared to cosmetic augmentation) due to thin tissue coverage, comorbidities, and chemotherapy/radiation. Can range in severity from requiring only oral antibiotics to removal and debridement.

Anaplastic Large Cell Lymphoma (ALCL) [12–15]—A Rare, Slow-Growing T-Cell Lymphoma That Is Associated with Textured Devices

(a) Typically, seen in the peri-prosthetic fluid, with treatment usually being explantation of the device with a complete capsulectomy.
(b) Some patients require chemotherapy or immunotherapy.
(c) Associated with textured implants.

Alternatives

(a) Ultimately, alternatives offered are dependent on patient goals and health, anatomy, and the surgeon's skill set.

(b) Some patients prefer no reconstruction, in which case the mastectomy flaps are closed primarily.
(c) Other commonly used options include autologous tissue breast reconstruction and fat augmentation, to name a few.

References

1. Cemal Y, Albornoz CR, Disa JJ, McCarthy CM, Mehrara BJ, Pusic AL, Cordeiro PG, Matros E. A paradigm shift in U.S. breast reconstruction: part 2. The influence of changing mastectomy patterns on reconstructive rate and method. Plast Reconstr Surg. 2013;131(3):320e–6e.
2. Albornoz CR, Bach PB, Mehrara BJ, Disa JJ, Pusic AL, McCarthy CM, Cordeiro PG, Matros E. A paradigm shift in U.S. breast reconstruction: increasing implant rates. Plast Reconstr Surg. 2013;131(1):15–23.
3. Hernandez-Boussard T, Zeidler K, Barzin A, Lee G, Curtin C. Breast reconstruction national trends and healthcare implications. Breast J. 2013;19(5):463–9.
4. Momeni A, Li AY, Tsai J, Wan D, Karin MR, Wapnir IL. The impact of device innovation on clinical outcomes in expander-based breast reconstruction. Plast Reconstr Surg Glob Open. 2019;7(12):e2524.
5. Sbitany H, Serletti JM. Acellular dermis-assisted prosthetic breast reconstruction: a systematic and critical review of efficacy and associated morbidity. Plast Reconstr Surg. 2011;128(6):1162–9.
6. Momeni A, Kanchwala SK. Improved pocket control in immediate microsurgical breast reconstruction with simultaneous implant placement through the use of mesh. Microsurgery. 2018;38(5):450–7.
7. Momeni A, Kanchwala S. Hybrid prepectoral breast reconstruction: a surgical approach that combines the benefits of autologous and implant-based reconstruction. Plast Reconstr Surg. 2018;142(5):1109–15.
8. Kanchwala S, Momeni A. Hybrid breast reconstruction-the best of both worlds. Gland Surg. 2019;8(1):82–9.
9. Suga H, Shiraishi T, Tsuji N, Takushima A. Risk factors for complications in expander-based breast reconstruction: multivariate analysis in Asian patients. Plast Reconstr Surg Glob Open. 2017;5(11):e1563.
10. Suga H, Shiraishi T, Shibasaki Y, Takushima A, Harii K. Predictive factors for drainage volume after expander-based breast reconstruction. Plast Reconstr Surg Glob Open. 2016;4(6):e727.
11. Xue DQ, Qian C, Yang L, Wang XF. Risk factors for surgical site infections after breast surgery: a systematic review and meta-analysis. Eur J Surg Oncol. 2012;38(5):375–81.
12. Mempin M, Hu H, Chowdhury D, Deva A, Vickery K. The A, B and C's of silicone breast implants: anaplastic large cell lymphoma, biofilm and capsular contracture. Materials (Basel). 2018;11(12):2393.
13. de Boer M, van Leeuwen FE, Hauptmann M, Overbeek LIH, de Boer JP, Hijmering NJ, Sernee A, Klazen CAH, Lobbes MBI, van der Hulst R, et al. Breast implants and the risk of anaplastic large-cell lymphoma in the breast. JAMA Oncol. 2018;4(3):335–41.
14. Cordeiro PG, Ghione P, Ni A, Hu Q, Ganesan N, Galasso N, Dogan A, Horwitz SM. Risk of breast implant associated anaplastic large cell lymphoma (BIA-ALCL) in a cohort of 3546 women prospectively followed long term after reconstruction with textured breast implants. J Plast Reconstr Aesthet Surg. 2020;73(5):841–6.
15. Clemens MW, Nava MB, Rocco N, Miranda RN. Understanding rare adverse sequelae of breast implants: anaplastic large-cell lymphoma, late seromas, and double capsules. Gland Surg. 2017;6(2):169–84.

Chapter 35
Autologous Breast Reconstruction

Corbin Muetterties

Introduction

- The lifetime incidence of breast cancer is approximately 1 in 8 for American women [1].
- Autologous breast reconstruction involves reconstruction of the breast using a patient's own tissue following mastectomy.
- Tissue flaps are elevated as either pedicled or free flaps and used to reconstruct the breast mound and replace skin deficiencies.
- The type of flap utilized is dependent on numerous factors, including the patient's body habitus, available donor tissue, and patient preference.

Benefits of Autologous Breast Reconstruction

- Allows reconstruction of the breast using a patient's own tissue.
- Natural appearance and feel of the reconstructed breast.
- Autologous reconstructions have long durability and less need for long-term surgical interventions than implant-based reconstructions.
- Allows avoidance of implant-related complications including capsular contracture, periprosthetic infections, and implant rupture.
- Avoids the need for implant monitoring.
- Allows for restoration of healthy skin and subcutaneous tissue in radiated tissue beds.

C. Muetterties (✉)
UCLA Medical Center, Los Angeles, CA, USA
e-mail: cmuetterties@mednet.ucla.edu

© The Author(s), under exclusive license to Springer Nature Switzerland AG 2025
J. Roostaeian et al. (eds.), *Plastic Surgery Clerkship*, Contemporary Surgical Clerkships, https://doi.org/10.1007/978-3-031-99098-4_35

- Numerous studies have demonstrated superior patient-reported outcomes with autologous breast reconstruction when compared to prosthetic reconstructive techniques [2–4].

Disadvantages of Autologous Breast Reconstruction

- Risk of flap loss or flap-related complications
- Donor site morbidity including risks of poor scarring, contour irregularities, seroma, wound dehiscence, and need for revisional procedures
- Breast size limited by amount of available donor tissue

Timing of Reconstruction

- Immediate reconstruction (at time of mastectomy)
    - Indicated for early-stage disease and patients with low risk for requiring post-op radiation therapy
    - Allows for greater preservation of mastectomy skin flaps (minimize size of skin paddle) at the time of reconstruction
- Delayed reconstruction (after cancer treatment is completed)
    - Indicated for advanced-stage disease or patients with high BMI or other factors precluding immediate reconstruction.
    - Autologous recon is commonly used to salvage complications related to implant-based reconstructions or sequelae of radiation therapy.
    - Typically should be completed 6 months after cessation of radiation therapy and 1 year in patients with advanced or inflammatory breast cancer [1].

History and Physical Exam

- Medical history
    - Hypertension, diabetes, pulmonary comorbidities, obesity
    - Current medications, including use of hormonal therapy (increases risk of thrombosis)
- Oncologic history
    - Neoadjuvant chemotherapy
    - Prior or planned radiation therapy
    - Tumor diagnosis, location, size

- Past surgical history, with close attention paid to surgical interventions which may affect donor flap or tissues, in particular:
  - Prior breast surgeries
  - Abdominal surgeries (including liposuction)
  - Prior axillary lymph node dissections
  - Coronary artery bypass grafting (CABG)
    The internal mammary vessels are commonly used as recipient vessels.
- Physical exam
  - Close attention should be paid to all prior scars, especially those which may affect the donor pedicle, perforators, or mastectomy skin flaps.
  - Breast width, volume, degree of nipple ptosis.
  - Skin laxity, stretch marks, skin thickness.
- Social history
  - Active smoking is a contraindication to most autologous breast reconstructions.
- Imaging
  - In the absence of concerning surgical scars, routine imaging is not required but may be obtained depending on the surgeon's preference.
  - Studies have demonstrated improved operative efficiency and lower surgical times with the use of preoperative computed tomographic angiography for perforator mapping [5].

Latissimus Dorsi Flap

- *Flap pedicle: thoracodorsal artery and vein.*
- The latissimus dorsi flap is most commonly used as a pedicled flap for salvage of failed implant-based reconstructions or patients with complications related to radiation therapy.
- The latissimus dorsi flap allows for transfer of a broad, well-vascularized muscle flap as well as an overlying skin paddle which can be used to replace irradiated breast skin.
- Due to the limited subcutaneous tissue and size of the flap, most commonly this flap is utilized with a tissue expander or small implant as a hybrid reconstruction in order to achieve adequate breast volume.
- Variations of the latissimus have been described, including perforator-based, muscle-sparing flaps (thoracodorsal artery perforator flap), and muscle-sparing latissimus flap (harvested on transverse or longitudinal branch of thoracodorsal artery).

- Most common complications of this flap include donor site complications, including poor scarring of the donor site, seroma, and wound dehiscence.
- Additionally, given this flap is most commonly used with an accompanying implant, patients additionally have the associated risks of implant-related complications.

Pedicled TRAM Flap

- Flap pedicle: superior epigastric artery/vein (continuation of internal mammary vessels).
- The transverse rectus abdominis myocutaneous flap (TRAM) is most commonly used as a pedicled flap for breast reconstruction.
- Prior to the development of modern perforator flap techniques, TRAM flaps were the workhorse flap for autologous breast reconstruction.
- However, with the advent of perforator flap techniques, these flaps are less frequently utilized due to the donor site morbidity associated with harvest of the entire rectus abdominis muscle and the smaller size of the superior epigastric vessels compared to the inferior vessels

    Higher chance of partial flap ischemia and fat necrosis with pedicled superior vessels

- This flap allows harvesting of the lower abdominal tissue and transfer of a large volume of skin, subcutaneous tissue, and muscle to reconstruct the breast. (Fig. 35.1)
- Unilateral or bilateral reconstructions can be performed using this flap, and flaps can be used to reconstruct the ipsilateral or contralateral breast.
- Complications include donor site wound healing complications, seroma, fat necrosis, flap loss (partial or complete), and, most notably, risk for abdominal hernia or bulge.
- Due to the need to harvest a large piece of abdominal fascia with the flap, reconstructions often require mesh reinforcement

Deep Inferior Epigastric Artery Perforator Flap (DIEP) Flap

- Flap pedicle: deep inferior epigastric artery/vein
- Pedicle length 14–18 cm
- Pedicle size: artery 2–4 mm, vein 2–4 mm
- The DIEP is a perforator flap, which has become the workhorse flap for autologous reconstruction in the microsurgery era. (Fig 35.2)

Fig. 35.1 Pedicle TRAM with implant placed beneath

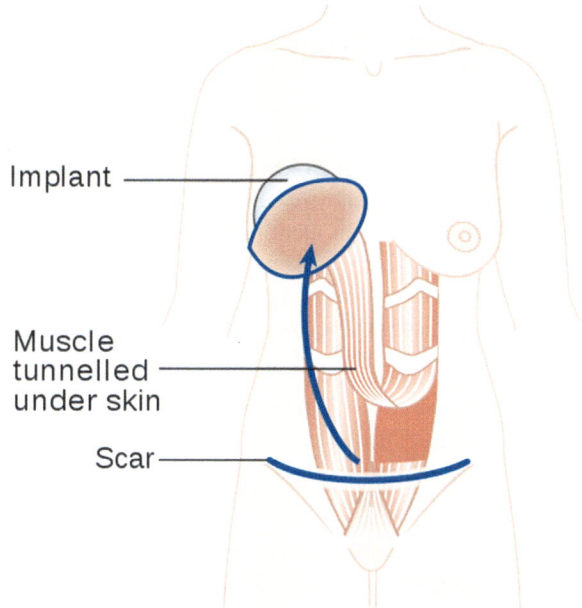

Fig. 35.2 Unilateral right DIEP flap reconstruction, preoperatively (above) and postoperatively (below)

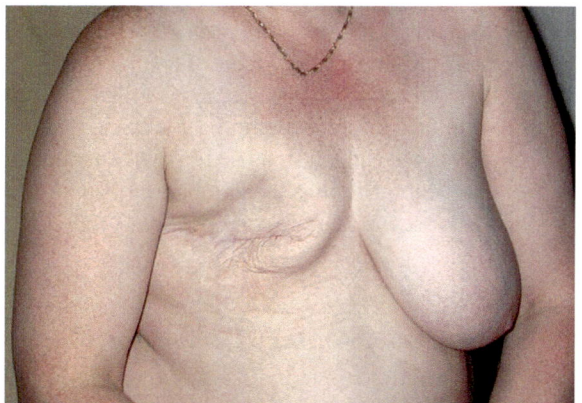

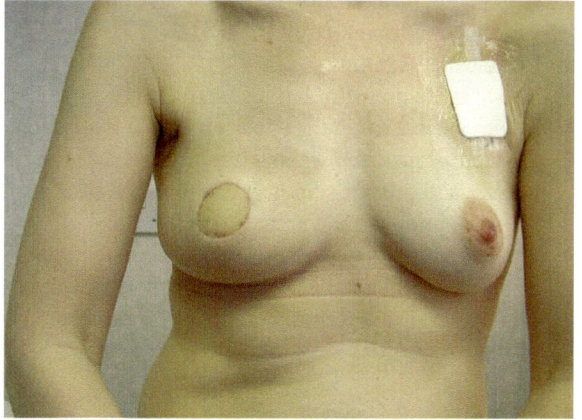

- Comparative studies have demonstrated high patient satisfaction scores for DIEP flaps when compared to latissimus dorsi flaps and implant-based reconstructions [3].
- This flap allows for harvesting of the tissue between the umbilicus and lower abdominal fold and can be utilized for unilateral or bilateral reconstructions.
- Abdominal donor site closure is similar to that of an abdominoplasty and typically well tolerated by patients.
- Flap harvest requires identification of abdominal perforators from the deep inferior epigastric artery system on the abdominal wall and subsequent isolation of the selected perforators by tracing them through the rectus abdominis muscle using microsurgical techniques.
    - Both medial and abdominal row perforators arise from the DIEA system to pierce the abdominal fascia and perfuse the overlying tissue.
    - Typically, DIEP flaps will be harvested on the medial or lateral row system; however, both can be harvested with sacrifice of a small portion of intervening muscle (muscle-sparing TRAM).
- The deep inferior epigastric artery and vein are then harvested in continuity with the isolated perforators by dividing them at their takeoff.
- The flap is then anastomosed to the chest utilizing either the internal mammary (most common) or thoracodorsal vessels as recipient vessels.
- The abdominal fascia is closed primarily, and the upper abdominal flap is elevated and closed similarly to an abdominoplasty.
- In cases where the entire abdomen is utilized to provide additional volume for a unilateral breast reconstruction, a bipedicle flap can be harvested based on both DIEA systems and anastomosed to two separate microvascular anastomoses.
- Common complications include fat necrosis (6%), abdominal seroma (3%), and donor site wound healing complications (10%) [6].

Superior Gluteal Artery Perforator Flap (SGAP)

- Flap pedicle: superficial branch of the superior gluteal artery/vein.
- Pedicle length: 5–8 cm.
- Pedicle size 1.5 mm.
- The SGAP allows for harvesting of excess gluteal adiposity from the upper gluteal crease based on the superior gluteal artery/vein.
- Dissection involves tracing captured perforators through the gluteus maximus muscle and greater sciatic foramen to the takeoff of the superior gluteal vessels from the internal iliac artery.
- Ideal candidates have excess buttock tissue relative to their lower abdomen and/or have an unavailable abdominal donor site due to prior surgery.
- Dissection of the terminal pedicle can prove tedious due to a dense network of friable veins.

- The resultant donor scar is hidden within the upper gluteal crease.
- Disadvantages of the SGAP flap are its increased firmness compared to abdominal tissue and requirement for flap harvest in the prone or lateral decubitus position, which limits efficiency when using a two-team approach.
- Most common complications include donor site seroma (15%) and donor site contour deformity requiring revision (20%) [7].

Lumbar Artery Perforator Flap

- Pedicle: third or fourth lumbar perforators (branch directly off abdominal aorta)
- Pedicle length 5 cm
- Pedicle size: artery 1.5 mm, vein 2 mm
- Flap: captures the hip roll of the lumbar back for use in breast reconstruction
- Advantages: avoids contour deformity of buttocks seen in SGAP flap
- Disadvantages: short pedicle length and small vessel size, requires harvest in the prone position and use of vessel grafts typically

Profunda Artery Perforator Flap

- Pedicle: perforators arising from the profunda femoris artery.
- Pedicle length 10 cm.
- Pedicle size 2 mm.
- Allows for harvest of a transversely or vertically oriented flap from the medial thigh tissue.
- Commonly, this flap is harvested as bilateral flaps, which are stacked to provide additional volume for a single breast as well as provide better symmetry for the thigh donor sites.
- Advantages: well-tolerated donor site.
- Disadvantages: limited donor tissue, often requires bilateral flaps to achieve sufficient volume for unilateral breast reconstruction.

References

1. LoTempio M, Allen R, Blondeel P. Alternative flaps for breast reconstruction. In: Nelligan P, editor. Plastic surgery. 3rd ed. London: Elsevier; 2013. p. 456–71.
2. Kamel G, Mehta K, Nash D, et al. Patient-reported satisfaction and quality of life in obese patients: comparison between microsurgical and prosthetic implant recipients. Plast Reconstr Surg. 2019;144(4):960e–6e.
3. Yueh J, Slavin S, Adesiyun T, et al. Patient satisfaction in post-mastectomy breast reconstruction: a comparative evaluation of DIEP, TRAM, latissimus flap, and implant techniques. Plast Reconstr Surg. 2010;125(6):1585–95.

4. Weichman K, Broer P, Thanik V, et al. Patient-reported satisfaction and quality of life following breast reconstruction in thin patients. Plast Reconstr Surg. 2015;136(2):213–20.
5. Haddock N, Nicholas T, Dumestre D, et al. Efficiency in DIEP flap breast reconstruction: the real benefit of computed tomographic angiography imaging. Plast Reconstr Surg. 2020;146(4):719–23.
6. Gagnon A, Blondeel P. Deep and superficial inferior epigastric artery perforator flaps. In: Wei F, editor. Flaps and reconstructive surgery. London: Elsevier; 2009. p. 501–22.
7. Chang E. Latest advancements in autologous breast reconstruction. Plast Reconstr Surg. 2021;127(1):111e–22e.

Chapter 36
Abdominoplasty and Body Contouring

Alexis L. Boson

Anatomy

Layers of the Abdominal Wall

- 7 layers
  - Skin
  - Subcutaneous fat
  - Scarpa's fascia–contiguous with the superficial fascial system throughout the body. Divides the thicker superficial layer of fat from the less dense deeper layer of fat.
  - Subscarpal fat—thicker and denser than Scarpa's fascia
  - Anterior rectus sheath
  - Muscle
  - Posterior rectus sheath
  - Arcuate line—transition point
    - Above the arcuate line: anterior and posterior rectus sheath
    - Below the arcuate line: anterior rectus sheath

Muscles of the Abdominal Wall

- Rectus abdominis
- External oblique

A. L. Boson (✉)
University of Texas, Medical Branch, Galveston, TX, USA
e-mail: alboson@utmb.edu

- Internal oblique
- Transverse abdominis

Hugger Zones Delineate the Vascular Supply of the Abdomen

- Zone 1—superior and inferior epigastric vessels
- Zone 2—circumflex iliac and external pudendal vessels
- Zone 3—intercostal vessels and external pudendal vessels

Sensory Innervation

- Derived from intercostal nerves T7–12

Umbilicus

- Anatomic location: midline at the level of the iliac crest
- Vascular supply: subdermal plexus, bilateral deep inferior epigastric arteries, ligamentum teres, median umbilical ligament

Evaluation

Patient Selection

- Body contouring.
    - Massive weight loss patients
        - History of gastric bypass or gastric sleeve
        - Will need further nutrition evaluation due to the nature of weight loss surgery
        - Must be weight stable for at least 6 months and 12–18 months from gastric surgery [1, 2]
        - May need to screen for nutritional labs and blood chemistry (iron, sodium, prealbumin) to ensure adequate healing potential
- Cosmetic.
    - Important to screen patients for body dysmorphia

- Patient expectations regarding scar placement, cosmetic outcome, need for possible revision surgeries, complications, and postoperative course should be discussed during the counseling appointment.

History [2, 3]

- Prior abdominal surgeries.
  - Bariatric surgery [4–6]
    - Restrictive procedures
      - Results in decreased caloric intake due to the smaller capacity of the stomach. Food continues to enter the duodenum and gets absorbed.
    - Combination (restrictive and malabsorptive)
      - Malabsorptive—foods bypass the duodenum, thereby decreasing absorption of calories and nutrients.
- Obstetric history—number of previous pregnancies, previous C-sections, or plans for further pregnancies.
  - If patient is planning on future pregnancies, advise the patient to complete childbearing prior to pursuing abdominoplasty in order to avoid recurrent laxity due to abdominal re-expansion.
- Exercise routine.
- History of weight loss or weight gain. If the patient is not weight stable or plans further weight loss, it is imperative to counsel the patient for optimal outcome, they should be stable for several months for the best aesthetic outcome.
  - If an abdominoplasty is performed and the patient continues to lose weight, will have recurrence of skin laxity.
- Known hernias.
- Comorbidities increase the risk of surgery and risk of complications. May require prior medical clearance prior to surgery.
  - Diabetes
  - History of DVT/PE
  - COPD/respiratory conditions. Patients with these conditions have a poor pulmonary baseline, which is further exacerbated by rectus plication, increasing restriction.
- Smoking history. If currently smoking, they should be counseled to discontinue smoking at least 4 weeks prior to surgery to minimize wound healing complications.

- Medications. Determine if the medications below are safe to temporarily discontinue.
  - Use of steroids impairs wound healing and increases the risk of dehiscence.
  - Hormones and blood thinners increase the risk of bleeding
- Unrealistic expectations or external motivators. It is important to discuss expectations during the initial consultation to manage expectations and determine if surgery is appropriate for the patient.

Physical Examination [2, 3]

- Scars
  - Demonstrate prior abdominal surgeries that could have affected the blood supply abdominal wall.
    - Midline scars can be tethered superiorly.
    - Patients with subcostal scars (e.g., Kocher incision for open gallbladder) are most likely to experience complications due to disruptions in the vascular supply of the abdominal wall, specifically Huger zone III.
    - McBurney incisions are not a contraindication to abdominoplasty—these are typically removed with the excised tissue.
- Presence of hernias or rectus diastasis
  - Identify location, size, and reducibility of hernias. Doing so will reduce the likelihood of bowel injury. Large hernias warrant consultation from a general surgeon.
  - Take note of the width of rectus diastasis as this will require rectus plication. Ask the patient to flex the rectus muscles and hold position with legs elevated off bed while palpating to feel the location of the muscles.
- Skin quality
  - Presence of stria indicates an attenuated or absent dermis.
  - Stria above the umbilicus cannot be removed and will become more obvious as the flap is stretched; however, stria present below can be removed. It is important to discuss this with the patient.
- Adiposity
  - It is important to determine if a patient's appearance is due to excess skin, subcutaneous tissue, or intra-abdominal fat.
    - If it is intra-abdominal in nature, the patient should be counseled to lose weight further for an optimal outcome.

- Prominent epigastric fat will not be resolved with abdominoplasty and will lead to poor cosmesis.
  - Assess thickness of subcutaneous fat with pinch test
    - Patient is asked to tense and relax the abdomen while standing with the Examiner pinching the abdomen. If the amount of tissue held in pinch decreases, the patient has significant myofascial laxity, which should be addressed.
  - Diver test
    - Patient is asked to stand upright and flex at the waist. Examiner evaluates Abdominal fullness in both positions. If fullness worsens when flexed, myofascial laxity is present.
- Rashes
  - Many patients with excess skin can experience intertrigo underneath the abdominal pannus.

Necessary Labs

- Body contouring patients. It is important to determine nutritional status in this patient population due to the increased risk of wound breakdown.
  - CBC, CMP, prealbumin, ferritin, iron panel
- Urine or blood nicotine test if a smoker.

Imaging (If Necessary)

- CT A/P if concerned about hernia

Types of Body Contouring

- Belt lipectomy—allows for resection of tissue from the trunk in a circumferential fashion. Can address laxity of buttocks and lateral thighs if a lower body lift is performed in conjunction [11].
- Panniculectomy—similar to abdominoplasty; however, rectus plication and umbilical transposition are not performed. Wedge excision only—used for patients with a protuberant panniculus.

- Abdominoplasty—removal of abdominal wall skin and fat below the umbilicus with rectus plication. Can address excess skin, fat, and myofascial laxity [3].
    - Types
        - Mini [2]
            - Ideal for those with infraumbilical excess skin, fat, and rectus diastasis.
            - Similar to traditional abdominoplasty except incision is smaller (12–16 cm).
            - There is no transposition of the umbilicus.
            - Rectus plication can be performed endoscopically in the supraumbilical region and under direct visualization in the infraumbilical region.
        - Traditional [3]
            - Ideal for excess skin, fat, and rectus diastasis, not limited to the infraumbilical region.
                - Umbilical transposition performed
                - Rectus plication is carried from xiphoid to pubis (Fig. 36.1)

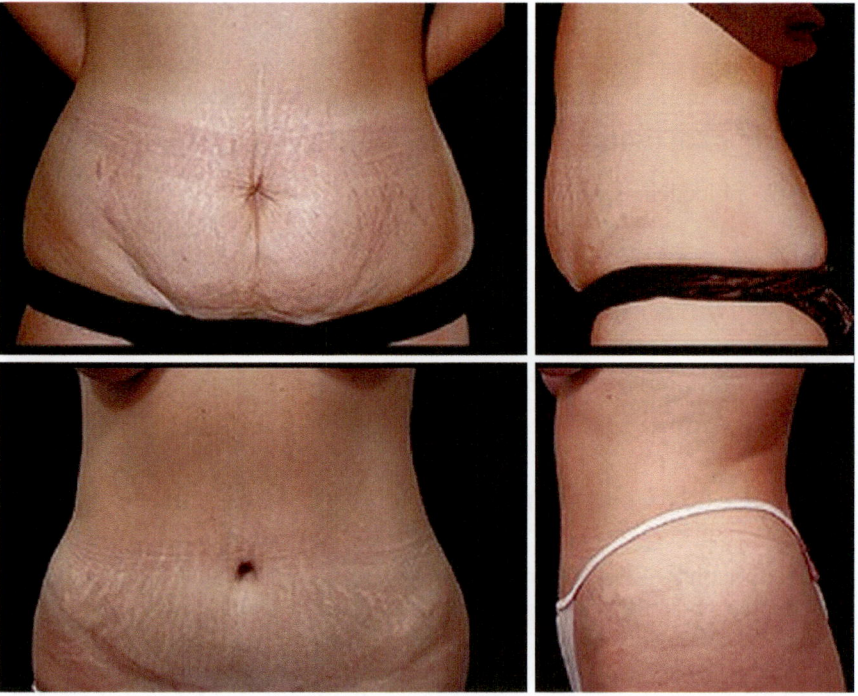

Fig. 36.1 Pre- and post-abdominoplasty

- Fleur-de-Lis (FDL) Abdominoplasty [7, 8]
  - Ideal for those with supraumbilical excess skin and horizontal (wide) component of skin laxity in addition to excess skin, fat, and rectus diastasis.
  - Vertical excision of supraumbilical skin is performed first. It is important to counsel patients regarding increased scars because they will have both a horizontal and vertical scar.

Complications [9, 10]

- DVT/PE. Inherent increased risk due to pulmonary restriction and decreased activity postoperatively.
  - Important to identify patients at increased risk: family history of VTE, personal history, multiple unexplained spontaneous abortions, known coagulopathy, etc.
  - Extended prophylaxis after surgery may be warranted.
- Loss/malposition/necrosis of the umbilicus.
- Can be done in combination with liposuction, typically safe if liposuction done conservatively. Greatest area of risk is supraumbilical (zone I).

Breast [1, 12, 13]

- After significant weight loss, characteristics of the breast are altered in that volume and breast tissue variably change. It is difficult to predict the effects of weight loss on the breast; however, ptosis and nipple medialization are common features.
- For breasts with poor skin envelope and volume loss, mastopexy augmentation is considered.
- For breasts with adequate skin envelope and significant volume loss, consider augmentation.
- Breasts with poor skin envelope and moderate volume loss require mastopexy.
- Breasts with poor skin envelope and no volume loss (i.e., macromastia) consider breast reduction.
- No breast reduction technique is superior to others in this patient population.

Brachioplasty [11, 14, 15]

- Removal of excess skin of the upper arms. Should upper arm fat remain after deflation, liposuction may be performed as a separate procedure prior to lipectomy.
- Contraindications:
  - Lymphedema
  - Neurologic or vascular disorders of the upper extremity
  - Connective tissue disorders
  - Rheumatoid arthritis
- Risk of injury to medial antebrachial cutaneous nerve—leave a small layer of fat over the fascia to minimize the chance of injury.
- Often has a risk of hypertrophic scarring, especially in medial incision (Fig. 36.2).

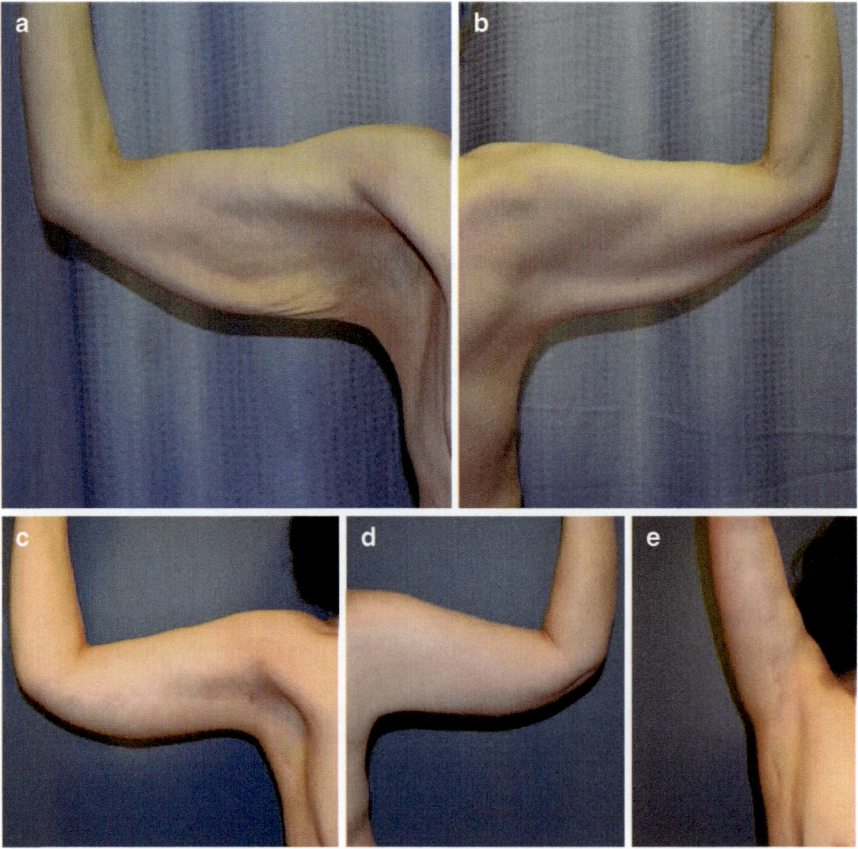

Fig. 36.2 Pre- and post-brachioplasty

Upper Body Lift [16]

- Removes skin and fat from the upper back.
- As the patient deflates, skin behaves as fabric does, draped upon a lamp. There is excess skin laxity in the lateral regions of the torso and descent of the lateral IMF.
- Can combine mastopexy (or gynecomastia in males), brachioplasty, back lift in surgery as appropriate to address patient concerns.

Liposuction—will be discussed in further depth in next chapter. Liposuction alone does not resolve skin laxity.

Thighplasty [1]

- Remove excess skin of thighs.
  - Can do medial and lower body lift however, should be staged due to excess tension if both performed at same time
  - Risk of injury to greater saphenous vein
- Contraindications:
  - Existing lymphedema
  - History of DVT
  - Presence of varicose veins (Fig. 36.3)

Complications of Body Contouring Procedures [9–12, 17]

- Seroma
- Dehiscence
- Infection
- Hematoma
- Wound healing complications

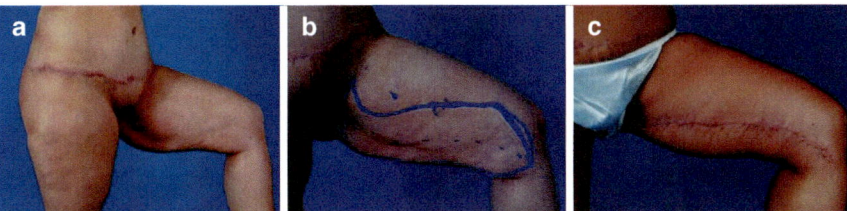

Fig. 36.3 Pre- and post-thighplasty with markings

References

1. Aly AS. Body contouring after massive weight loss. St Louis: Quality Medical Publishing; 2006.
2. Nahai F. The art of aesthetic surgery: principles & techniques. St. Louis: Quality Medical Publishing; 2005.
3. Janis JE. Essentials of plastic surgery. 2nd ed. St. Louis, Boca Raton: Quality Medical Publishing CRC Press/Taylor & Francis Group; 2014. xxv, 1336 p.
4. Gilbert EW, Wolfe BM. Bariatric surgery for the management of obesity: state of the field. Plast Reconstr Surg. 2012;130(4):948–54.
5. Hamad GG. The state of the art in bariatric surgery for weight loss in the morbidly obese patient. Clin Plast Surg. 2004;31(4):591–600. vi
6. A review of bariatric surgery procedures. Plast Reconstru Surg. 2006;117:S8–S13.
7. Dellon AL. Fleur-de-lis abdominoplasty. Aesth Plast Surg. 1985;9(1):27–32.
8. Friedman T, O'Brien Coon D, Michaels VJ, Purnell C, Hur S, Harris DN, et al. Fleur-de-Lis abdominoplasty: a safe alternative to traditional abdominoplasty for the massive weight loss patient. Plast Reconstr Surg. 2010;125(5):1525–35.
9. Bunting H, Lu KB, Shang Z, Kenkel J. Vertical abdominoplasty technique and the impact of preoperative comorbidities on outcomes. Aesthet Surg J Open Forum. 2021;3(1):ojaa043.
10. Buck DW, Mustoe TA. An evidence-based approach to abdominoplasty. Plast Reconstr Surg. 2010;126(6):2189–95.
11. Aly AS, Cram AE, Heddens C. Truncal body contouring surgery in the massive weight loss patient. Clin Plast Surg. 2004;31(4):611–24. vii
12. Taylor J, Shermak M. Body contouring following massive weight loss. Obes Surg. 2004;14(8):1080–5.
13. Losken A. Breast reshaping following massive weight loss: principles and techniques. Plast Reconstr Surg. 2010;126(3):1075–85.
14. Strauch B, Greenspun D, Levine J, Baum T. A technique of brachioplasty. Plast Reconstr Surg. 2004;113(3):1044–8; discussion 9.
15. Gusenoff JA, Coon D, Rubin JP. Brachioplasty and concomitant procedures after massive weight loss: a statistical analysis from a prospective registry. Plast Reconstr Surg. 2008;122(2):595–603.
16. Soliman S, Rotemberg SC, Pace D, Bark A, Mansur A, Cram A, et al. Upper body lift. Clin Plast Surg. 2008;35(1):107–14. discussion 21
17. Rubin JP, Nguyen V, Schwentker A. Perioperative management of the post-gastric-bypass patient presenting for body contour surgery. Clin Plast Surg. 2004;31(4):601–10, vi.

Chapter 37
Liposuction

Patrick R. Keller

Introduction

- Suction-assisted lipectomy, often referred to as liposuction, is a safe and effective procedure for the removal of excess subcutaneous fat in most parts of the body.
- Nearly all surgeons tumesce with wetting solution to reduce blood loss and improve pain control.
- The most common complication is contour irregularity, which can be prevented by adhering to proper technique.
- Zones of adherence are areas of fibrous attachment of deep fascia to dermis and should not routinely be suctioned due to the high risk of contour deformity.

Anatomy [1–3]

Adipose Tissue of Trunk and Lower Extremities

- Subcutaneous adipose tissue (Fig. 37.1)
  - Superficial (Camper's) adipose tissue is dense, with organized septae.
    - Suctioning here will likely cause contour irregularities.
  - Deep (Scarpa's) adipose tissue is loose and areolar with disorganized septae.

P. R. Keller (✉)
Department of Plastic and Reconstructive Surgery, Johns Hopkins University School of Medicine, Baltimore, MD, USA
e-mail: patrick.keller@jhmi.edu

Fig. 37.1 Subcutaneous adipofascial layers of the trunk. (Taken from Markman and Barton [1])

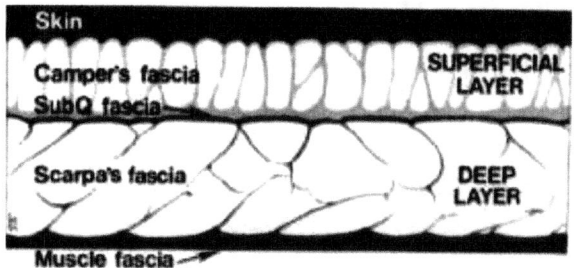

- Separated from superficial fat by superficial/subcutaneous fascia ("Scarpa's fascia").
- Differences in thickness of layers in anteroposterior and superoinferior dimensions (Fig. 37.2).
- Fibrous septae travel deep to superficial, frequently contain nutrient perforating vessels. These are generally preserved in liposuction.

Fig. 37.2 Relative distribution of superficial vs deep layers of fat as they change depending on region. (Taken from Markman and Barton [1])

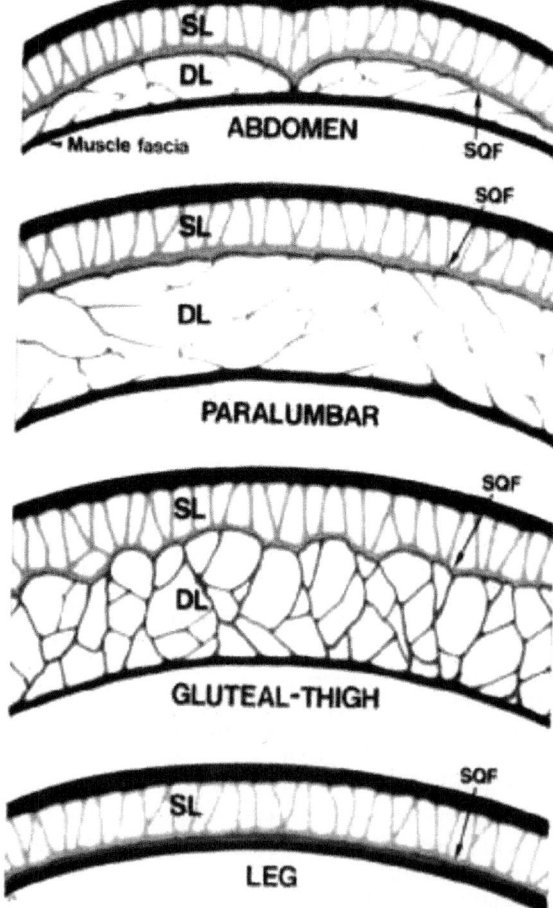

Fig. 37.3 The five zones of adherence: lateral gluteal depression, gluteal crease, distal posterior thigh, mid medial thigh, and inferolateral iliotibial tract. These zones are highly susceptible to contour irregularities if suctioned. (Taken from Rohrich et al. [3])

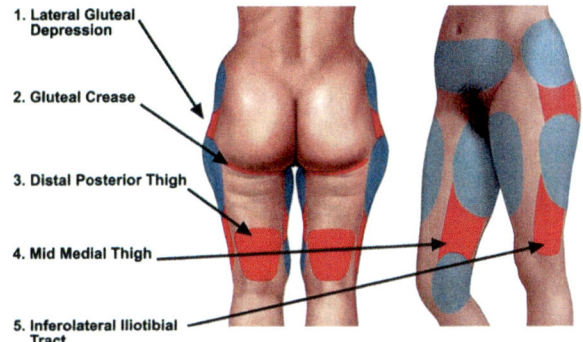

1. Lateral Gluteal Depression
2. Gluteal Crease
3. Distal Posterior Thigh
4. Mid Medial Thigh
5. Inferolateral Iliotibial Tract

Zones of Adherence

- Zones of adherence (Fig. 37.3)
    - Five areas of fibrous attachment of dermis to the underlying deep fascia.
        - Lateral gluteal depression, gluteal crease, distal posterior thigh, mid medial thigh, inferolateral iliotibial tract
    - Define normal curves and contours of body.
    - Disruption causes contour deformities.

Evaluation [4, 5]

History

- Patient goals
- Weight stability
- History of blood clots, Caprini score
- Surgical history, anesthetics, childbirth, hernias
- Current medications
- Nutritional status (especially if history of bariatric surgery)
- Evidence of body dysmorphic disorder

Physical Exam

- Quality of skin and dermis
    - Determine if skin is likely to contract, or if some excision is necessary.

- Presence of visceral fat or rectus diastasis
  - May limit the ability to get a flat abdomen.
- Body mass index (BMI)
  - Current recommendation: patient should be within 30% of ideal BMI.
- Bulges and scars
  - Clues as to possible underlying abdominal hernias.
  - Consider a CT scan if hernia is suspected.
- Appropriate consent and photo documentation

Treatment [3–9]

Preoperative Considerations

- Stop all nonessential medications (e.g., herbal supplements) to reduce the risk of bleeding complications.
- Caution with SSRI—can increase risk of lidocaine toxicity. Consider stopping drug or using less lidocaine.
- Smoking cessation ≥4 weeks before surgery.
- For diabetics: tight glycemic control perioperatively
- Caprini risk assessment to stratify for VTE risk
- Caution with beta-blockers—can cause hypertensive crisis due to unopposed alpha agonist actions from epinephrine in tumescent.
- Location: hospitals vs free-standing ambulatory surgical center vs office-based.
- Inpatient vs outpatient decision:
  - 2011 ASPS task force guidelines identified patients suitable for outpatient surgery: lipoaspirate volume <5 L, case lasts <6 hours and finishes by 3p, BMI is <35, and ASA class is 1–2, not combining with other procedures.
- Pre-op counseling: advise on possible need for skin excision if there is skin excess.

General Technique

- Place access incisions in locations that allow access to the same area from multiple directions to allow for cross-hatching.
- One hand on the cannula handle, one on the patient's skin, feeling for depth and location of the cannula tip.
- Move the cannula in and out over its near-whole length, constantly changing tunnel, moving in a fan-like motion.

- Frequent pinching of skin and fat to assess for areas that need more suctioning and to compare sides.
- Plane of suctioning is usually within deep or intermediate fat. Superficial or subdermal plane only under select circumstances.
- Do not suction or disrupt zones of adherence.
- Cannula choice:
  - Blunt tip lessens perforation risk.
  - Mercedes tip cannulas in 3–5 mm range are most commonly used.
  - Multiport cannulas are more efficient at aspiration than Mercedes tips.
- SAFElipo technique
  - Multistep approach to body contouring aimed at preventing contour irregularities.
  - Involves four main steps: (1) tumescing, (2) fat separation via pre-tunneling, (3) lipoaspiration, and (4) fat equalization via post-tunneling.

Wetting Solutions

- Solution that is injected subcutaneously into treatment areas prior to suctioning
- Contents: lidocaine, epinephrine, crystalloid
  - E.g., 1 L LR, 50 cc 1% lido, 1 amp epi
- Purpose: improve pain control, reduce blood loss
- Max dose of subcutaneous lidocaine in tumescent: 35–55 mg/kg
- Allow 25 minutes to pass for the maximum vasoconstrictive effect of epinephrine
- Endpoint: tissue blanching, moderate turgor
- Wetting solution types:
  - Differ in terms of the amount of solution injected and expected blood loss (EBL) as a percentage of the volume of aspirate
  - Dry
    - Rarely used.
    - No solution is infused.
    - EBL as a percentage of the aspirated volume: 20–45%.
  - Wet
    - Rarely used
    - 100–300 ml of solution into each site
    - EBL percentage: 4–30%
  - Superwet

- 1 cc of solution per 1 cc aspirate
- Most common
- EBL percentage: 1–4%

– Tumescent

- 2–3 cc solution per 1 cc aspirate
- EBL percentage: 1%.

Adjuncts

- Suction-assisted liposuction (SAL)

  – Use of vacuum suction
  – More efficient than the use of a simple 60 cc syringe held under suction

- Power-assisted liposuction

  – Motor vibrates the cannula, increases the speed of fat removal
  – Reduces surgeon fatigue

- Water-assisted liposuction

  – Dual-purpose cannula that simultaneously emits jet of tumescent from one port, suctions adipose tissue with the other
  – No thermal energy emitted
  – Unclear benefits

- Ultrasound-assisted liposuction

  – Uses vibration amplification of sound energy resonance (VASER) to generate heat energy
  – More seromas
  – Small increase in skin tightening

- Laser-assisted liposuction (LAL)

  – Combines SAL with a laser of varying wavelengths, energy absorbed by tissue predominantly as heat.
  – Questionable benefits over SAL.
  – Skin burns can occur—typically use lubrication to help prevent burns.
  – Avoid skin resection when using LAL, as heat can damage skin edges.

- Radiofrequency-assisted liposuction

  – Uses RF to heat tissues, including dermis
  – Improved skin tightening
  – Requires transcutaneous skin temperature monitoring

Fluid Management

- Avoid under- or over-resuscitation.
- Replace fluids lost before (e.g., pre-op fasting) and during surgery (e.g., insensible losses).
  - No accepted standard
  - Low-volume liposuction (lipoaspirate <5 L):
    - Maintenance fluids only, based on intraoperative hemodynamics
  - High-volume liposuction (>5 L):
    - Inpatient admission, strict I/O's (foley if needed), frequent vitals
    - Fluid replacement
      - Common range is 1.2:1–2:1 of total volume of fluid administered (including tumescent, fluids via IV, etc.) to total volume of aspirate.
      - Alternative is 0.25 cc of IV fluids per 1 cc of lipoaspirate >5 L.

Post-Operative Care

- Bruising is expected, resolves in several weeks.
- VTE prophylaxis: use Caprini risk score assessment to determine need. Very important, as VTE and pulmonary embolism are the most common causes of death after liposuction.
- Compression garments are typically used, and some use foam compression.
- Edema can last for months and is expected.

Outcomes and Complications [4, 7–9]

- Lidocaine toxicity
  - Signs and symptoms appear at different plasma levels for different patients. Peak levels occur 6–12 hours post-op.
  - Early signs: perioral numbness, drowsiness, tinnitus.
  - Intermediate: shivering, muscle twitches, AV dissociation, death.
  - Late: seizure, coma.
  - Treatment: benzodiazepines, supportive care.
    - If bupivacaine toxicity or cardiac symptoms, add lipids.
- Fluid overload
- Contour deformity

- Prevent by using a small cannula, pinch test, and cross tunneling
 - Treat with fat grafting (either at time of surgery or ≥6 months post-op), revision liposuction, skin removal, SAFElipo technique
- Fluid collections
 - Prevent with compression garments, avoidance of over-suctioning
 - Can percutaneously drain postoperatively if they are significant
- Skin necrosis or thermal injury
- Infection
- Venous thromboembolism or fat embolism
- Mortality is 19 per 100,000
 - Most common: pulmonary embolism. Also, fat embolism, sepsis, necrotizing fasciitis, and rarely, organ perforation.

References

1. Markman B, Barton FE. Anatomy of the subcutaneous tissue of the trunk and lower extremity. Plast Reconstr Surg. 1987;80:248–54.
2. Lockwood TE. Superficial fascial system (SFS) of the trunk and extremities: a new concept. Plast Reconstr Surg. 1991;87:1009–18.
3. Rohrich RJ, Smith PD, Marcantonio DR, Kenkel JM. The zones of adherence: role in minimizing and preventing contour deformities in liposuction. Plast Reconstr Surg. 2001;107:1562–9.
4. Chia CT, Neinstein RM, Theodorou SJ. Evidence-based medicine: liposuction. Plast Reconstr Surg. 2017;139:267e–74e.
5. Hunstad JP, Aitken ME. Liposuction: techniques and guidelines. Clin Plastic Surg. 2006;33:13–25.
6. Wall SH, Lee MR. Separation, aspiration, and fat equalization: SAFE liposuction concepts for comprehensive body contouring. Plast Reconstr Surg. 2016;138:1192–201.
7. Iverson RE, Lynch DJ. Practice advisory on liposuction. Plast Reconstr Surg. 2004;113:1478–90.
8. American Society of Plastic Surgeons (ASPS). Pathways to preventing adverse events in ambulatory surgery in 2011.
9. Mendez BM, Coleman JE, Kenkel JM. Optimizing patient outcomes and safety with liposuction. Aesthet Surg J. 2019;39:66–82.

Chapter 38
Facial Analysis

Sean Saadat

Principles [1]

- The face is commonly divided into subunits when discussing facial aesthetic analysis (Fig. 38.1).
- Symmetry is a key principle in human's perception of beauty, specifically in a horizontal midline plane when looking at the face.
  - However, perfect symmetry is not considered ideal, small discrepancies are expected and appreciated as beauty.
- Facial analysis is not only important for beauty but also for function—interpersonal cues, facial expressions, ocular function, mastication, and respiration.
  - A beautiful face is a functional face.
- Facial analysis has two components: soft tissue and skeletal.
  - It is important to understand these two components both not only as separate entities but also as two factors that work in harmony to establish the human facial appearance and function as we observe it.
- Learning to analyze the facial apparatus can also be crucial in helping to diagnose multiple medical problems, such as paralytic disease (stroke, Bell's palsy), endocrine/metabolic disorders (Graves induced proptosis), congenital disorders, and much more.
- When analyzing a patient's facial structure, it is also important to know, if possible, what the baseline appearance of the patient's face is and if either the patient

S. Saadat (✉)
UCLA Plastic Surgery, Los Angeles, CA, USA
e-mail: ssaadat@mednet.ucla.edu

Fig. 38.1 Facial aesthetic subunits

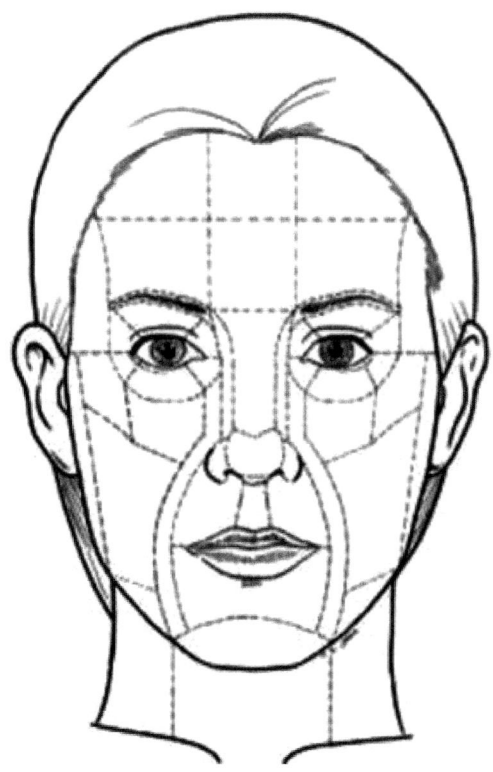

or anyone familiar to the patient can describe any changes that may have occurred over time.

Anatomic Considerations

- The facial skeleton is formed in utero by the convergence of multiple facial prominences.
  - Disruption of the union of the prominences is what results in facial clefts, most commonly observed as a cleft lip or palate, although many other facial cleft patterns exist (i.e., Tessier clefts).
- The soft tissue layers of the face include an intricate structure of nerves, blood vessels, dynamic muscles, and fat compartments that give the face its overall shape and function.
  - Understanding these layers is crucial before any facial operation, since the slightest error in anatomic understanding can have devastating effects on the patient.

38 Facial Analysis

- With facial aging, it is important to note that the aged appearance of the face is a result of two key factors:
    - Gravitational descent of tissues over time over the skeletal structure
    - Volume loss throughout the face that results in a deflated and saggy appearance, which can also result in functional problems such as visual blockage from excess eyelid or brow skin
- Most commonly, the face is divided into three horizontal vectors and five vertical vectors.
    - This allows for a more universal idea of understanding the standard facial makeup and helps any medical practitioner to pick up on any abnormalities that may exist on the human face.
    - Vertically, the distances from menton to subnasale, from subnasale to brow, and from brow to hairline should be roughly equal.
    - Horizontally, the distances lateral to the lateral canthus should be roughly equal to the length of the eyes should be roughly equal to the intercanthal distance on frontal view.

Imaging

- Specific imaging for facial analysis depends on what component of the face you are trying to better understand.
- Standard photography:
    - Photographic imaging of the face is a key component of facial analysis in any situation.
    - The face is made up of many convex and concave points, so it is imperative that any individual photographing the face for aesthetic analysis be very meticulous about lighting, positioning, and the consistency of any variables through all images.
    - Many plastic surgeons will have special rooms or areas that are designed for taking optimal preoperative photographs of a patient's face from every angle.
    - The standard facial photographs are taken from the frontal view, side views, oblique views, bird's-eye view, and basal view.
    - A consistent background is also very important as this removes any question of possible confounding variables when analyzing the intricate light reflexes and contours of the human face through images.
    - 3-D imaging has also become a very popular component of facial analysis as this allows the surgeon to visualize a patient's facial structure in a more comprehensive manner prior to planning any operation
- Advanced medical imaging [3]:
    - CT scan

- CT scan is often the most common and first-line imaging modality for the face when any skeletal or traumatic injuries are being considered.
- Maxillofacial protocols typically allow for 1 mm thickness cuts to see more detailed skeletal anatomy and allow for 3D reconstruction.
- CT imaging is not necessary for pure aesthetic surgery but is useful if there is concern for traumatic disruption of the facial structure.
- Can be used for virtual surgical planning [2, 5].

– MRI

- Focuses on soft tissue, useful in tumor reconstruction.

Facial Reconstruction

- A key component of plastic surgery practice is often in the setting of trauma or neoplastic destruction of normal facial appearance and function.
- Understanding the structural forces that affect the face is crucial when planning facial reconstruction.

  – Coordination with oncologic surgical services (often ENT or OMFS) for a stepwise approach to operative technique [4].
  – A crucial component of planning of facial reconstruction is the presence of or plan for future radiation.

    - Radiation has several negative effects on tissue quality, wound healing, and surgical outcomes.
    - Radiated tissue will often need to be excised and included in the reconstruction and creating a larger defect.

Facial Aesthetic Enhancement

- Cosmetic surgery of the face has been on the rise year after year for several decades.
- It is important to discuss thoroughly with a patient what their aesthetic goals are prior to planning any operation.
- During the exam and evaluation, it is advised that the facial appearance is discussed openly with the patient so that they understand not only what would be addressed by the requested operation but also what may not be addressed and asymmetries that may persist even after the operation.
- Much of facial aesthetics is to counteract the aging face.

Ethnic Considerations

- Ethnic variations in beauty standards often exist, and it is important to consider these when determining the goals of an aesthetic (or reconstructive) operation with a patient.

Effects of Aging on the Face

- Causes of aging
    - Sun damage
    - Weight changes
    - Alcohol and tobacco use
    - Medical comorbidities
- Key effects of aging on the face (Fig. 38.2)
    - Decrease in elasticity of skin and thinning of subcutaneous tissue results in sagging
    - Loss of volume and increased laxity of retaining ligaments
    - Loss of bone mass and facial height
    - Prominent rhytides
    - Ptosis of submandibular glands
    - Dermatochalasis and ptosis of the lacrimal gland
- Goals of surgical intervention are to [6]:
    - Improve skin quality and laxity
    - Address volume loss
    - Restore the anatomic position of tissue
    - Excise redundant tissue

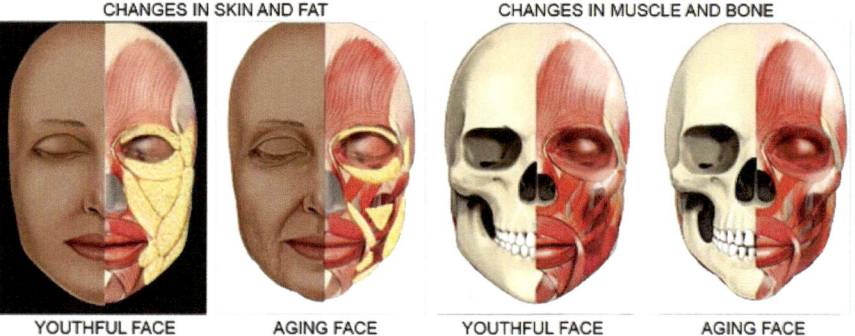

Fig. 38.2 Anatomy of an aging face

References

1. Fitzgerald R, Graivier MH, Kane M, Lorenc ZP, Vleggaar D, Werschler WP, Kenkel JM. Facial aesthetic analysis. Aesthet Surg J. 2010;30 Suppl:25S–7S. https://doi.org/10.1177/1090820X10373360. PMID: 20844297.
2. Chan TJ, Long C, Wang E, Prisman E. The state of virtual surgical planning in maxillary reconstruction: a systematic review. Oral Oncol. 2022;133:106058. ISSN 1368-8375. https://doi.org/10.1016/j.oraloncology.2022.106058.
3. Papel ID, Jiannetto DF. Advances in computer imaging/applications in facial plastic surgery. Facial Plast Surg. 1999;15:119–25. https://doi.org/10.1055/s-2008-1064308.
4. Furukawa M, Mathes DW, Anzai Y. Evaluation of the facial artery on computed tomographic angiography using 64-slice multidetector computed tomography: implications for facial reconstruction in plastic surgery. Plast Reconstr Surg. 2013;131:526–35. https://doi.org/10.1097/PRS.0b013e31827c6f18.
5. Vyas KS, Gibreel WO, Mardini S. Virtual surgical planning (VSP) in craniomaxillofacial reconstruction. Facial Plast Surg Clin North Am. 2022;30(2):239–53.
6. Baker TJ, Stuzin JM. Personal technique of face lifting. Plast Reconstr Surg. 1997;100(2):502–8. https://doi.org/10.1097/00006534-199708000-00038. PMID: 9252622.

Chapter 39
Nonsurgical Facial Rejuvenation

Emily L. Geisler

Introduction

The demand for nonsurgical facial rejuvenation has grown in recent years. There exists a wide array of treatment techniques for the plastic surgeon to have at hand, as isolated treatment or an adjunct to surgical management. Most methods require repeat sessions to improve and maintain results and do not typically provide the same degree or longevity of improvement as surgical intervention. However, these techniques can be effective in restoring a youthful facial appearance. Additionally, these practices have gained popularity in recent years due to their lack of permanence, allowing patients to "trial" rejuvenation procedures with reduced recovery time. These interventions are also typically less expensive for patients than surgery.

Causes of Facial Aging

Causes

A. Sun exposure: collagen decreases, elastin becomes disorganized, and skin becomes laxer and dyschromic; associated with fine rhytids and skin malignancies.
B. Chronologic: dermis/epidermis thinning, decreased collagen and elastin, decreased subcutaneous fat, rhytids form at dynamic areas, and those prone to gravitational pull.

E. L. Geisler (✉)
Division of Plastic Surgery, The University of Texas Medical Branch, Galveston, TX, USA
e-mail: elgeisle@UTMB.EDU

(a) Static Rhytids: wrinkles that are present without facial animation
(b) Dynamic Rhytids: wrinkles that exist during muscular contraction

C. Smoking: systemic hypoxia and local irritants can cause fine rhytids.

Patient Evaluation

A full history and facial exam aids in selecting the appropriate and desired treatment for each patient. Patients will have specific requests and identified problems. Patients should be evaluated at rest and while animating to assess dynamic and static rhytids. Areas of volume deficiency should be noted, and the patient skin type should be noted.

Fitzpatrick Skin Types

I. Extremely fair, never tans, burns easily/severely
II. Burns, difficult to tan
III. Burns/tans moderately
IV. Tans moderately and easily, minimal burns
V. Dark brown skin, rarely burns
VI. Dark brown/black skin; never burns

Methods of Treatment [1–4]

Lasers

Cause selective tissue damage by using light with a single wavelength to target specific chromophores. The different chromophores have different applications (hemoglobin, vasculature; melanin, skin pigment, hair follicles; water, epidermis, dermis).

A. Ablative (water chromophore): vaporize superficial epidermis and coagulates deeper tissues, causing progenitor cell proliferation and eventual re-epithelialization, increased collagen synthesis, and reorganization of elastin. Used for facial resurfacing.

   1. CO_2 (10,600 nm):
      - Treatment: fine lines and deep rhytids
      - Chromophore: water

- Mechanism: greatest effect in papillary dermis where collagen is replaced with organized bundles; reepithelialization occurs in 8–10 days.
- Risks: can cause hypopigmentation, especially in Fitzpatrick I/II, erythema, scarring, and infection.

2. Erbium YAG (2940 nm):
    - Treatment: superficial fine lines
    - Chromophore: water
    - Mechanism: less thermal diffusion than with CO2, although depth and effect are comparatively decreased; useful for thinner skin

B. Non-ablative: epidermis is not vaporized, so recovery is significantly faster; causes dermal heating, which leads to inflammation, and collagen generation/remodeling, which tightens the skin.

1. Fractional Resurfacing (1.5 μm wavelength, 300 μm depth)
    - Treatment: dyschromia, fine lines.
    - Chromophore: blue dye applied onto the skin.
    - Mechanism: blue dye pattern provides microscopic thermal zones of treatment with surrounding tissue left untreated, usually only treating 13–17% of the skin at one time and repeating treatments once a week for four to five total sessions with minimal downtime for each.

2. Nd:YAG (1064 nm)
    - Treatment: telangiectasia, fine lines
    - Chromophore: nonspecific—red blood cells, blood vessels, melanin, water
    - Mechanism: greatest effect at 1–2 mm depth within dermis, causes collagen generation and reorganization, leading to skin tightening.

Intense Pulsed Light (IPL)

IPL is not a laser and emits photons in 500–1300 nm range, targeting specific chromophores at different ranges:

- 550–80 nm: water, hemoglobin.
- 550–570 nm: superficial pigment.
- 590–755 nm: deep pigment.
- IPL can treat hypervascularity and hyperpigmentation and improve texture/decrease pore size.
- It requires several treatment sessions, and realistic expectations must be established with the patient.
- Contraindicated in pregnancy, isotretinoin use, Fitzpatrick types V and VI, and photosensitivity.
- Side effects include erythema, scabbing, pigmentation changes, and scarring.

Dermabrasion and Microdermabrasion

Method of mechanical resurfacing that uses a rotary device to remove superficial layers of skin, promoting improved skin contour and quality.

1. Dermabrasion: it uses a rotary device at a controlled angle, speed, and direction to abrade the superficial layers of the skin until pinpoint bleeding is reached, indicating the papillary dermis has been reached.
   - Indications: scars, rhytids, telangiectasia, actinic keratoses, nevi, rhinophyma
   - Contraindications: isotretinoin use, herpes outbreak, hypertrophic or keloid scarring, anticoagulation.
   - Reepithelialization occurs in 7–10 days; however, skin may remain pink for several months.
   - Hypopigmentation occurs in 10–20% of patients
2. Microdermabrasion: it uses a device that uses suction to pull the skin into the device, then sends a stream of inert particles (aluminum oxide, sodium chloride) onto the skin to remove dirt, oil, and the stratum corneum. Does not require physician oversight.
   - Indications: photoaging, superficial rhytids, shallow acne scars, stretch marks, actinic keratoses
   - Contraindications: current isotretinoin (Accutane) use or use within 1 year, history of facial radiation, hypertrophic or keloid scarring, rosacea

Chemical Peels

Chemical peels involve applying a chemical exfoliant to produce a controlled epidermal and/or dermal wound. They are generally used for dyschromias and fine rhytids, depending on the depth of the peel.

Preparation: skin is cleansed, +/− sedation depending on depth and size of treatment, and acyclovir prophylaxis for herpes simplex.

1. Superficial Peels:
   - Depth: superficial epidermis
   - Indications: mild dyschromia, melasma, fine wrinkles
   - Agent: alpha hydroxy acid (AHA), Jessner's solution, salicylic acid
     - AHA peels require neutralization with water or a basic solution.
   - Overall safe and unlikely to cause injury, may require multiple treatments to achieve the desired effect

2. Medium Depth Peels
   - Depth: epidermis and superficial dermis.
   - Indications: fine wrinkles, dyschromia.
   - Agent: TCA.
   - Appropriate depth of penetration noted when white frost with erythematous strikethrough appears.
   - Requires up to a week of recovery time for swelling and erythema to resolve.
   - TCA does not require neutralization, naturally neutralizes with keratin in skin.
3. Deep Peels
   - Depth: papillary dermis.
   - Indications: coarse wrinkles, acne scars.
   - Agents: Phenol.
   - Appropriate depth of penetration reached when a solid white frosting without background erythema appears.
   - Patients must be put on cardiac monitoring during treatment due to the risk of arrhythmia with phenol. IV access should be obtained.

Botulinum Toxin

Botulinum toxin is a naturally derived protein from the *Clostridium botulinum* bacteria. It is commonly used to treat facial wrinkles, hyperhidrosis, and migraines.

- Mechanism: protein consists of two parts, a heavy chain that binds to presynaptic axon terminal cell surfaces, and a light chain that gets translocated across the cell membrane to prevent acetylcholine release at the neuromuscular junction, temporarily paralyzing the muscle.
- Effect: initial effect seen within 1 week and lasts up to 6 months.
- Contraindications: disorders of the neuromuscular junction (Lambert-Eaton syndrome, myasthenia gravis, multiple sclerosis, amyotrophic lateral sclerosis), pregnant/breastfeeding, use of aminoglycosides or calcium channel blockers.
- Targets: forehead lines (frontalis), glabella (corrugator supercilii, procerus, orbicularis oculi), crow's feet/lateral eyelid (orbicularis oculi), bunny lines (nasalis, procerus), nasolabial folds (levator labii superioris, zygomaticus minor and major, levator anguli oris), perioral wrinkles (orbicularis oris), marionette lines (depressor anguli oris), cobblestone chin (mentalis), platysmal bands (platysma) (Fig. 39.1).
- Note: rarely, if the toxin migrates through the orbital septum fascia to the levator palpebrae superioris, it may cause blepharoptosis (eyelid droop). This is temporary and can be managed with alpha-adrenergic ophthalmic solutions to contract the Muller muscle, which elevates the lid.

Fig. 39.1 Muscular schematic of muscles in the face. (Author's own work)

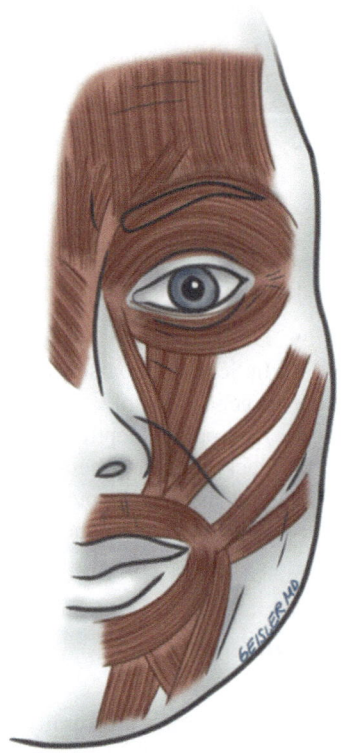

Volume Restoration

Injectables consist of a wide array of substances and are useful for volume restoration or redistribution.

1. Absorbable

    (a) Fat: harvested from liposuction, processed, and injected to enhance subcutaneous volume commonly in the temporal, infraorbital, and malar regions, nasolabial folds, and chin. Requires a surgical procedure. Must be overfilled to account for resorption (40–80% take).
    (b) Hyaluronic acid: most commonly used filler due to enzymatic reversibility. Degree of cross-linking determines viscosity and duration, and therefore, the indications are as follows—higher cross-linking means higher viscosity, used for deeper injections, and lower cross-linking means less viscosity, used for more superficial injections. Last for 6–12 months. If there is difficulty with the injection, then this is a reversal agent. First-line nonsurgical intervention. Brand names include: Restylane, Juvederm.

(c) Poly-L-lactic acid (PLLA): lactic acid microparticles in cellulose matrix, primarily used to treat nasolabial folds and deeper wrinkles. Causes fibroblasts to generate collagen. Lasts for 2 years. Brand names include Sculptra.
(d) Calcium hydroxylapatite: microparticles in polysaccharide gel that promote collagen formation. Primarily used for deep facial wrinkles, cheek, and chin augmentation. Lasts 6–18 months.

2. Nonabsorbable:

(a) Polymethyl methacrylate (PMMA): synthetic polymer microspheres in bovine collagen solution, which promotes collagen generation. Primarily used to treat nasolabial folds.

3. Collagen injections are no longer utilized due to the risk of allergic cross-reaction.

Care must be taken when injecting to avoid inadvertent entry into a blood vessel, which could cause the filler to migrate. A rare but devastating complication is injection of filler into an ophthalmic artery branch, which causes retrograde flow into the ophthalmic artery, causing blindness. This can be avoided with careful injection and aspiration prior to injection.

Conclusion

Nonsurgical facial rejuvenation provides many tools to the plastic surgeon to treat a wide array of aesthetic concerns. Their therapies are generally very safe and effective. Most require repeat treatments to maintain results. With thoughtful assessment and application of these techniques, plastic surgeons can achieve excellent results for their patients with minimal downtime.

References

1. Brown DL, et al. Michigan manual of plastic surgery. 2nd ed. Beaverton: Ringgold, Inc; 2015.
2. Janis JE. Essentials of plastic surgery. 2nd ed. Boca Raton: CRC Press; 2014.
3. Thorne C, Chung KC, Gosain A, Guntner GC, Mehrara BJ. Grabb and Smith's plastic surgery. 7th ed. Philadelphia: Wolters Kluwer/Lippincott Williams & Wilkins Health; 2014.
4. Farber SE, Epps MT, Brown E, Krochonis J, McConville R, Codner MA. A review of nonsurgical facial rejuvenation. Plast Aesthet Res. 2020;7:72.

Chapter 40
Face and Neck Lift

Edward H. Nahabet

Anatomy

Fascial Layers

- The relevant layers of the face from superficial to deep include the skin, the subcutaneous fat, the superficial musculoaponeurotic system (SMAS) that envelopes the facial mimetic musculature, and the deep fascia.
- The superficial fascia, or SMAS, is continuous with the temporoparietal fascia (aka superficial temporal fascia) in the temporal region and the platysma in the neck.
- The deep fascia in the face is known as the parotidomasseteric fascia and is continuous with the deep temporal fascia in the temporal region and the deep cervical fascia in the neck.

Motor and Sensory Nerves

- The facial nerve exits the calvarium through the stylomastoid foramen, courses anteriorly to pierce the parotid gland, branches into the upper and lower divisions, and subsequently into the five terminal branches
  - Temporal/frontal
  - Zygomatic
  - Buccal

E. H. Nahabet (✉)
UCLA Plastic Surgery, Los Angeles, CA, USA
e-mail: edwardnahabet@mednet.ucla.edu

- Marginal mandibular
- Cervical

- The five branches exit the parotid gland and pierce the deep fascia before traveling anteriorly to innervate the mimetic muscles.
  - The facial nerve is therefore present in the surgical field on medial dissection if dissecting under the SMAS—most facelift techniques are not deep to the deep fascia.
- The frontal branch and the marginal mandibular branches are most at risk for injury during face/neck lifting.
- The frontal branch crosses the zygomatic arch and courses more superficially along the undersurface of the temporoparietal fascia, traveling superiorly along Pitanguy's line—a line drawn from 0.5 cm below the tragus to 1.5 cm superolateral to the lateral brow [1].
- The facial mimetic muscles are all innervated on their deep surface except for the mentalis, levator anguli oris, and buccinator muscles.
- The marginal mandibular branch travels superficial to or within the deep cervical fascia and follows the mandibular border before perforating the deep cervical fascia, crossing the facial vessels, and traveling superiorly above the mandibular border, where it is most at risk for injury.
- The sensory innervation to the face is provided by the three branches of the trigeminal nerve (ophthalmic, maxillary, mandibular) and cervical spinal nerves.
- The greater auricular nerve (GAN) arises from cervical spinal nerves C2 and C3 and provides sensation to the ear lobule.
- The GAN emerges superficially at the posterior border of the sternocleidomastoid muscle (SCM) and crosses the midpoint of the SCM at McKinney's point, which is located 6.5 cm inferior to the external auditory canal (Fig. 40.1).

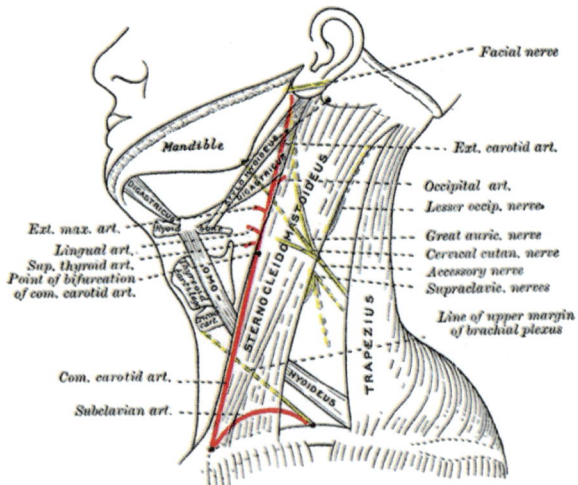

Fig. 40.1 Anatomy of the head and neck

Facial Fat Pads (Fig. 40.2)

- The subcutaneous fat of the face is divided into various anatomical compartments.
- Key fat pads in facial rejuvenation include the superficial nasolabial, superficial lateral cheek, superficial medial cheek, and the deep medial cheek compartments [2].

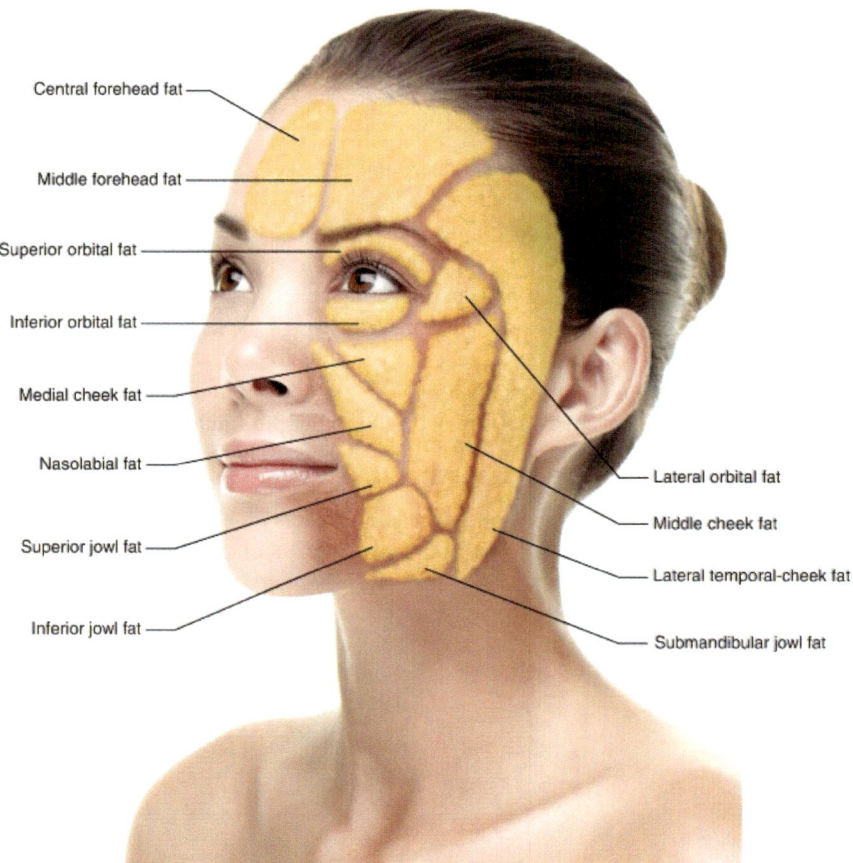

Fig. 40.2 Facial fat pads

Patient Evaluation

- Features of the aging face include the following: increased skin laxity, animation and resting rhytids or wrinkles, deepening of the nasolabial fold, descent of soft tissues, volume loss, fat accumulation in the lower third of the face resulting in jowling and blunting of the cervicomental angle, and bony atrophy.
- Preoperative evaluation includes obtaining a complete history and identifying any active smokers, patients with poorly controlled hypertension, diabetics, other comorbidities, and use of antiplatelet agents, anticoagulants, or NSAIDs.

Incision

- The typical facelift/neck lift incision contains three segments: supra-auricular, preauricular, and postauricular components.
- The supra-auricular component of the incision can be placed either in the temporal hair-bearing region or along the hairline of the sideburn—in patients with a short and narrow sideburn, a hairline incision appears more natural (Fig. 40.3).
- The preauricular incision is marked at the junction of the auricle and facial skin, traveling at the most posterior aspect of the tragus for the intratragal component and then coursing anteriorly again along the lobule-face junction posteriorly.
- In males, the pre-auricular incision is placed in the pre-tragal sulcus so as not to relocate any male sideburn or hair onto the non-hair-bearing tragal region (Fig. 40.4).
- The postauricular component of the incision travels along the posterior lobule, superiorly along the retroauricular sulcus, and then courses posteriorly about the midpoint of the auricle and travels inferiorly either within the hair-bearing occipital scalp or at the hairline [3] (Fig. 40.5).

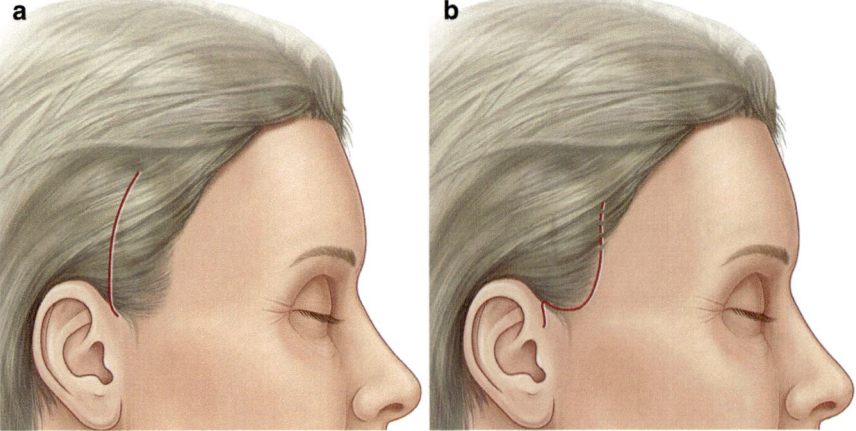

Fig. 40.3 Temporal Incision Patterns

Fig. 40.4 Pre-auricular incision patterns

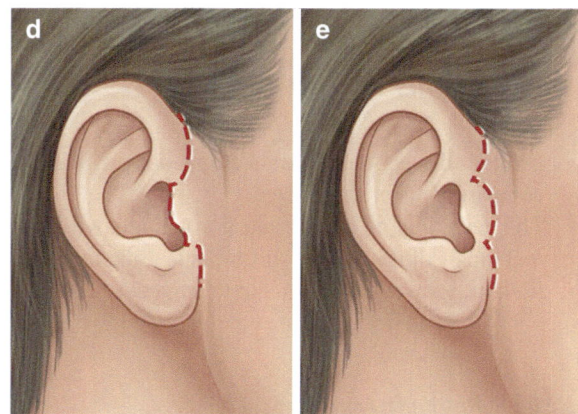

Fig. 40.5 Post-auricular incision patterns

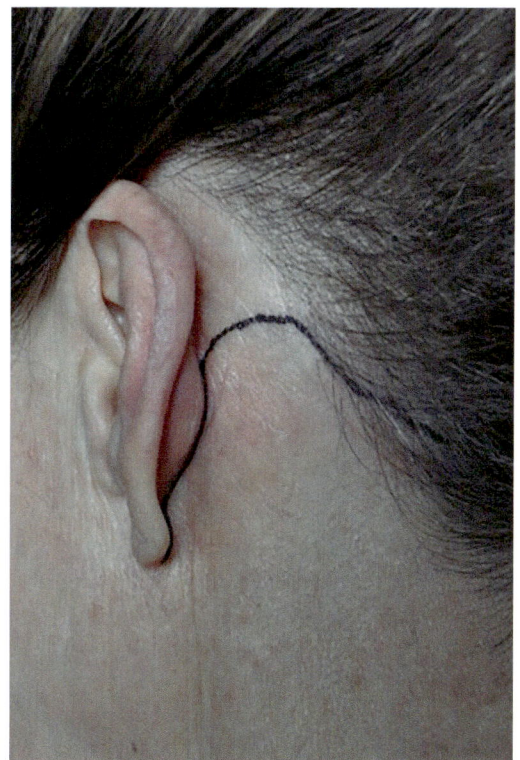

Operative Techniques: Facelift

Subcutaneous Facelift

- Involves dissection in the subcutaneous plane and does not elevate the deeper fat compartments or the SMAS.
- This technique is appropriate for patients with significant skin laxity, but minimal ptosis of the deeper soft tissues of the face.
- Risk of devascularization and telangiectasias of the face.

SMAS Procedures

- The above technique can be performed in conjunction with techniques to address the SMAS.
- Addressing the SMAS separately allows for differing vectors of pull between the skin (generally more posterior) and the SMAS (more superior).
    - SMAS plication—involves elevation of a subcutaneous skin flap followed by direct plication sutures within the SMAS to lift the deeper structures of the face
    - SMASectomy with imbrication—involves elevation of a subcutaneous skin flap followed by incision of the SMAS with elevation and advancement or resection of a strip and suture repair

Deep Plane (aka sub-SMAS) Facelift

- Involves dissection in a plane deep to the SMAS, elevating a SMAS flap, and is also known as the deep plane facelift.
- This can be performed in conjunction with a subcutaneous facelift, or the skin and subcutaneous fat can be lifted with the SMAS as a composite flap.
- Benefits of raising the subcutaneous layer and SMAS separately include maintaining different vectors of pull.
- The facial nerve branches are present in this subSMAS plane medially after they pierce the deep fascia.

Operative Techniques: Neck Lift

Neck Lift

- Evaluation of the neck involves assessing skin quality and excess, presence of subcutaneous and preplatysmal fat, presence of subplatysmal fat, resting or dynamic platysmal bands, presence of prominent submandibular glands, and prominence of the anterior digastric muscles.
- Neck rejuvenation can be performed through a full-length face/neck lift incision or alternatively through a direct submental incision measuring approximately 3 cm either in or posterior to the submental crease—direct incision allows more optimal visualization.
- The procedure typically involves a subcutaneous dissection with clear visualization of the platysma.
- Avoid excessive resection of subcutaneous fat and excessive skin tightening, as that can blunt the cervicomental angle.
- Interplatysmal or subplatysmal fat can be excised directly.
- Platysmaplasty is used to address any platysmal diastasis and can be performed by suturing the medial edges of the platysma to each other to the level of the hyoid bone.
- Additional procedures to optimize the neckline include submandibular gland and anterior digastric excision if these structures adversely affect an ideal neck and jaw contour.

Adjunct Procedures

Fat Grafting

- As age-related fat atrophy is a well-known finding, facial fat grafting can help restore volume that has been lost—commonly targeted areas include the nasolabial fold and the malar fat pads [4].

Complications

Hematoma

- The most common early complication following facelift is a hematoma, with an incidence of approximately 3% in non-hypertensive patients and approximately 8% in hypertensive patients
- Males are at a greater risk than females [5].

- The most common cause is uncontrolled acute postoperative hypertension.
- Nausea and poor pain control can also contribute to increased blood pressure and hematoma.

Nerve Injury

- The most commonly injured symptomatic nerve during rhytidectomy is the great auricular nerve (GAN), with an incidence of 6–7% and can result in anesthesia of the lower ear [6].
- The buccal branch of the facial nerve is the most commonly injured nerve; however, due to significant arborization and redundancy, there is usually minimal consequence.
- Injury to the marginal mandibular nerve results in an inability to evert or pucker the lip on the affected side.
- Subplatysmal dissection in the neck can cause a cervical branch injury which would result in an asymmetric lower lip when the patient is in a full smile, with less tooth show on the affected side [7].
- Typically, nerve palsy postoperatively is managed with observation. Acute changes may be due to the local anesthetic. Even if it persists past the immediate postoperative period, often it is a neuropraxia that will resolve with time.

Skin Necrosis

- The risk for skin necrosis remains low but is raised in the setting of active smokers or high tension on the flaps.
- The most common area of skin necrosis is the retro-auricular skin flap.
- If there is any concern for compromise, sutures may be released to relieve tension on the skin flap.

References

1. Trussler AP, Stephan P, Hatef D, Schaverien M, Meade R, Barton FE. The frontal branch of the facial nerve across the zygomatic arch: anatomical relevance of the high-SMAS technique. Plast Reconstr Surg. 2010;125(4):1221–9.
2. Rohrich RJ, Pessa JE. The fat compartments of the face: anatomy and clinical implications for cosmetic surgery. Plast Reconstr Surg. 2007;119(7):2219–27.
3. Chang DS, Janis JE, Garvey PB. Chapter 8. Basics of microsurgery. In: Janis J, editor. Essentials of plastic surgery. St. Louis: Quality Medical Publishing; 2014.
4. Rohrich RJ, Ghavami A, Constantine FC, Unger J, Mojallal A. Lift-and-fill face lift: integrating the fat compartments. Plast Reconstr Surg. 2014;133(6):756–67.

5. Derby BM, Codner MA. Evidence-based medicine: face lift. Plast Reconstr Surg. 2017;139(1):151e–67e.
6. Lefkowitz T, Hazani R, Chowdhry S, Elston J, Yaremchuk MJ, Wilhelmi BJ. Anatomical landmarks to avoid injury to the great auricular nerve during rhytidectomy. Aesthet Surg J. 2013;33(1):19–23.
7. Daane SP, Owsley JQ. Incidence of cervical branch injury with "marginal mandibular nerve pseudo-paralysis" in patients undergoing face lift. Plast Reconstr Surg. 2003;111(7):2414–8.

Chapter 41
Rhinoplasty

Sean Saadat

Anatomy [1, 2]

- The external nose can be divided into nine different subunits (Fig. 41.1):
  - Dorsum
  - Two lateral sidewalls
  - Tip
  - Two alar lobules
  - Columella
  - Two soft triangles
- Structurally, the nose is made up of two paired lower lateral cartilages, two paired upper lateral cartilages, and two nasal bones superiorly that merge with the maxilla to create the lateral nasal sidewalls.
  - The attachment points of these respective cartilages are important to know when performing rhinoplasty.
    - Keystone region
      - Where the nasal bones and upper lateral cartilages meet to separate the bony and cartilaginous components of the nasal complex
    - Scroll ligament
      - The fibrous union connecting the upper and lower lateral cartilages to one another

---

S. Saadat (✉)
UCLA Plastic Surgery, Los Angeles, CA, USA
e-mail: ssaadat@mednet.ucla.edu

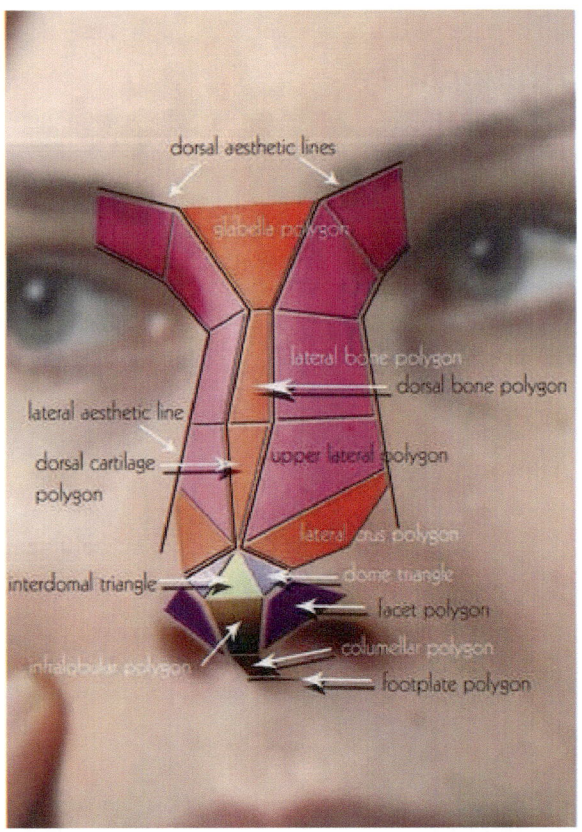

Fig. 41.1 Aesthetic components of the nose

- Pitanguy's ligament
    - Ligamentous attachment of the anterior septal angle to the nasal tip skin
- The septum is oriented perpendicular to the external nasal structural complex, and at the nasal tip, this structure has been described in an "M-Arch" shape.
    - External nasal valve refers to the nostril.
    - Internal nasal valve is the junction between the septum and upper lateral cartilage, where the angle is the narrowest.
        - This is typically the point of the most constricted airflow.
        - The internal valve should be about 10–15° at minimum to allow for optimal nasal airflow. Anything less will lead to valve collapse and difficulty with nasal breathing.
- The nasal septum consists of a caudal cartilaginous component, known as the quadrangular cartilage.
    - The cartilaginous component is posteriorly attached to the perpendicular plate of the ethmoid bone superiorly and the vomer bone inferiorly.

- The most anterior projecting point of the cartilaginous septum is referred to as the anterior septal angle.
- Within the nose, there are three sets of turbinates from the lateral wall-oriented inferior, middle, and superior in relation to the nasomaxillary floor and are designed to help create turbulent and humidified airflow through the nose for optimal airway function.
  - Turbinates will often hypertrophy as a result of trauma or inflammation, leading to nasal airway obstruction.
- There are also several ducts that drain into the nasal passage, and knowing where they are within the airway is crucial when performing a rhinoplasty safely.
  - Below the Inferior turbinate
    - Nasolacrimal duct
  - Below the middle turbinate
    - Frontonasal duct
    - Anterior and middle ethmoid sinus ostia
    - Maxillary sinus ostium
  - Below the superior turbinate
    - Posterior ethmoid sinus ostia

Imaging

- Not typically needed for rhinoplasty.
- CT maxillofacial is the gold standard for evaluation of nasal airway anomaly.
- For airway concerns, nasal endoscopy can be a helpful component of visualizing the exact cause of airway obstruction in a patient.
- If there is concern for soft tissue neoplasia, MRI may be ordered additionally to help visualize the soft tissue structures rather than bone.

Nasal Analysis

- Aesthetic and functional analysis of the nose is best done in a stepwise and sequential fashion.
- Keywords for Aesthetic Exam
  - Dorsal Aesthetic Lines [4]

- Defined as the light reflex on frontal view originating on the supraorbital ridges, traversing medially along the glabellar area, converging at the medial canthal ligaments, diverging at the keystone area, and terminating at the nasal tip.
- Ideally should be symmetric and linear on exam.

– Tip Defining Points
- The outermost projected points of the lower lateral cartilage genu and visible with frontal lighting.
- The ideal distance between these light reflex points is approximately 6–8 mm.

– Nasal Tip Projection
- Determined on lateral view by the distance from the maxilla to the most outward projecting point of the nasal tip.

– Nasal Tip Rotation
- Determined on lateral view by the position of the outermost projected point of the nasal tip in relation to the Frankfurt horizontal line.
- Ideal rotation is between 90–95° in men and 95–100° in women.

– Alar Base Width
- The width of the nostril complex was measured on frontal and basal views from the most lateral point of the nostril to the midline columella.

- Keywords for Functional Exam [3]

– Internal Valve Collapse
- Upon maximum nasal inspiratory effort, there will be noted collapse of the nasal complex at the level of the upper lateral cartilages, indicating weakness or narrowing of the internal nasal valve.
- The Cottle test is used to confirm the presence of internal valve collapse
    – Put fingers on cheeks and pull laterally, and if it improves, the airflow is positive.

– External Valve Collapse
- Upon maximum nasal inspiratory effort, there will be noted collapse of the nasal ala, indicating weakness of the nostril leading to nasal airflow obstruction.

– Septal Deviation
- Based on the frontal and basal views of the nose.
- Deviation is described in the direction to which the septum is bowing.
- Deviation of the nasal septum can lead to uneven airflow and airway obstruction that is often worse on the side to which the septum is deviated.

- Turbinate Exam
    - Using a nasal speculum, the inferior turbinate can be easily visualized on the basal view.
    - The middle and superior turbinates are usually visualized with endoscopy, given their more posterior and superior position.
    - Inferior turbinate hypertrophy is described as either mucosal or bony in nature.
        - CT scan can help to differentiate the etiology, although mucosal hypertrophy will be evident with the presence of a "boggy" and inflamed mucosal surface on visual exam.

Presentation

- Acute Fracture
    - Patients will often present with a nasal bone fracture to the emergency department, often caused by blunt force trauma to the face.
    - Septal hematoma.
        - A crucial component of the exam in acute nasal trauma
        - Collection of blood between the cartilaginous septum and the nasal mucosal lining.
            - If untreated will lead to pressure-induced necrosis of the nasal septum and external nasal collapse or fistula formation, also known as a saddle nose deformity.
    - Always ask the patient if they notice any changes to the aesthetic or function of their Nasal complex after the trauma occurred.
        - Aesthetic changes may be obscured due to edema, depending on how soon the patient presents after the trauma.
- Chronic Issues
    - May be from previous trauma, congenital, or allergy induced
    - Always ask the patient about history of allergies and any medications they may use to try and alleviate the symptoms of nasal obstruction (i.e., Afrin or Steroid sprays).
    - In the setting of chronic airway obstruction, nasal endoscopy can be an important tool to ensure the etiology is not located deeper within the nasal cavity, such as middle turbinate hypertrophy, nasal polyps, or sinus obstruction.

Operative Overview [5]

- Rhinoplasty can be performed in either a closed or an open fashion, depending on the goals of surgery.
  - The open approach will often allow for much better visualization of the nasal complex and increased control of the outcome.
- Closed
  - Performed fully endonasal with no incision across the external columella
  - Incisions
    - Septal
      - Hemitransfixion
        - Incision along the anterior septal angle in order to expose the entirety of the nasal septum through a closed approach.
      - Killian
        - Incision placed parallel to the dorsum 0.5–1.5 cm posterior to the anterior septal angle.
        - Designed to avoid exposure of the anterior septal angle and disturbance of crucial tip structures and ligaments when there is no indication for changes to the nasal tip
    - Nasal (Fig. 41.2)
      - Marginal
        - Incision along the caudal rim of the lower lateral cartilages to expose the entirety of the lower lateral cartilage
      - Intercartilaginous
        - Incision made at the level of the scroll ligament between the upper and lower lateral cartilages
      - Transcartilaginous
        - Incision made in the center of the lower lateral cartilage leading to a splitting of the lateral crus of the cartilage
        - Only indicated when planning for reduction of the lower lateral cartilage width (aka cephalic trim)
        - Rarely used as it can be destabilizing in nature
  - Open
    - Incision
      - Transcolumellar incision carried horizontally across the columella at the midpoint and carried out endonasally in a marginal fashion for full exposure of the nasal tip and dorsum

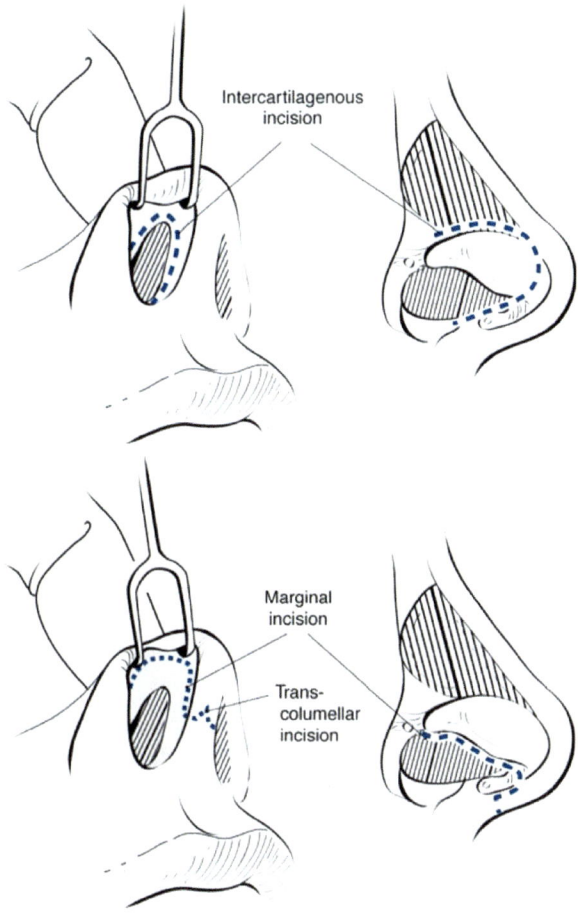

Fig. 41.2 Common incisions for access to the septum (upper) and lower lateral cartilage (lower)

- Grafts
    - Grafts are a key component of rhinoplasty that allow the surgeon to redefine structural components of the nose and address any irregularities.
    - Most commonly, the septal cartilage is used for designing grafts in a primary rhinoplasty.
        - Revision rhinoplasty will often have the septum harvested, so alternative sources of cartilage must be used for structural modification.
            - Rib cartilage
            - Ear cartilage
            - Cadaveric rib cartilage
        - Septal harvest pearls:
            - L-strut design is crucial to maintaining nasal support by the septum.

- The septum is harvested posteriorly from its bony attachment, noting that an "L-strut" of at least 1 cm width must be left behind to ensure adequate structural support.
- Common Grafts
  - Spreader Graft (Fig. 41.3)
    - Cartilage placed between the upper lateral cartilage and the nasal septum to address internal valve collapse and widen the angle of the internal nasal valve
  - Dorsal Onlay Graft
    - Cartilage placed along the nasal dorsum for increased projection or dorsal height
    - Commonly used in patients of Asian descent due to the lack of a nasal bridge
  - Lateral Crural Strut Graft
    - Extension of the lateral limb of the lower lateral cartilage when there is a need for increased nasal sidewall support and repositioning of the lower lateral cartilage
  - Columellar Strut
    - Single piece of cartilage placed inferior to the caudal septum between the medial crus of the lower lateral cartilages to help increase tip projection and rotation
  - Septal Extension graft
    - Cartilage secured to the anterior septal angle to help control tip position, projection, and rotation

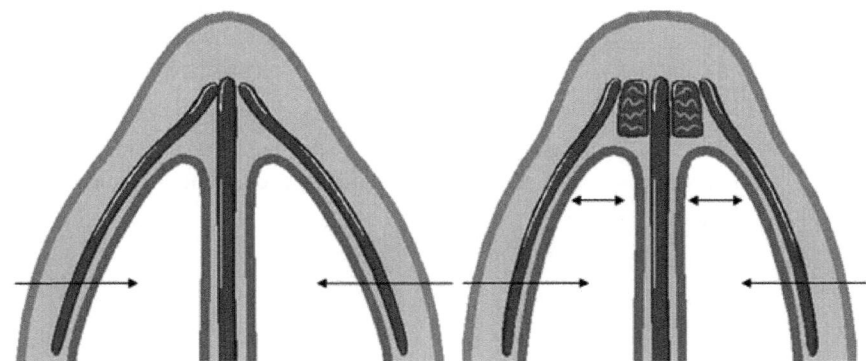

Fig. 41.3 Spreader grafts

- Most structurally sound tip graft when compared to the columellar strut, given its more secured nature
- Tip Graft
  - Piece of cartilage placed over the nasal tip to help blunt any contour irregularities
- Alar Rim Graft
  - Cartilage graft placed along the nostril rim in order to increase alar support, address any alar notching, and correct external valve collapse.

Complications [6]

- The most common complication to counsel patients on prior to undergoing rhinoplasty is the lack of nasal airway improvement postoperatively as well as continued concerns about nasal appearance
- Uncontrolled bleeding is a rare complication of rhinoplasty, but nevertheless should be something that is discussed with the patient.
  - Uncontrolled bleeding can often be due to violation of the posterior ethmoidal artery on septal harvest.
  - Treatment of postoperative nasal bleeding should include tilting of the patient's head forward to prevent swallowing of blood and packing of the nasal airway to tamponade the active bleeder.
    - DDAVP may also be given to help with increased platelet aggregation.
- It is also important to ask the patient about the history of facial fractures.
  - If there is a history of facial fractures or serious facial trauma, a CT scan will be important to determine if there is any aberrant anatomy resulting from an undiagnosed skull base fracture (i.e., cavernous sinus syndrome).
- Another rare complication also includes CSF leak due to dural tear when harvesting the bony septum posteriorly from the perpendicular plate of the ethmoid bone.
  - Should maintain suspicion if the patient presents with persistent clear drainage from the nose more than 1 week after rhinoplasty.
  - Fluid can be tested for beta 2-transferrin to rule out CSF leak.

References

1. Fichman M, Piedra Buena IT. Rhinoplasty. [Updated 2022 Jun 21]. In: StatPearls [Internet]. Treasure Island: StatPearls Publishing; 2022. Available from: https://www.ncbi.nlm.nih.gov/books/NBK558970/.
2. Burget GC, Menick FJ. The subunit principle in nasal reconstruction. Plast Reconstr Surg. 1985;76(2):239–47. https://doi.org/10.1097/00006534-198508000-00010. PMID: 4023097.
3. Adamson PA, Litner JA, Dahiya R. The M-Arch model: a new concept of nasal tip dynamics. Arch Facial Plast Surg. 2006;8(1):16–25. https://doi.org/10.1001/archfaci.8.1.16. PMID: 16415443.
4. Mojallal A, Ouyang D, Saint-Cyr M, Bui N, Brown SA, Rohrich RJ. Dorsal aesthetic lines in rhinoplasty: a quantitative outcome-based assessment of the component dorsal reduction technique. Plast Reconstr Surg. 2011;128(1):280–8. https://doi.org/10.1097/PRS.0b013e318218fc2d.
5. Park SS. Fundamental principles in aesthetic rhinoplasty. Clin Exp Otorhinolaryngol. 2011;4(2):55–66. https://doi.org/10.3342/ceo.2011.4.2.55. Epub 2011 May 31. PMID: 21716951; PMCID: PMC3109328.
6. Rettinger G. Risks and complications in rhinoplasty. GMS Curr Top Otorhinolaryngol Head Neck Surg. 2007;6:Doc08. Epub 2008 Mar 14. PMID: 22073084; PMCID: PMC3199839.

Chapter 42
Blepharoplasty

Edward H. Nahabet

Anatomy

- The orbicularis oculi is a thin, sphincter-type muscle located just below the skin surface and is divided into three parts—the orbital, preseptal, and pretarsal components.
- The orbital division allows forced eye closure, the preseptal division is responsible for voluntary blinking and the lacrimal pump mechanism, and the pretarsal division contributes to involuntary lid closure.
- The eyelid consists of the anterior, middle, and posterior lamella.
- The anterior lamella consists of the skin and the orbicularis muscle.
- The middle lamella consists of the orbital septum, pre-septal, and post-septal fat.
- The posterior lamella is formed by the tarsus (or tarsal plate) and the conjunctiva.
- The upper and lower lid tarsal plates attach to the medial and lateral orbital rim via the medial and lateral canthal tendons [1].

Upper Eyelid

- The levator palpebrae superioris is the primary upper eyelid elevator and originates at the orbital apex from the annulus of Zinn and travels anteriorly as the tendinous aponeurosis and fuses with the orbital septum just above the tarsus.

E. H. Nahabet (✉)
UCLA Plastic Surgery, Los Angeles, CA, USA
e-mail: edwardnahabet@mednet.ucla.edu

© The Author(s), under exclusive license to Springer Nature Switzerland AG 2025
J. Roostaeian et al. (eds.), *Plastic Surgery Clerkship*, Contemporary Surgical Clerkships, https://doi.org/10.1007/978-3-031-99098-4_42

- The upper eyelid contains the orbital septum, which originates from the superior orbital rim and joins the levator aponeurosis just superior to its insertion on the tarsus.
- Caudally, the levator has attachments to the dermis, which forms the crease known as the supratarsal crease
- In occidental patients, the supratarsal crease is located approximately 7 mm above the lash margin for males and 8–10 mm above the lash margin in females
- In Asian patients, the supratarsal crease is located 4–6 mm above the lash margin as the levator fuses with the septum more inferiorly.
- Mueller's muscle, which has sympathetic innervation, originates from the undersurface of the levator and inserts onto the tarsus.
- The lacrimal gland is also located in the upper eyelid in the superolateral orbit, deep to the anterior rim [2].

Lower Eyelid

- The lower eyelid anatomy is analogous to the upper eyelid.
- The primary lower lid retractor is the capsulopalpebral fascia, which originates from the inferior rectus fascia and envelopes the inferior oblique muscle; it retracts the inferior eyelid with inferior rectus contraction and downward gaze.
- The inferior tarsal muscle is also a lower lid retractor and analogous to Mueller's muscle of the upper eyelid.

Fat Pads

- Anterior to the septum, the fat is called the SOOF (suborbicularis oculi fat) on the inferior lid and ROOF (retro-orbicularis oculi fat) on the superior lid.
    - These are of minor importance compared to the fat pads below.
- The upper and lower eyelids contain periorbital fat pads that lie posterior to the septum.
- The upper eyelid has two fat pads—the medial (or nasal) and central, which are separated by an interpad septum.
    - The location of the upper lateral fat pad is occupied by the lacrimal gland instead.
    - The nasal fat pad is usually a paler color than the central one, which helps differentiate them
- The lower eyelid has three fat pads—the medial (or nasal), central, and lateral.
- The inferior oblique muscle separates the medial and central fat pads.

- The central and lateral fat pads are separated by a fascial extension from Lockwood's ligament known as the arcuate expansion [3].

Patient Evaluation

- There are numerous periorbital changes that occur with aging, including most notably:
  - Brow ptosis
  - Excess skin of the upper or lower eyelids known as dermatochalasis.
  - Herniation of the upper and lower eyelid fat pads through a weakened septum [4, 5]
    - Herniation of fat under the inferior lid and tethering of skin from the oribomalar ligament causes the bags under the eyes known as the tear trough or nasojugal groove
- Comprehensive blepharoplasty evaluation requires assessment of the frontalis, brow position, upper and lower eyelid skin, resting position of the upper eyelid margin, visual field, eyelid fat pads, and the lid-cheek junction.
- If the upper eyelid margin covers more than 1–2 mm of the upper limbus (junction of iris and white sclera), this is defined as eyelid ptosis and should be evaluated and addressed by ptosis repair surgery.
- The brow should rest at the level of the superior orbital rim in men, or up to 1cm higher in women, and any inferior displacement is considered brow ptosis and should be evaluated and addressed prior to blepharoplasty.
- The frontalis muscle should be evaluated, as resting forehead creases may indicate a hyperdynamic frontalis compensating for brow ptosis.
- The upper and lower eyelids should then be evaluated for any excess skin and for evidence of fat pad herniation.
- The integrity of the lower lid should be tested for with the lower lid distraction test and the snapback test.
- Lower lid distraction test—performed by pinching the lower eyelid skin and distracting it away from the patient.
- Distraction >6 mm indicates a lax lower lid.
- Snapback test—performed by gently pinching the lower lid skin away from the patient and allowing it to snap back.
- A 3–4 s recoil on the snapback test indicates poor ability to recoil.
- The lid-cheek junction, aka the tear trough or nasojugal groove, should be evaluated.
- A loss of midface or mid-cheek volume in combination with herniating orbital fat can result in the appearance of "bags under the eyes," commonly known as the tear trough deformity [8].

- The midface should also be evaluated in profile view for the position of the malar eminence relative to the eye; if it is posterior, it is considered a negative vector and a higher risk for ectropion.
  - Ectropion is an outward contracture of the lower eyelid with increased scleral show and is one of the primary concerns to avoid when performing a lower blepharoplasty.
- Lastly, a visual field test should be performed and documented prior to any periorbital procedures.

Treatment (Fig. 42.1)

Upper Eyelid Procedures

- Patient should be evaluated and treated according to the findings of their upper eyelid.
- Excess skin, also known as dermatochalasis, is treated with a skin-only excision.
- Some surgeons will also take a strip of orbicularis muscle, particularly if it is bulky or hypertrophic.
- If the patient demonstrates any fat herniation of the medial or central fat pads, a partial fat pad excision can be performed—care must be taken not to hollow out the upper eyelid.

Lower Eyelid Procedures

- The lower eyelid can be approached through a subciliary skin incision just below the lash margin or through a transconjunctival incision on the inside of the eyelid.
- A transconjunctival incision is made in the conjunctivae of the lower eyelid and carries a lower risk for ectropion.
- Through either of these incisions, the lower eyelid fat pads can be accessed.

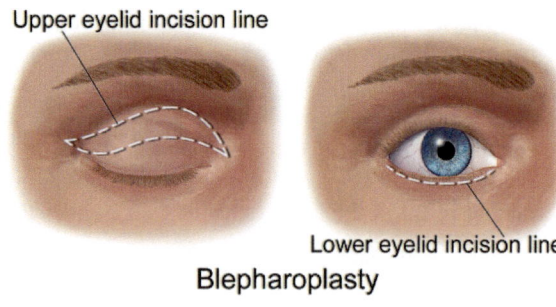

Fig. 42.1 Common incisions for upper and lower blepharoplasty

- If there is herniation or bulging of these fat pads, a fat resection or fat repositioning can be performed [6, 7].
- In the case of a patient with a tear trough deformity, the orbicularis muscle is dissected off the orbital septum, the tear trough ligament (orbitomalar ligament) is released so the fat can be repositioned or resected to alleviate the deformity [8].
- If the lower lid has excess skin or dermatochalasis, the skin can be excised as well.
    - In a subcilliary approach, the skin is excised directly incorporating the subciliary incision.
    - In a transconjunctival approach, the skin can be excised via a separate incision subciliary incision.

Adjunct Procedures

Canthal Procedures

- Patients with a lax lower lid defined by >6 mm distraction or a snapback test that reveals poor recoil may benefit from a canthal procedure to prevent ectropion.
- Additionally, a negative vector may benefit from increased suspension.

Canthoplasty

- A canthopexy allows tightening of the lower lid to minimize the risk of scleral show.
- This can be performed through the lateral aspect of an upper eyelid blepharoplasty incision.
- Dissection is carried through the orbicularis down to the lateral orbital rim.
- A suture, often double armed, is passed through the lateral canthal tendon and secured to the periosteum of the orbital rim.
- Alternatively, the lateral canthal tendon can be cut and resuspended—this is often reserved for cases of severe lower lid laxity [7].

Chemical Peels

- In patients with minimal skin laxity of the lower eyelid, a chemical peel can be a powerful adjunct, helping rejuvenate the lower eyelid skin.

Complications

Lagophthalmos

- Lagophthalmos is defined as the incomplete closure of the eyelids.
- An excessive skin resection of the upper eyelid can cause lagophthalmos and should be avoided at all costs
    - If it does occur, it often improves with symptom management (lubricating eye drops) and massage and time.

Chemosis

- Edema of the conjunctivae is known as chemosis and can occur in the postoperative period.
- Treatment consists of lubrication with ophthalmic drops or ointment.

Ectropion

- Ectropion is an eversion of the lower eyelid, more common with transcutaneous approaches versus transconjunctival approaches.
- Treatment in the postoperative period involves lid massage and lubricating drops.
- If no improvement after 6 months, patients require operative intervention.

Retrobulbar Hematoma

- A retrobulbar hematoma is a progressive collection of blood in the retrobulbar space (behind the eye).
- This complication is considered an emergency as the pressure can compress the optic nerve and result in blindness.
- Patients will present with pain, proptosis, and periorbital ecchymosis.
- Treatment consists of performing a lateral canthotomy, which can be done at bedside to decompresses the orbit and relieve the pressure, followed by hematoma evacuation [9].

References

1. Chang DS, Janis JE, Garvey PB. Chapter 8. Basics of microsurgery. In: Janis J, editor. Essentials of plastic surgery. St. Louis: Quality Medical Publishing; 2014.
2. Neligan P. Chapter 8. Blepharoplasty. In: Plastic surgery, vol. 2. London: Elsevier; 2018.
3. Cohen AJ, Nguyen Burkat C. Oculofacial, orbital, and lacrimal surgery. Cham: Springer; 2019.
4. Codner MA, Kikkawa DO, Korn BS, Pacella SJ. Blepharoplasty and brow lift. Plast Reconstr Surg. 2010;126(1):1e–17e.
5. Oh S-R, Chokthaweesak W, Annunziata CC, Priel A, Korn BS, Kikkawa DO. Analysis of eyelid fat pad changes with aging. Ophthalmic Plast Reconstr Surg. 2011;27(5):348–51.
6. Goldberg RA. Transconjunctival orbital fat repositioning: transposition of orbital fat pedicles into a subperiosteal pocket. Plast Reconstr Surg. 2000;105(2):743–51.
7. Fagien S. Algorithm for canthoplasty: the lateral retinacular suspension: a simplified suture canthopexy. Plast Reconstr Surg. 1999;103(7):2042–53.
8. Wong C-H, Hsieh MKH, Mendelson B. The tear trough ligament. Plast Reconstr Surg. 2012;129(6):1392–402.
9. Friedland JA, Lalonde DH, Rohrich RJ. An evidence-based approach to blepharoplasty. Plast Reconstr Surg. 2010;126(6):2222–9.

Chapter 43
Brow Lift

Irene A. Chang and Michael W. Wells

Introduction

The surgical approach to brow lift has changed and evolved in the past several decades. Effective rejuvenation of the upper face results from effective brow repositioning and maintenance of the brow shape. Currently, there are many well-described surgical approaches to address brow aesthetics, with benefits and limitations to each technique.

Anatomy

Musculature

- Frontalis muscle
  - Origin: galea aponeurotica
  - Insertion: supraorbital dermis by interdigitating with orbicularis oculi
    - Loose connective tissue underneath the frontalis allows for movement
    - Muscular and periosteal adhesions limit brow movement (important in surgical release)

I. A. Chang (✉)
Division of Plastic and Reconstructive Surgery, UC Davis, Sacramento, CA, USA
e-mail: irechang@health.ucdavis.edu

M. W. Wells
Division of Plastic and Reconstructive Surgery, UCLA, Los Angeles, CA, USA

- Innervation: temporal (more commonly referred to as "frontal") branch of the facial nerve
- Action: elevates the brow; creates transverse forehead rhytids
- Galea aponeurosis: extends to the periosteum at the superior orbital rim; encapsulates the frontalis

- Corrugator supercilii muscle
  - Paired small, pyramidal muscles
  - Medial to the eyebrow, deep to the frontalis, and superior to the orbicularis oculi
  - Transverse head
    - Origin: superomedial orbital rim
    - Insertion: dermis superior to medial eyebrow
    - Innervation: temporal (Frontal) branch of the facial nerve
    - Action: moves the brow medially; creates oblique and vertical glabellar lines
  - Oblique head
    - Origin: superomedial orbital rim
    - Insertion: medial eyebrow dermis
    - Innervation: zygomatic branches of the facial nerve
    - Action: depresses brow; creates oblique glabellar lines
  - Depressor supercilii muscle
    - Deep to the corrugator supercilii; facilitates similar action as the oblique head of the corrugator supercilii
    - Origin: superomedial orbital rim
    - Insertion: medial eyebrow dermis
    - Innervation: zygomatic vs temporal branches of the facial nerve
    - Action: Depresses brow; creates oblique glabellar lines

- Procerus muscle
  - Small, triangular muscle in the glabella
  - Origin: nasal bone, superior lateral nasal cartilage
  - Insertion: medial eyebrow dermis, occipitofrontalis muscle
  - Innervation: zygomatic vs temporal branches of the facial nerve
  - Action: depresses brow; creates oblique glabellar and transverse nasal root lines

- Orbicularis oculi
  - Innervated by the zygomatic branch of facial nerve.
  - Medial orbital portion causes medial brow depression.
    - Insignificant contributor to glabellar rhytids
  - Lateral orbital portion can cause lateral brow depression.
    - Creates lateral orbital rhytids (crow's feet) with smiling

Innervation

- Motor
  - Temporal branches of the facial nerve
    - Located underneath the temporoparietal fascia (superficial temporal fascia, continuation of galea and SMAS in zygomatic region) 1 cm inferior and lateral to the sentinel vein.
    - Track path by Pitanguy's line: 1 cm inferior to tragus to 1.5 cm above the lateral brow.
    - Crosses over the zygomatic arch at its middle third, just superficial to the periosteum, and continues superiorly to run on the underside of the TPF, a location for injury as it is more superficial here.
    - Avoidance of excessive upward traction and cautery in this region during coronal and endoscopic dissection will lessen the risk of injury to the nerve branches.
- Sensory (Branches of V1)
  - Zygomaticotemporal nerve
  - Supratrochlear nerve [1]
    - Exits the orbit medially and arborizes
    - Enters the corrugator and then the frontalis to supply sensation to the forehead
  - Supraorbital nerve [2, 3]
    - Exits through the foramen lateral to the supratrochlear nerve
    - Superficial branch: enters frontalis above the orbital rim, supplies the forehead
    - Deep branch: travels laterally just medial to the temporal crest; supplies the scalp posterior to the hairline
      - Transection with subgaleal dissection and coronal incisions may cause postoperative scalp paresthesia [2].

Major Vessels

- Sentinel Vein.
  - Medial of two zygomaticotemporal communicating veins (between superficial and deep systems) [4].
  - 1.5 cm above and lateral to the lateral canthus.
  - Temporal branch of the facial nerve is about 1 cm above the vein.
- Supraorbital and supratrochlear vessels travel with their nerves.

Brow Retaining Ligaments

- Orbital ligament: fibrous sheath connecting the periosteum of the orbital rim and the superficial temporal fascia to the lateral canthus [5]
- Temporal and supraorbital ligamentous adhesions, lateral brow and lateral orbital thickening of the periorbital septum: Periorbital attachments released for brow elevation [6]
  - The sentinel vein is a landmark for the temporal line of fusion, which is released to allow brow elevation.
- Brow-retaining ligament and upper lid-retaining ligament: zones of adhesion from bone to skin that are released for brow elevation [7]

Preoperative Evaluation

- Brow shape and position
- Rhytids
  - Transverse and vertical
  - Present at rest or with animation
    - Deep static rhytids may require extensive subcutaneous dissection.
- Skin quality and color
  - Dyschromia and skin texture influence the surgical result.
  - Adjunctive skin care should be considered.
- Measurement Guidelines
  - Anterior hairline to brow: typically about 5-6 cm in women; 7-8 cm in men.
  - Eyebrow position at lateral limbus: on orbital rim in men; 1 cm above orbital rim in women.

- Medial brow club-shaped and lateral brow tapers; ends lie at approximately the same level, but the lateral end may be slightly elevated.
- Gentle arch: peak at junction of the medial two-thirds and lateral one-third, lying halfway between the lateral limbus and the lateral canthus
- Medial brow: lies in a vertical line with the medial orbital fissure and the alar base
- Lateral brow: lies on the oblique line from the alar base through the lateral orbital fissure
- In midpupillary line

  - Anterior hairline to brow: 5–6 cm in women
  - Brow to superior orbital rim: 1 cm (in women)
  - Brow to supratarsal crease: 1.6 cm
  - Brow to midpupil: 2.5 cm

Indications and Patient Assessment

- Brow ptosis
- Deep rhytids and/or furrows traversing the forehead, glabella, and/or nasal radix
- The appearance of a heavy or redundant forehead or temporal skin
- Pseudo-blepharoptosis and/or visual field restriction
- Integrity of lateral canthal support, lid tone, and lid position
- Upper lid position

Operative Approaches

Coronal [8]

- Universal option, fallen out of favor because of the extent of dissection and the ability to achieve similar results with less invasive techniques.
- Incision can be beveled to allow hair to grow through the scar.
- Coronal, modified coronal, or anterior hairline incision.
- Incision placed at least 3 cm posterior to hairline for better scar camouflage.
- Useful for low hairline because excised skin is hair bearing: 1.5 mm of anterior hairline retrodisplacement required for every 1 mm of eyebrow elevation.

Risks of scarring, alopecia, numbness, and overcorrection. Poor choice for bald individuals or high hairline.

Anterior Hairline Incision

- Useful if hairline is high (hairline on oblique portion of forehead from lateral view)
- Incision 1–2 mm posterior to hairline
- Risk of scar visibility
- Greater scalp excision performed laterally to preferentially correct lateral brow descent

Endoscopic

- Several incisions placed inconspicuously just posterior to the hairline to optimize traction on the scalp and forehead
- Needs adequate release of periorbital septa and adhesions
- Less invasive method
- Less scarring, numbness, patient acceptance, and edema
- Challenging: high hairline or acutely sloped forehead

Lateral Temporal [3]

- Limited extension of a traditional facelift incision over temporalis muscle
  - More medial places supraorbital nerve at risk
  - Dissection plane above deep temporal fascia to prevent temporal nerve injury
- Corrects lateral orbital hooding that may not be corrected with upper blepharoplasty alone
- May be performed in conjunction with or independent of the endoscopic lift

Transpalpebral/Transblepharoplasty

- Lateral brow tacking to periosteum or deep temporal fascia to obtain a mild lateral lift
- Internal browpexy for stabilization of the lateral brow and excision of the corrugator muscles to treat glabellar rhytids
- Limits scars to the blepharoplasty incision alone
- Corrects lateral orbital hooding that may not be corrected with upper blepharoplasty alone

Direct

- Useful in men with thick skin, deep rhytids to conceal the scar, or those with alopecia
- Supraciliary
  - Removal of the ellipse of skin and subcutaneous tissue only at the supraorbital rim to conceal the scar above the eyebrow
- Midbrow
  - Removal of midforehead skin strip to conceal incision in transverse rhytid
  - Advances the hairline downward

Plane of Dissection

- Subcutaneous
  - Preserves posterior scalp sensation by avoiding the deep supraorbital branch
  - Useful for improving deep transverse rhytids by disconnecting dermal adhesions
  - Decreases flap vascularity and can be associated with increased wound complications
  - Tedious dissection
  - Difficult to perform medial brow depressor muscle excision
- Subgaleal
  - Rapid, easy dissection.
  - Allows direct excision or scoring of muscle.
  - Some surgeons argue that fixation of the galea to the periosteum is quicker than periosteum to bone, which may improve the durability of the lift.
  - Risk of injuring the temporal nerve as it becomes superficial.
- Subperiosteal
  - Requires release of arcus marginalis for effective lift.
  - Should be avoided in the medial brow area if medial brow elevation is not desired.
  - Some surgeons believe it provides a more sustained lift [9].
- Biplanar
  - Subcutaneous with endoscopic subperiosteal approach
  - Improves forehead rhytids with suprabrow muscle excision

Muscle Weakening

- Direct muscle excision
    - Removal of the corrugators and portions of frontalis
        - Must preserve sufficient muscle to maintain brow animation
    - Fat grafting to the glabella after corrugator removal corrects depression deformities [10].
- Muscle scoring
    - Frontalis, corrugators, and lateral orbicularis
- Chemical paralysis with botulinum toxin
    - Paralysis of frontalis can result in worsening of brow ptosis, although can correct dynamic rhytids

Complications

- Sensory nerve deficits: due to injury of the supraorbital or supratrochlear nerves; requires careful preservation during corrugator excision.
- Posterior scalp dysesthesias: from the transection of the deep branch of the supraorbital nerve.
- Frontalis muscle paralysis: from frontal branch injury in temporal dissection.
- Skin necrosis: from excessive tension.
- Alopecia: from excessive tension or thermal injury; keep anterior hairline incision 1–2 mm posterior to hairline to prevent damage to anterior hair follicles; bevel and zigzag coronal incision to minimize disruption of hair follicles.
- Infection.
- Hematoma and bleeding.
- Abnormal hair part or visible scar: excessive tension.
- Chronic pain: supraorbital nerve dysesthesias; more likely if history of migraines.
- Permanent overcorrection: from traction and excessive scalp excision.
- Abnormal soft tissue contour: can occur with muscle excision.
- Asymmetry, poor cosmesis, or lateral displacement of brow: excessive corrugator excision.
- Dimpling.

Conflicts of Interest All Authors have no conflicts of interest or sources of funding to disclose

References

1. Janis JE, et al. Anatomy of the supratrochlear nerve: implications for the surgical treatment of migraine headaches. Plast Reconstr Surg. 2013;131(4):743–50.
2. Knize DM. Reassessment of the coronal incision and subgaleal dissection for foreheadplasty. Plast Reconstr Surg. 1998;102(2):478–89; discussion 490–2.
3. Janis JE, et al. The anatomy of the corrugator supercilii muscle: part II. Supraorbital nerve branching patterns. Plast Reconstr Surg. 2008;121(1):233–40.
4. Nahai F. The art of aesthetic surgery: principles & techniques. St. Louis: Quality Medical Publishing; 2005.
5. Knize DM. Limited-incision forehead lift for eyebrow elevation to enhance upper blepharoplasty. Plast Reconstr Surg. 1996;97(7):1334–42.
6. Moss CJ, Mendelson BC, Taylor GI. Surgical anatomy of the ligamentous attachments in the temple and periorbital regions. Plast Reconstr Surg. 2000;105(4):1475–90.
7. Knize DM. Anatomic concepts for brow lift procedures. Plast Reconstr Surg. 2009;124(6):2118–26.
8. Ellenbogen R. Transcoronal eyebrow lift with concomitant upper blepharoplasty. Plast Reconstr Surg. 1983;71(4):490–9.
9. Troilius C. A comparison between subgaleal and subperiosteal brow lifts. Plast Reconstr Surg. 1999;104(4):1079–90; discussion 1091–2.
10. Guyuron B, Knize DM. Corrugator supercilii resection through blepharoplasty incision. Plast Reconstr Surg. 2001;107(2):606–7.

Chapter 44
Botox/Filler

Kaylee B. Scott and Laurel D. Ormiston

Botox

Introduction

- Botulinum neurotoxin functions by blocking the presynaptic release of acetylcholine at the neuromuscular junction, inhibiting the action of the corresponding muscle [1].
  - Botox is used to turn a muscle or function "off"—any condition caused by hyperstimulation can be treated with botulinum toxin.
- The most common formulations of botulinum toxin, approved by the US Food and Drug Administration, are type A, which include onabotulinumtoxinA (Botox), abobotulinumtoxinA (Dysport), and incobotulinumtoxinA (Xeomin).
- Botulinum toxin is commonly used for facial rejuvenation, specifically for the treatment of dynamic rhytides, but has many other off-label uses (Table 44.1).
- These products are diluted with sterile saline prior to use. Dilution varies by specific product and can be adjusted depending on the desired concentration (Table 44.2).
- The decision to use one product or another is typically related to practitioner preference and product cost.

Table 44.1 FDA approvals granted to commercially available type A botulinum toxins [2–4]

Indication	FDA approval		
	Botox	Dysport	Xeomin
Moderate to severe glabellar lines	✔	✔	✔
Moderate to severe lateral canthal lines	✔		
Chronic migraine	✔		
Cervical dystonia	✔	✔	✔
Blepharospasm	✔		✔[a]
Strabismus	✔		
Chronic sialorrhea			✔
Upper limb spasticity	✔	✔	✔
Severe primary axillary hyperhidrosis	✔		
Neurogenic detrusor overactivity	✔		
Lower limb spasticity		✔	

[a]With prior Botox treatment

Table 44.2 Sample dilutions for selected type A botulinum toxins

Product	Volume of diluent per vial	Resulting dose units per 0.1 mL
Botox	2.5 mL per 100 U vial	4 Units
Dysport	2.5 mL per 300 U vial	12 Units
Xeomin	2.5 mL per 100 U vial	4 Units

0.9% sodium chloride diluent is recommended for reconstitution. Resulting dose units can be altered by using alternative amounts of diluent [2–4]

- These products differ in their relative strengths [5]:
    - 1 U of Botox is equivalent to 2–3 U of Dysport (1:2 or 1:3)
    - 1 U of Botox is equivalent to 1 U of Xeomin (1:1)
- Strength of the product will also vary by treatment area, technique, and dilution.
- Dysport may have a wider area of diffusion than Botox and faster onset as well [6].

Patient Evaluation

- When evaluating the patient, it is important to gather a history of previous treatments, allergic reactions, and history of neuromuscular disease and discuss goals and desires.
- Botulinum toxin is considered a class C drug in pregnancy; thus, it may be preferential to delay treatment until after birth [2–4].

- The patient seeking treatment of facial rhytides should be examined in an upright position, noting the position of the brow and eyes both at rest and when instructed to frown.

Common Uses

Forehead and Glabellar Lines

- Elevation of the brow through the action of the frontalis muscle contributes to the development of transverse forehead lines.
- Activity of the corrugators and procerus muscles moves the brow inferiorly, contributing to vertical/oblique (corrugator), transverse (procerus) lines.
  - Orbicualris oculi has some contribution but often is not treated for this indication.
- These areas are typically treated as a functional unit, as their actions are antagonistic. Treatment of the frontalis without addressing muscles of the glabellar region may result in unwanted brow ptosis, while treatment of the glabellar muscles without treatment of the frontalis may result in a surprised or quizzical expression, especially if the frontalis is not treated laterally [1].
- Avoid injection into the levator palpebrae superioris when treating the glabellar region, which results in eyelid ptosis. Injection should occur at least 1 cm above the brow to avoid this complication (Fig. 44.1).

Lateral Canthal Lines (Crow's Feet)

- Contraction of the lateral aspect of orbicularis oculi contributes to the formation of "crow's feet" or lateral canthal lines.
- Injection should occur in a superficial subdermal plane and should be at least 1.5 cm away from the lateral canthus. Injection in this position prevents diffusion of the product into the extraocular muscles, which could result in diplopia (Fig. 44.1) [7].

Bunny Lines

- Contraction of the nasalis and procerus muscles can produce lines on the side of the nose, which radiate downward, and are coined "bunny lines."
- These can be treated with superficial injections into this area, evenly spaced along the area of contraction (Fig. 44.1).
- Avoid injection and diffusion into muscles which elevate the upper lip which may cause lip drooping [8].

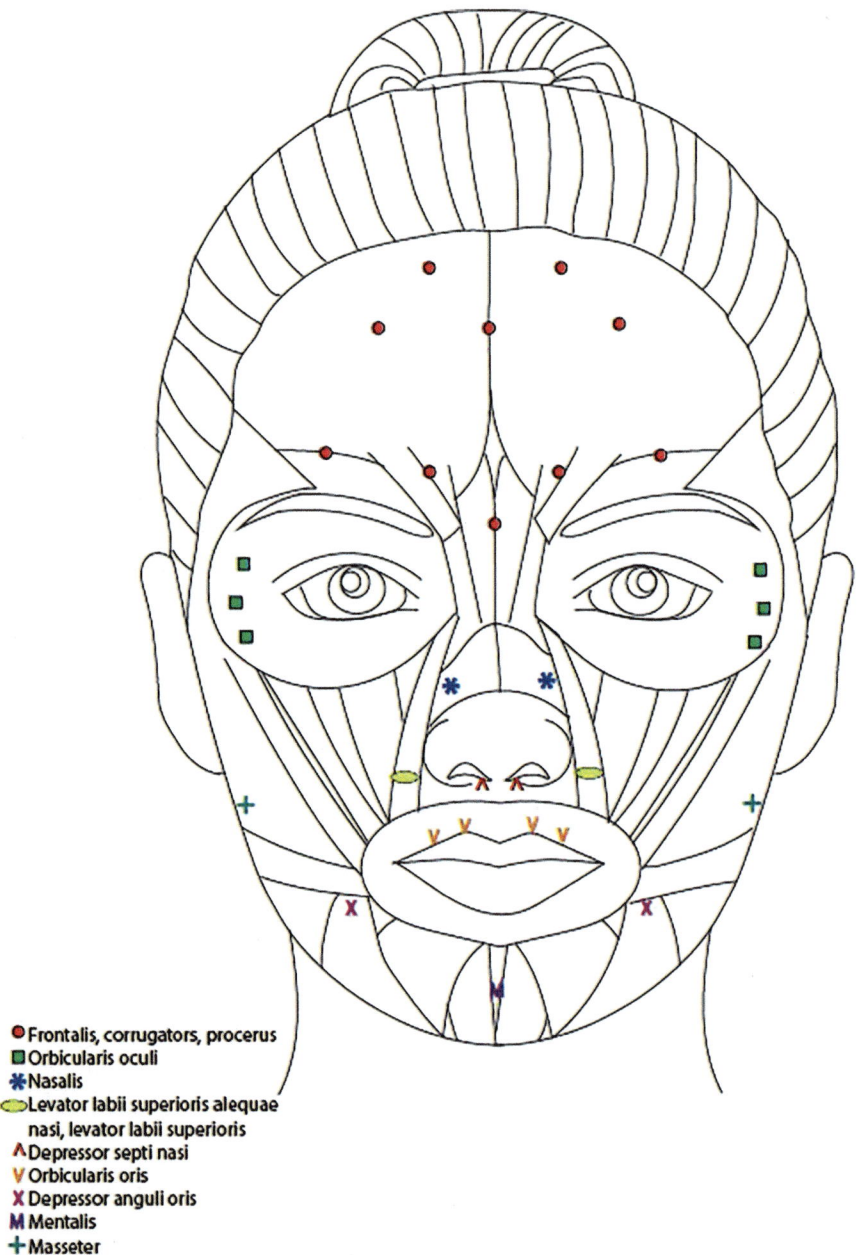

Fig. 44.1 Common injection points for facial rejuvenation through the use of botulinum toxin

Perioral Rhytides (Smoker's Lines)

- Contraction of the orbicularis oris can lead to vertical perioral rhytides ("smoker's lines") along the vermillion border.
- If there is a dynamic component to these rhytides with pursing of the lips, they can be amenable to treatment with botulinum toxin, though treatment with filler or resurfacing (dermabrasion, laser, or peel) is generally recommended for static lines [1].
- Injection occurs along the vermillion border, taking care to avoid the commissures and midline, to avoid drooping and lip flattening (Fig. 44.1) [1, 8].

Melomental Folds (Marionette Lines)

- Melomental folds ("marionette lines") may be in part related to the action of the depressor anguli oris, a muscle used in frowning.
- To target this muscle, injection is recommended 1 cm lateral and inferior to the oral commissures on each side of the mouth (Fig. 44.1) [8, 9].
- Care must be taken to avoid injection into the surrounding muscles, which are important for smile.

Dimpled Chin

- Dimpling of the skin may occur with contraction of the mentalis muscle, which can be treated with injection 1 cm inferior to the mental sulcus, avoiding injection into the orbicularis muscle of the lower lip (Fig. 44.1) [10].

Gummy Smile

- Injection into the levator labii superioris and levator labii superioris alaeque nasi can reduce excessive gingival display when smiling, often referred to as a "gummy smile."
- Injection is recommended adjacent to the alar bases of the nose to target these muscles (Fig. 44.1) [11].

Dynamic Nasal Tip Ptosis

- Action of the depressor septi nasi can cause complaints of nasal tip ptosis and excessive upper lip shortening with smile.
- This can be treated with injection into this muscle, located at the nasal base and/or just beneath the nasal tip (Fig. 44.1) [12, 13].

Masseter

- Patients with masseter hypertrophy may have the appearance of a square face. This is sometimes accompanied with symptoms of headache and teeth grinding or bruxism.
- Botulinum toxin injection can improve both facial appearance and symptoms related to bruxism [14].
- Care must be taken to avoid the parotid gland, marginal mandibular nerve, and other facial nerve branches [15].
- A line drawn from the tragus to the lateral commissure helps to delineate an area of treatment, which should occur inferior to and at approximately the midpoint of this line (Fig. 44.1) [1].

Hyperhidrosis (Excessive Sweating)

- Injection into the axilla, hands, and feet can be used for the treatment of hyperhidrosis of these regions.
- Some authors describe the use of an iodine-starch test to identify the areas of greatest concern. This involves applying iodine to the area, waiting for it to dry, then applying starch. The areas with hyperhidrosis develop a darkened color [16].
- Typical treatment doses include 50 units for axilla, 100 units for the palm, and 150 units for the plantar surface of the foot [16].

Migraine Therapy

- Botulinum toxin has shown promise in the treatment of patients with chronic migraine.
- Though the exact mechanism of effect is unknown, studies have shown improved response compared to placebo at 3 months, as well as improved patient quality of life [17].
- Muscles that are targeted include the corrugators, procerus, frontalis, temporalis, occipitalis, cervical paraspinals, and the trapezius [18].

Vasospastic Disorders

- In conditions such as Raynaud syndrome, perivascular injection in the palm can help reduce vasospasm and allow for good distal blood flow.

Cerebral Palsy

- Patients with spastic cerebral palsy often have botulinum injections to release muscles and prevent contracture-related difficulties.

Facial Palsy

- Patients with unilateral facial palsy can have contralateral Botox to improve dynamic symmetry.

Complications

- Botulinum toxin is generally considered a safe and effective product when properly used; however, complications can occur.
- Side effects of botulinum toxin include brow ptosis, eyelid ptosis, diplopia, ectropion, oral incompetence, drooling, xerostomia, loss of full smile, weakness with chewing, ecchymosis, tenderness, and headache [2–4].
- Function gradually recovers over time; however, temporizing measures can improve patient comfort as the product loses its effect. In the case of eyelid ptosis, alpha-adrenergic ophthalmic solutions, such as apraclonidine, can be prescribed to relieve symptoms by activating the Muller muscle. Lubricating drops can be helpful to protect the eye in cases of ectropion. Sialogogues can help enhance salivary gland function in instances of xerostomia from accidental salivary gland injection [19].
- Other rare though serious complications of botulinum toxin include anaphylactic reaction and diffuse spread of the toxin, resulting in systemic symptoms of botulism. These phenomena are more common when higher doses of the product are administered [19].

Filler

Introduction

- "Filler" encompasses a wide range of autologous, biologic, and synthetic materials used for soft tissue augmentation.
- Autologous materials include fat, dermis, fascia, cartilage, and tissue culture products.
- Biologic fillers include hyaluronic acid (Restylane, Juvederm, Perlane, Belotero Balance) and collagen products. These are semi-permanent.

- Semi-permanent synthetic fillers include calcium hydroxyapatite (Radiesse) and poly-L-lactic acid (Sculptra).
- Polytetrafluoroethylene and polymethylmethacrylate are synthetic permanent fillers.
- Physical properties that must be considered when selecting a filler include elasticity, viscosity, particle size, degree of cross-linking (HA fillers), and concentration.
- Particle size is an important consideration when determining injection depth—in general, products with smaller particles can be injected more superficially, while those with larger particles are injected into deeper layers of the soft tissue [20, 21].
- Fillers are generally FDA-approved for injection in the cheeks, lips, and lower face.

Injection Technique

- Aspiration before product injection is recommended to avoid intravascular injection, which can lead to soft tissue necrosis and other severe complications.
- Injection into more superficial layers is typically done with a fanning technique to evenly disperse the product, while deeper injection into subcutaneous or super-periosteal planes can be done with layering [20].
- Local anesthetic nerve blocks can increase patient comfort during injection.
- If lumps or nodules are appreciated at the time of injection, the product should be massaged to evenly disperse.
- Injection of HA filler too superficially can lead to bluish discoloration of the skin, referred to as the Tyndall effect.

Common Uses

Lip Augmentation

- Filler can be used to create fuller, more symmetric, and youthful-appearing lips in the appropriate patient.
- An infraorbital and mental nerve block can be performed prior to injection.
- Injection into the perioral deep dermal or intradermal plane at the vermillion border and philtral columns can improve the appearance of vertical perioral rhytides [20].
- Injection into a plane superficial to the orbicularis oris can also be performed for the creation of fuller lips [20].

Malar Augmentation

- Malar augmentation with filler can be used to combat midfacial volume loss, which occurs with aging.
- Injection is performed in the supraperiosteal plane, using a stacking technique [20].
- It is important to avoid the infraorbital nerve, located about 1 cm below the inferior orbital rim, between the medial third and central portion of the rim [22].

Nasolabial Folds

- Fillers can be used to soften prominent nasolabial folds, a consequence of facial aging and loss of malar volume.
    - Generally, some degree of nasolabial fold is present during animation; the injector must evaluate whether the deformity is static or dynamic.
- Injection should occur medial to the fold, and with a goal of softening rather than complete effacement, in the superficial or deep subcutaneous plane [20].

Tear Trough

- Midfacial aging can result in periorbital fat atrophy and laxity of the orbicularis retaining ligament.
- Injection occurs in the supraperiosteal plane at the medial orbital rim to correct this deformity [20].
- Care should be taken to aspirate prior to injection to avoid intravascular injection and occlusion.

Liquid Rhinoplasty

- Minor contour corrections of the nasal structure can be addressed with fillers rather than traditional rhinoplasty.

Additional Uses

- Filler can also be used to augment the appearance of temple hollowing, which can occur with aging as well as HIV lipodystrophy from protease inhibitors [23].
- Filler has demonstrated utility in treating and/or temporizing lagophthalmos, eyelid malposition, and orbital volume loss [24].

Complications

- Intravascular injection can lead to focal soft tissue necrosis.
- It is thought that retrograde flow after intravascular injection can result in filler material entering the retinal artery, which can cause vision loss [25].
- Other complications include overcorrection, asymmetry, nodules, ecchymosis, dermatitis, and infection [25].
- Intralesional hyaluronidase is used to correct asymmetries and in instances of vascular compromise due to HA filler use.
- Retrobulbar injection of hyaluronidase can be used in attempt to reverse iatrogenic filler blindness.

References

1. Janes LE, Connor LM, Moradi A, Alghoul M. Current use of cosmetic toxins to improve facial aesthetics. Plast Reconstr Surg. 2021;147(4):644e–57e.
2. Allergan I. Highlights of prescribing information: BOTOX (onabotulinumtoxinA). Allergan, Inc; 2010. Available from: https://www.accessdata.fda.gov/drugsatfda_docs/label/2011/103000s5236lbl.pdf.
3. Ipsen Biopharmaceuticals Inc. Highlights of prescribing information: DYSPORT (abobotulinumtoxinA). Ipsen Biopharmaceuticals, Inc.; 2016. Available from: https://www.accessdata.fda.gov/drugsatfda_docs/label/2016/125274s107lbl.pdf.
4. Merz Pharmaceuticals LLC. Highlights of prescribing information: XEOMIN (incobotulinumtoxinA). Merz Pharmaceuticals; 2019. Available from: https://www.accessdata.fda.gov/drugsatfda_docs/label/2019/125360s074lbl.pdf.
5. Karsai S, Raulin C. Current evidence on the unit equivalence of different botulinum neurotoxin A formulations and recommendations for clinical practice in dermatology. Dermatol Surg. 2009;35(1):1–8.
6. Trindade de Almeida AR, Marques E, de Almeida J, Cunha T, Boraso R. Pilot study comparing the diffusion of two formulations of botulinum toxin type A in patients with forehead hyperhidrosis. Dermatol Surg. 2007;33(1 Spec No.):S37–43.
7. Matarasso SL, Matarasso A. Treatment guidelines for botulinum toxin type A for the periocular region and a report on partial upper lip ptosis following injections to the lateral canthal rhytids. Plast Reconstr Surg. 2001;108(1):208–14; discussion 15–7.
8. Carruthers J, Carruthers A. Aesthetic botulinum A toxin in the mid and lower face and neck. Dermatol Surg. 2003;29(5):468–76.
9. Choi YJ, Kim JS, Gil YC, Phetudom T, Kim HJ, Tansatit T, et al. Anatomical considerations regarding the location and boundary of the depressor anguli oris muscle with reference to botulinum toxin injection. Plast Reconstr Surg. 2014;134(5):917–21.
10. Rohrich RJ, Janis JE, Fagien S, Stuzin JM. The cosmetic use of botulinum toxin. Plast Reconstr Surg. 2003;112(5 Suppl):177S–88S; quiz 88S, 92S; discussion 89S–91S.
11. Suber JS, Dinh TP, Prince MD, Smith PD. OnabotulinumtoxinA for the treatment of a "gummy smile". Aesthet Surg J. 2014;34(3):432–7.
12. Dayan SH, Kempiners JJ. Treatment of the lower third of the nose and dynamic nasal tip ptosis with Botox. Plast Reconstr Surg. 2005;115(6):1784–5.
13. Ghavami A, Janis JE, Guyuron B. Regarding the treatment of dynamic nasal tip ptosis with botulinum toxin A. Plast Reconstr Surg. 2006;118(1):263–4.

14. Wu WT. Botox facial slimming/facial sculpting: the role of botulinum toxin-A in the treatment of hypertrophic masseteric muscle and parotid enlargement to narrow the lower facial width. Facial Plast Surg Clin North Am. 2010;18(1):133–40.
15. Trevidic P, Sykes J, Criollo-Lamilla G. Anatomy of the lower face and botulinum toxin injections. Plast Reconstr Surg. 2015;136(5 Suppl):84S–91S.
16. Freeman MD, Margulies IG, Sanati-Mehrizy P, Burish N, Taub PJ. Nonaesthetic applications for botulinum toxin in plastic surgery. Plast Reconstr Surg. 2020;146(1):157–70.
17. Bruloy E, Sinna R, Grolleau JL, Bout-Roumazeilles A, Berard E, Chaput B. Botulinum toxin versus placebo: a meta-analysis of prophylactic treatment for migraine. Plast Reconstr Surg. 2019;143(1):239–50.
18. Nahabet E, Janis JE, Guyuron B. Neurotoxins: expanding uses of neuromodulators in medicine--headache. Plast Reconstr Surg. 2015;136(5 Suppl):104S–10S.
19. Witmanowski H, Blochowiak K. The whole truth about botulinum toxin – a review. Postepy Dermatol Alergol. 2020;37(6):853–61.
20. Wilson AJ, Taglienti AJ, Chang CS, Low DW, Percec I. Current applications of facial volumization with fillers. Plast Reconstr Surg. 2016;137(5):872e–89e.
21. Attenello NH, Maas CS. Injectable fillers: review of material and properties. Facial Plast Surg. 2015;31(1):29–34.
22. Wilhelmi BJ, Mowlavi A, Neumeister MW, Blackwell SJ. Facial fracture approaches with landmark ratios to predict the location of the infraorbital and supraorbital nerves: an anatomic study. J Craniofac Surg. 2003;14(4):473–7; discussion 8–80.
23. Shuck J, Iorio ML, Hung R, Davison SP. Autologous fat grafting and injectable dermal fillers for human immunodeficiency virus-associated facial lipodystrophy: a comparison of safety, efficacy, and long-term treatment outcomes. Plast Reconstr Surg. 2013;131(3):499–506.
24. Tan P, Kwong TQ, Malhotra R. Non-aesthetic indications for periocular hyaluronic acid filler treatment: a review. Br J Ophthalmol. 2018;102:725–35.
25. Sclafani AP, Fagien S. Treatment of injectable soft tissue filler complications. Dermatol Surg. 2009;35(Suppl 2):1672–80.

Chapter 45
Brazilian Butt Lift

Patrick R. Keller

Overview

- Gluteal augmentation fat grafting (GFG, a.k.a. Brazilian Butt Lift or BBL) involves large volume harvest of subcutaneous fat from undesired areas and subsequent large volume grafting of that fat into the buttocks and thighs to improve aesthetic contours.
- BBL has been reported to have the highest mortality rate of any cosmetic surgical procedure. This is secondary to fatal pulmonary fat embolism (PFE), which results from intramuscular injection combined with inferior gluteal vein injury.
- Multiple task forces have been created to better understand the etiology of PFE in BBL. Their key recommendation is to inject fat only superficially in the subcutaneous plane, and never intramuscularly.
- Poor technique, improper instrumentation, and surgeon fatigue are factors thought to be associated with intramuscular injection.
- Adjunctive ultrasound use is now required by law in some areas.

Anatomy [1–3]

Female Thigh and Buttock Contour

- The thigh-buttock region can be defined using a lateral thigh-to-buttock ratio and a posterior thigh-buttock junction angle (Figs. 45.1 and 45.2).

P. R. Keller (✉)
Department of Plastic and Reconstructive Surgery, Johns Hopkins University School of Medicine, Baltimore, MD, USA
e-mail: patrick.keller@jhmi.edu

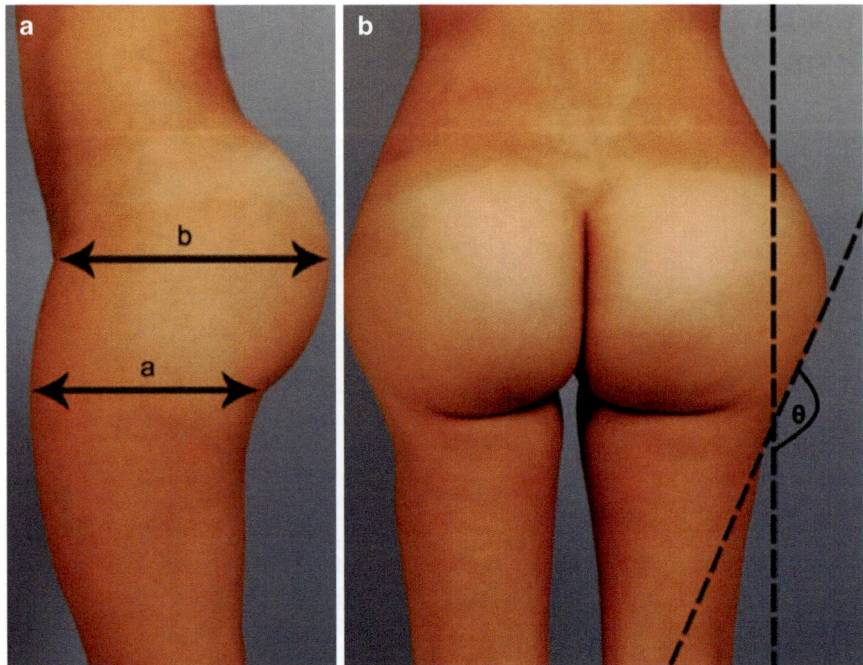

Fig. 45.1 Lateral and posterior views of the thigh and buttock region. Lateral thigh-to-buttock ratio is defined as a/b, where a and b are the horizontal distances at the levels of infragluteal crease and point of maximal buttock projection, respectively. Posterior view shows the thigh-buttock angle (the angle between vertical meridian and an oblique line drawn from the most lateral buttock projection to the thigh-buttock junction). (Taken from Vartanian et al. [1])

- The most attractive posterior thigh-buttock junction angle is 170° and becomes less attractive as the angle becomes more acute.
  - Exception: Those identifying as Middle Eastern felt the angle of 140° most attractive.
- Most attractive lateral thigh-to-buttock ratio is less clear, but the most preferred ratio id 0.8 or 0.6.

Regional Neurovascular Anatomy

- Knowledge of buttock anatomy is critical to avoiding PFE (Fig. 45.3a–c).
- Danger triangle defined by PSIS, greater trochanter, and ischial tuberosity. Injections in this space are at high risk for neurovascular injury and fat embolism (Fig. 45.4).

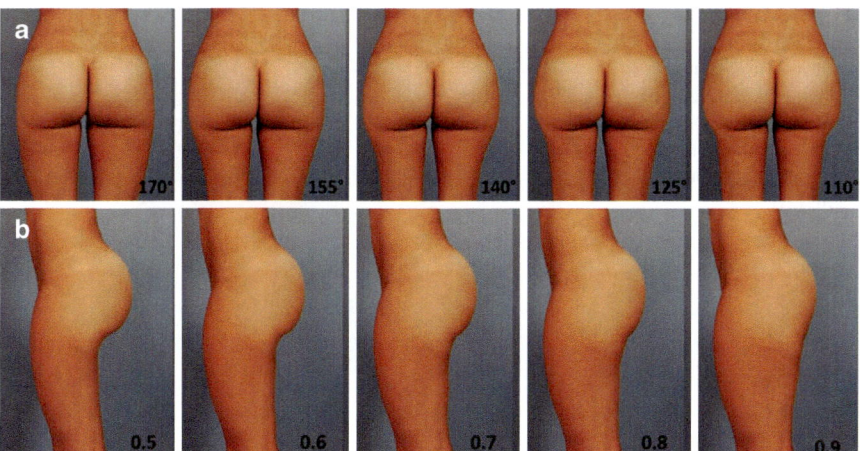

Fig. 45.2 Various lateral thigh-to-buttock ratios and posterior thigh-buttock angles. (Taken from Vartanian et al. [1])

- Superficial muscles: gluteus maximus, medius, and minimus, tensor fascia lata.
- Deep muscles: piriformis, obturator internus, gemellus superior and inferior, quadratus femoris.
- Superior gluteal artery and vein exit the greater sciatic foramen above the piriformis muscle, dividing into superficial and deep branches. Superficial branch passes deep to gluteus maximus, and deep branch passes between gluteus medius and minimus.
- Inferior gluteal artery and vein exits the greater sciatic foramen inferior to piriformis and descends as single trunk deep to gluteus maximus and into the posterior thigh.
- Sciatic nerve exits greater sciatic foramen inferior to piriformis and runs deep to the superficial gluteal muscles.

Fig. 45.3 (**a–c**) Gluteal muscular and neurovascular anatomy. (**a**) Superficial muscles. (**b**) Deep muscles. (**c**) Neurovascular bundles. (Taken from Villanueva et al. [2])

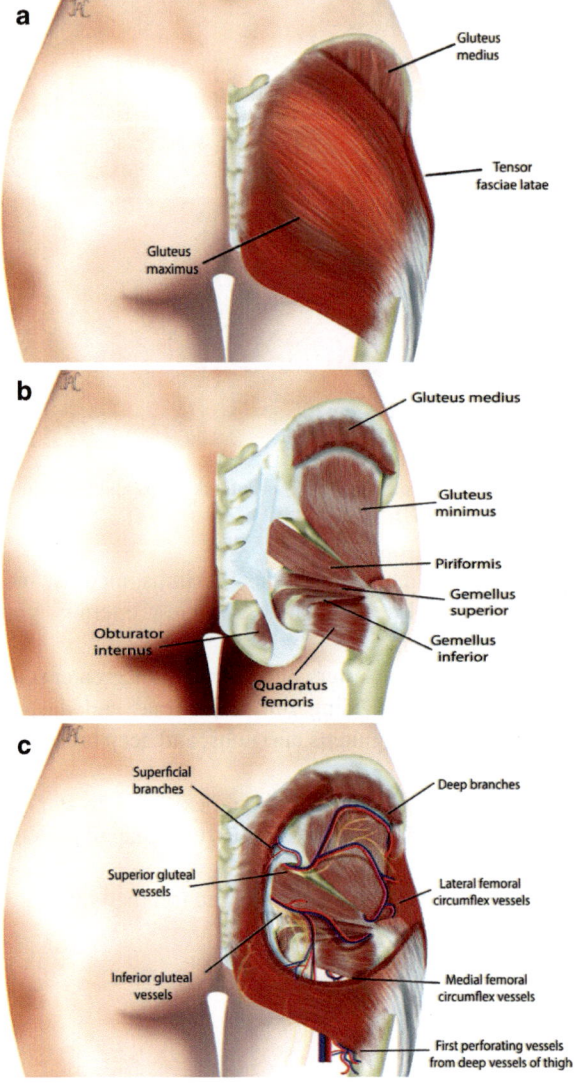

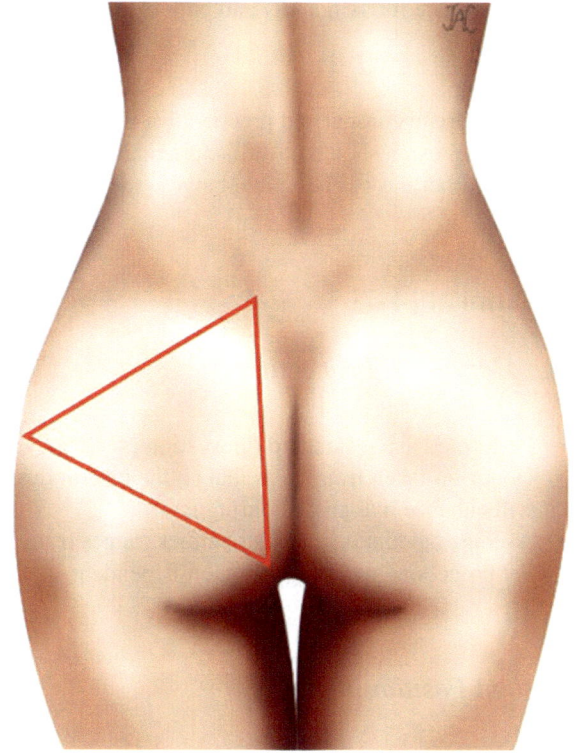

Fig. 45.4 Buttock danger zone. Defined by PSIS, greater trochanter, and ischial tuberosity. (Taken from Villanueva et al. [2])

Evaluation [4]

History

- Patient goals.
- Weight stability.
- History of blood clots, Caprini score.
- Surgical history, anesthetics.
- Current medications.
- Nutritional status.
- Evidence of body dysmorphic disorder.
- Evaluation should include factors related to liposuction (see Chap. 37).

Physical Exam

- Locations of excess fat, with focus on areas bothersome to patient.
- Quality of skin and dermis.

- Evaluate for skin laxity and buttock ptosis.
- BMI.
- Scars.
- Appropriate consent and preoperative photo documentation.
- Physical exam should cover factors related to liposuction, for example, the presence of hernias or abdominal bulges (see Chap. 37).

Treatment [4–7]

Fat Harvest & Processing

- Performed using standard liposuction practices.
- Donor fat taken from areas that (i) the patient desires to be reduced and (ii) that will enhance overall contouring goals.
- Average amount injected per buttock ranges from 500 to 1000 g of processed fat.
- Fat processing method is surgeon-dependent.

Patient Positioning

- Supine, prone with hips flexed, jackknife, and lateral decubitus are commonly used positions.

Injection Techniques

- Critical point: staying superficial reduces the risk of fascial perforation.
- Syringe-based techniques:
  - Utilize the Coleman technique (1 cc syringes) or modified Coleman "large syringe" technique (up to 60 cc syringes).
  - Use handheld syringes loaded with dehydrated fat.
  - Cannula tips are in the 3–4 mm range, typically non-exploded tip, of varying lengths and thicknesses.
  - One hand injects fat in reciprocating axial motion; the other hand palpates exact location of the cannula tip.
  - Cons: increased surgeon fatigue.
- Precise injection technique (PIT)
  - Variation of syringe-based technique

- Injection technique:
  - Visual and palpable verification of the cannula tip just underneath the dermis (with notable pop as going through reticular dermal septae).
  - Microdroplet Coleman technique: retrograde injection of 1–2 cc aliquots, using shorter, 2.4 mm Tulip cannulas.
  - Avoid over-injecting.
  - Keep strict track of the amount injected in each of the four zones (Fig. 45.5).
- Pros: safe, effective. Uses smaller boluses, less fat necrosis, lumps, and bumps.
- Cons: long operative time (6 h).
  - IV sedation used to mitigate increased risks of prolonged general anesthesia (DVT, pulmonary complications, and theoretical increased risk of IGV perforation due to muscle relaxation and venous engorgement).
  - Increased surgeon fatigue.
  - Limited ability to perform combined procedures.

- Expansion vibration lipofilling
  - Injection technique:
    - Extension of the SAFELipo principle. Utilizes power-assisted liposuction (PAL) pump-propulsion mechanics, but the circuit is reversed.
      - Fat lobules, 1–4 mm in diameter, are pushed from the cannister, through the tip, into the subcutaneous space.
      - The vibration of PAL coupled with an exploded tip cannula allows for simultaneous expansion and backfilling with fat in a theoretically homogenous distribution.
    - Cannula: angled, exploded tip, 4–5 mm diameter, 40 cm long.

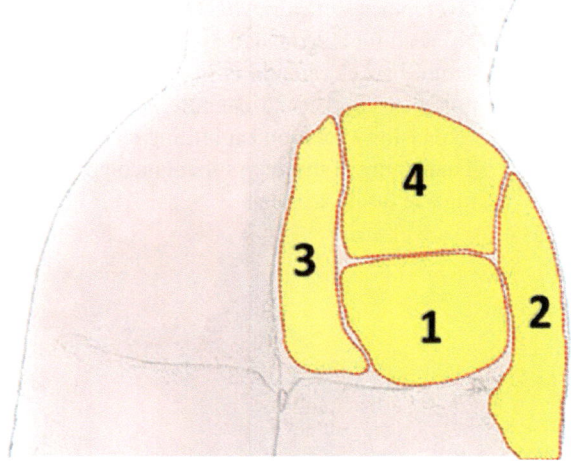

Fig. 45.5 Locations and order of injections using the Precision Injection Technique method. (Taken from Rodriguez et al. [5])

- Pros:
    - Shorter operative time (1–2 h).
    - Decreased surgeon fatigue, potentially allowing for maintained proprioception and increased cannula-tip awareness.
    - Aggressive expansion of subcutaneous spaces allows for greater reshaping of the buttock contour.
- Cons:
    - Grafting larger fat lobules: theoretical increased risk of fat necrosis, lumps, and bumps.
    - Some surgeons believe that exploded tip cannulas increase the risk of tearing of muscle fascia, allowing for migration of fat along pressure gradients.

- Ultrasound-assisted technique
    - Ultrasound can be utilized as an adjunct to any type of cannula-based fat grafting.
    - Injection technique, according to original description:
        - Decanted fat is injected with a 3 mm blunt cannula.
        - Ultrasound probe is held by the assistant, placed on the skin of the gluteal region, and tracks the cannula depth (Fig. 45.6).
        - The real-time image is projected to a screen for the surgeon and assistant to view.
        - Pros: believed to be the safest way to perform BBL.
        - Cons: increased operative time, purchase cost of ultrasound device, need for training on use of ultrasound, and need for an assistant to hold the probe and follow the cannula.
    - (ULTRA) BBL technique:
        - Overcomes some drawbacks of the original ultrasound technique.
        - No need for a dedicated assistant.
        - 4 mm basket cannula is inserted into the correct plane under ultrasound guidance. Probe and cannula are held still, and fat is instilled using the Expansion Vibration Lipofilling technique.
        - Thickening of the deep subcutaneous layer and downward migration of the muscle fascia are seen.

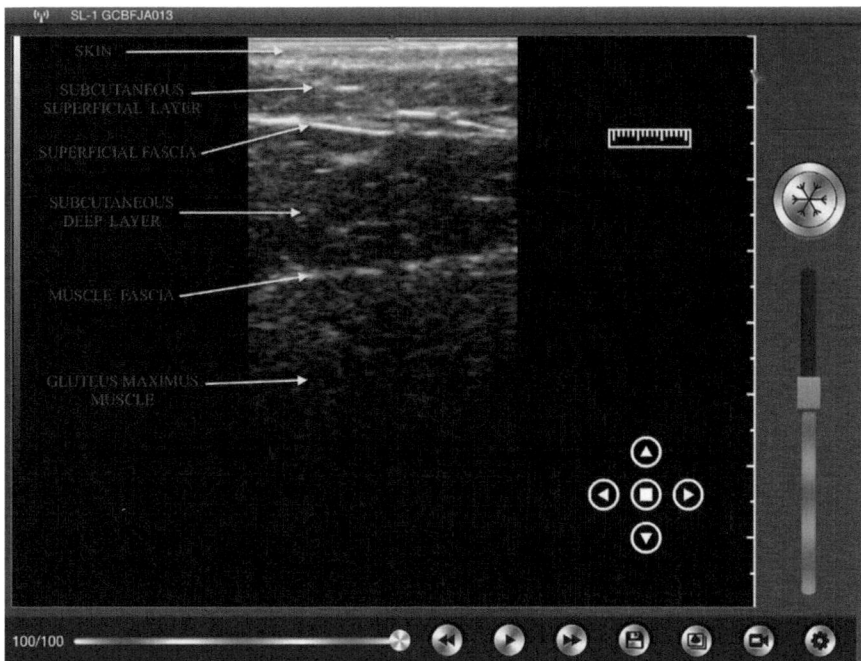

Fig. 45.6 Ultrasound image of the buttock. Layers are: skin, superficial subcutaneous fat, superficial fascia, deep subcutaneous fat, muscle fascia, gluteus maximus muscle. (Taken from Cansancao et al. [7])

Post-Operative Care

- Hydration (inpatient vs outpatient, depending on volume of lipoaspirate)
- Compression garments and foam compression
- No sitting for at least 3 weeks

Outcomes and Complications [2, 4–6]

- BBL mortality rate is as high as 1:3000, the highest of any cosmetic surgery procedure.
- Death is uniformly caused by fatal pulmonary fat embolism.
  - Macro-fat embolism:
    - Characterized by the accumulation of fat in the pulmonary circuit, which causes electromechanical dissociation (EMD). Symptoms include tachycardia, hypoxemia, and hypotension not responsive to pressors or fluids. Death occurs intraoperatively, soon after the onset of EMD.
    - Caused by fat entering the venous circulation in conjunction with injury to the gluteal veins.

- Cannulation injection theory: large vein accidentally cannulated, fat injected.
    - Laceration siphon theory: large vein is accidentally injured or torn, and the high-pressure fat flows into the low-pressure venous system.
  - Micro-fat embolism:
    - Inflammatory condition from free fatty acid damage to pulmonary endothelial cells
    - Onset 24–48 h post-op
    - Range of symptoms: mild dyspnea to ARDS
    - Treatment: supportive care. Possibly: steroids, ethanol, albumin.
  - In all cases of death, fat has been found outside of the subcutaneous plane (i.e., below muscle fascia).
  - There have been many techniques proposed to avoid intramuscular injection and hence PFE. Most techniques focus on ensuring the surgeon has constant knowledge of the exact location of the cannula tip. Some examples:
    - Decrease surgeon fatigue leads to increased proprioception and decreased thenar fatigue and hence increased tip awareness.
    - Use of smaller cannulas and Coleman technique to feel cannula tip pop through reticular fibers in the subdermis.
    - Use ultrasound to visualize the cannula tip.
- Areas of lumpiness and hardness
  - Unclear if mitigated with the use of the Coleman technique
- Contour irregularities, under/overfilling
- Infection/abscess
- Complications associated with liposuction

References

1. Vartanian E, et al. The ideal thigh: a crowdsourcing-based assessment of ideal thigh aesthetic and implications for gluteal fat grafting. Aesthet Surg J. 2018;38:861–9.
2. Villanueva NL, Del Vecchio DA, Afrooz PN, Carboy JA, Rohrich RJ. Staying safe during gluteal fat transplantation. Plast Reconstr Surg. 2018;141:79–86.
3. Turin SY, et al. Gluteal vein anatomy: location, caliber, impact of patient positioning, and implications for fat grafting. Aesthet Surg J. 2020;40:642–9.
4. Del Vecchio D, Kenkel JM. Practice advisory on gluteal fat grafting. Aesthet Surg J. 2022;42:1019–29. https://doi.org/10.1093/asj/sjac082.
5. Rodriguez RL, D'Amico RA, Rubin JP. Gluteal augmentation: avoidance of intramuscular injection using precise superficial fat graft technique. In: Kalaaji A, editor. Plastic and aesthetic regenerative surgery and fat grafting. Springer International Publishing; 2022. p. 1373–84. https://doi.org/10.1007/978-3-030-77455-4_91.
6. Del Vecchio D, Wall S. Expansion vibration lipofilling: a new technique in large-volume fat transplantation. Plast Reconstr Surg. 2018;141:639e–49e.
7. Cansancao AL, Condé-Green A, Vidigal RA, Rodriguez RL, D'Amico RA. Real-time ultrasound–assisted gluteal fat grafting. Plast Reconstr Surg. 2018;142:372–6.

Chapter 46
Hand Anatomy, Function, and Exam

Nirbhay S. Jain

Terminology

- The hand is a unique structure and thus has unique terminology used to describe it.
- Axes are not anterior and posterior but volar (or palmar) and dorsal.
- Lateral structures are described as radial, and medial structures are described as ulnar.
- Metacarpals are numbered from 1 to 5 from radial to ulnar.
- Fingers are described as thumb, index, long (or middle), ring, and small.
  - Shorthand T, IF, LF, RF, and SF.
  - Fingers are never given numbers.
- It is important to understand the language of hand surgery to understand what is occurring during a consultation or an operation.

Anatomy and Function

- General principles
  - The hand surgeon is typically responsible for anything distal to the elbow.
  - The hand is only one part of the whole; understanding the context of the hand anatomy in the greater whole is critical [1].

N. S. Jain (✉)
Division of Plastic Surgery, Department of Surgery, University of California, Los Angeles, Los Angeles, CA, USA
e-mail: nsjain@mednet.ucla.edu

- Form begets function; it is impossible to discuss hand function without knowing the anatomy, and it is impossible to do an exam without knowing function [2, 3].
- Bones
  - Bone and joints form the framework upon which the rest of the hand is structured.
  - Elbow articulation is made of the radial head, the ulnar olecranon, and the humerus.
  - Critical ligament structures include the ulnar collateral ligament.
  - Wrist is composed of several articulations (Fig. 46.1).
    - Proximal: distal radioulnar joint (DRUJ)
      - Made up of the ulnar head, distal radius, and triangular fibrocartilage complex.
      - Allows for pronation/supination of the forearm with the radius rotating around the fixed ulna.
    - Distal
      - Radiocarpal joint: radius interacting with two bones in the proximal row of carpus (lunate, scaphoid).
      - Midcarpal joint: proximal row of carpus (radial to ulnar: scaphoid, lunate, triquetrum, pisiform), which is mobile, interacts with the fixed unit of distal row (trapezium, trapezoid, capitate, hamate).
  - Carpus
    - Two rows: proximal and distal.
    - Proximal is "mobile"; distal is fixed to metacarpals.

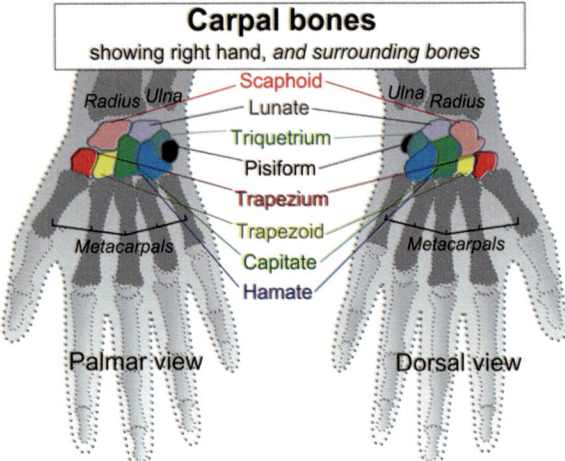

Fig. 46.1 Carpal bones

- Trapezium interacts with the thumb.
- Normal alignment: capitate is collinear with lunate and third metacarpal.
- On XR forms three arcs, known as Gilula's lines (Fig. 46.2).

– Fingers

- Each finger has a metacarpal (numbered 1 through 5).

  – Key insertions

  - 1st metacarpal: Abductor Pollicis Longus (APL), opponens
  - 2nd metacarpal: Extensor Carpi Radialis Longus (ECRL), Flexor Carpi Radialis (FCR)
  - 3rd metacarpal: Extensor Carpi Radialis Brevis (ECRB)
  - 5th metacarpal: Extensor Carpi Ulnaris (ECU), Flexor Carpi Ulnaris (FCU)

- The thumb has two phalanges; the other fingers have three.

  – Phalanges are called proximal, middle, distal, or P1, P2, P3.
  – Thumb only has proximal, distal, or P1, P2.
  – Joint between P1 and P2 is the Proximal Interphalangeal Joint (PIPJ).

Fig. 46.2 Gilula's lines

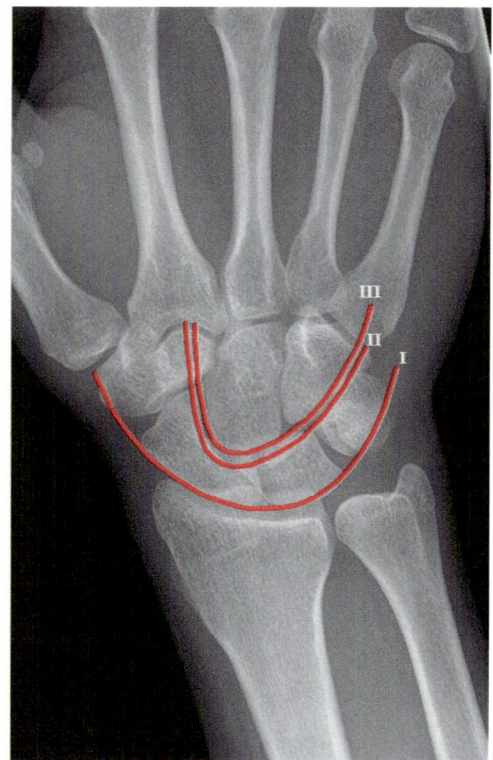

- Joint between P2 and P3 is the Distal Interphalangeal Joint (DIPJ).
- Joint between P1 and P2 in the thumb is the Interphalangeal Joint (IPJ).

- Key ligaments are the ulnar collateral ligament of the thumb and the volar plate.
- Intrinsic plus position:
  - Common position when splinting.
  - Flexion at the metacarpophalangeal joint (MCP) and extension of the interphalangeal joints.
  - Keeps collateral ligaments at the most stretched position and the extensor mechanism lax to prevent contractures when the hand is fixed in this position for a period of time.
- Typical ranges of motion (ROM):
  - MPJ 90° flexion to 30° extension.
  - PIPJ 100° flexion to 0° extension.
  - DIPJ 80° flexion to 0° extension.
  - Wrist 75° flexion to 75° extension.
  - The thumb carpometacarpal joint is a saddle joint that allows for opposition and a high degree of function of the thumb/hand.
- Finger tendon insertions:
  - Flexor
    - Flexor digitorum profundus inserts on P3 and flexes PIPJ and DIPJ.
    - Flexor digitorum superficialis inserts on P2 and flexes PIPJ but not DIPJ.
  - Extensors
    - Extensor tendons divide into the central slip, which inserts on dorsal P2, and the lateral bands that combine with lumbrical and interossei muscle tendons to form the terminal tendon that inserts on P3.

- Vessels
  - Two main blood supplies, ulnar > radial (Fig. 46.3)
    - Radial is typically more dominant to thumb.
  - Forms two main arches in hand, superficial and deep.
  - Dorsal metacarpal arteries form another arch from radial and ulnar and interossei, not needed to repair if cut (redundant).
  - Kaplan's cardinal line.
    - Line formed from the first webspace to the hook of the hamate, path of the superficial palmar arch.
  - Venous drainage is mainly dorsal, deep, and superficial drainage.

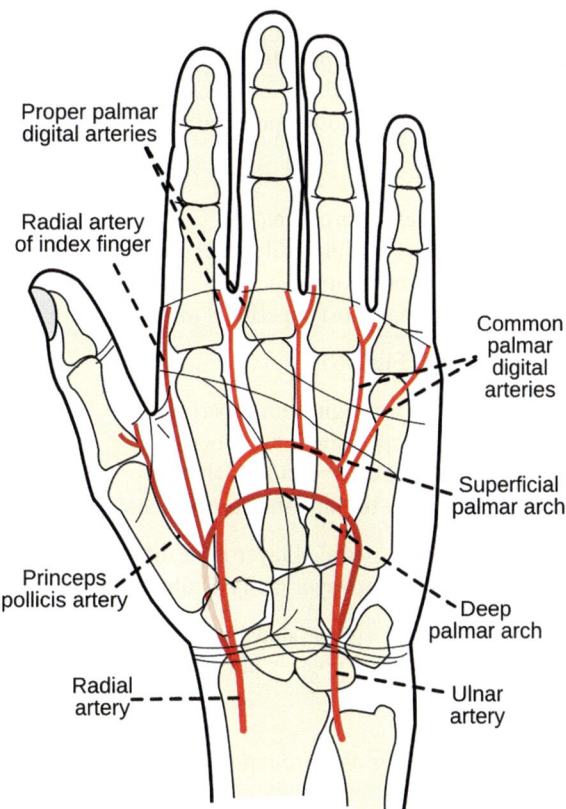

Fig. 46.3 Vascular supply to the hand

- Deep from venae comitantes, superficial from cephalic (radial) and basilic (ulnar).
  - Arteries volar to nerves in palm, dorsal in fingers.
  - Can be examined with Allen's test.
- Muscles of the forearm
  - Five compartments
  - Superficial volar (innervated by median nerve, ulnar for FCU)
    - PT
      - Pronator teres
      - Main role is to pronate the wrist (moves radius around ulna)
    - PL
      - Palmaris longus
      - Absent in about 20% of people
      - Tenses palmar fascia

- FCR
    - Flexor carpi radialis
    - Flexes, radially deviates wrist
    - Radial-most superficial muscle
- FCU
    - Flexor carpi ulnaris
    - Flexes, ulnarly deviates wrist
    - Stronger muscle
    - Ulnar-most superficial muscle
- FDS (Fig. 46.4)
    - Flexor digitorum superficialis
    - Independent muscle bellies
    - Flexes PIP (but not DIP)
    - Runs through the carpal tunnel superficially in two layers
        - Superficial layer is RF/MF ulnar/radial.
        - Deep layer is SF/IF, ulnar/radial.

- Deep Volar (innervated by anterior interosseous nerve; FDP is split in half (radial is AIN, ulnar is ulnar))

    - FDP
        - Flexor digitorum profundus

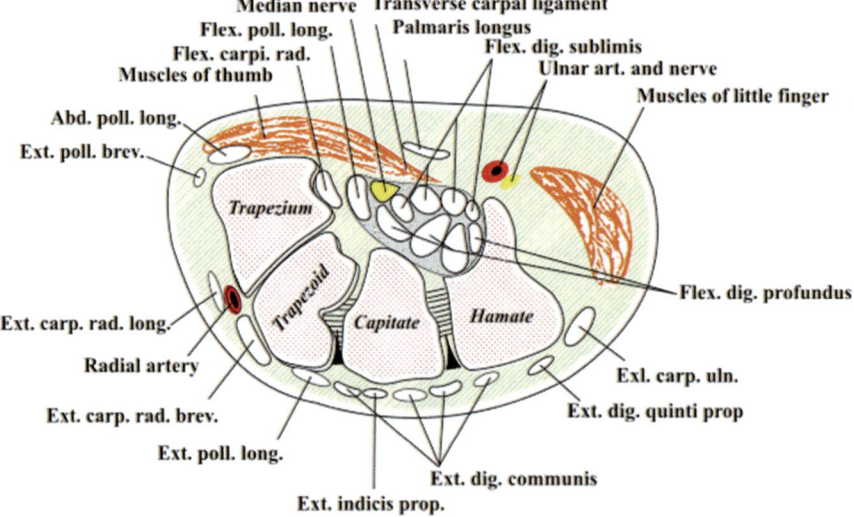

Fig. 46.4 Cross-section of the wrist at the carpal tunnel

- Common muscle belly (all fingers flex together; index sometimes can be separate)
- Flexes DIP (and PIP)
- Runs through carpal tunnel in one layer
- Goes through split in FDS to reach DIP via Camper's chiasm

- FPL
  - Flexor pollicis longus
  - Flexes interphalangeal joint (IP) of thumb
  - Runs through the carpal tunnel
  - Most distal testable muscle

- PQ
  - Pronator quadratus
  - On the radius distally
  - Minor pronator of the wrist

- Mobile Wad (innervated by radial nerve)

  - BR
    - Brachioradialis.
    - Flexes the elbow when the forearm is in neutral.
    - Inserts on distal radius—does not flex/extend wrist.

  - ECRL
    - Extensor carpi radialis longus
    - Radial structure
    - Extends, radially deviates the wrist

  - ECRB
    - Extensor carpi radialis brevis
    - Extends the wrist
    - Central stabilizer of the wrist

- Superficial dorsal (innervated by the posterior interosseous nerve (PIN))

  - EDC
    - Extensor digitorum communis
    - Extends fingers at MCP joints
    - Common muscle belly, conjoined function through junctura

  - ECU
    - Extensor carpi ulnaris
    - Extends wrist, ulnarly deviates

  - EDM

- Extensor digiti minimi
- Extends SF independently of other fingers
- Deep Dorsal (PIN)
  - APL
    - Abductor pollicis longus
    - Abducts the thumb at the metacarpal
  - EPB
    - Extensor pollicis brevis
    - Extends thumb at P1
  - EPL
    - Extensor pollicis longus
    - Extends thumb at P2
  - EIP
    - Extensor indicis proprius.
    - Extends the index independently.
    - Ulnar to EDC tendon (can be used to identify EIP vs EDC during surgery).
    - Most distal muscle (can be used to identify EIP vs EDC during surgery).
    - Redundancy of EIP and EDC to index allows sacrifice of EIP for tendon transfers (see Chap. 54).
- Muscles of the Hand (Intrinsic)
  - Lumbricals [4, 5]
    - Originate on the radial side of the FDP tendons
    - Innervated by the corresponding FDP nerve (median 1 and 2, ulnar 3 and 4)
    - Provide flexion at MCP, extension of PIPJ and DIPJ
  - Thenar Muscles
    - ADP
      - Adductor pollicis
      - Ulnar innervated (most distal ulnar muscle)
      - Adducts thumb (key pinch)
    - OP, FPB, APB
      - Opponens pollicis, flexor pollicis brevis, abductor pollicis brevis
      - Thenar muscles, innervated by the median nerve directly (most distal)
      - FPB with dual innervation from the ulnar nerve
      - Insert on the thumb proximal phalanx
  - Hypothenar

- Opponens digiti minimi (ODM)
- Flexor digit minimi (FDM)
- Abductor digiti minimi (ADM)
- Palmaris brevis (PB)
- Innervated by the ulnar nerve
- Provide an independent function of the small finger

  – Interossei

  - Palmar adduct fingers, dorsal abduct
  - Three palmar, four dorsal
  - All ulnar innervated

- Nerves

  – Nerves have two different innervation patterns: dermatomal/myotomal and peripheral.

  - Understanding the different patterns allows for ID of different injuries.
  - Dermatomes:
    – C5 is the radial shoulder.
    – C6 is the radial forearm.
    – C7 is the central hand.
    – C8 is the ulnar hand.
    – T1 is the medial arm.
  - Myotomes:
    – Progresses from proximal to distal

  – Sensory Nerves

  - Major sensory nerves of the forearm are the lateral brachial cutaneous nerve (continuation of the musculocutaneous, runs with the cephalic vein) and the medial antebrachial cutaneous nerve (MABC from the plexus, runs with the basilic vein).

  – Motor/Mixed

  - Radial:
    – Enters the forearm between the BR and ECRL/ECRB.
    – Dives deep, gives off PIN at supinator, which ends in wrist capsule and SRN, which arises between BR and ECRL.
    – SRN gives sensation to the dorsal radial fingers.
  - Median:
    – Enters the forearm lateral to the brachial artery between PT.
    – Branches with AIN diving deep to the wrist capsule.

- Remainder runs between FDS and FDP, gives palmar cutaneous branch 5 cm proximal to wrist and then enters the carpal tunnel.
- Ulnar
  - Enters the forearm around the medial epicondyle at the cubital tunnel
  - Travels under FCU with dorsal sensory branch 6–8 cm proximal to ulnar head
  - Enters the Guyon canal and branches again
- Normal variant nerve connections
  - Martin Gruber: median to ulnar connection in the palm
  - Riche-Cannieu: ulnar to median connection in the palm

Examining the Hand

- General Principles
  - The hand is only a part of the whole; it needs to do it in the context of greater injuries going on.
  - Every patient should receive an XR.
  - Basic principles remain the same: inspect, palpate, and test.
  - The exam is simple: know the function of muscles and nerves, and piece together the injury pattern.
- Testing Flexors
  - FDP vs FDS
    - FDP is tested by blocking the PIPJ and isolating the DIPJ.
    - FDS is tested by blocking the other fingers in extension (to eliminate the contribution of the FDP since it is a common muscle belly) and flexing the PIPJ.
  - FCR vs FCU
    - Flex wrist, observe any deviation
    - Tested by deviating wrist as well (ulnarly deviated wrist, flex tests FCU)
  - PL
    - Tested by palpating the tendon while flexing the wrist
  - FPL
    - Tested by flexing the IPJ of the thumb
- Testing Extensors
  - EPL (Fig. 46.5)

- Lay hand flat and retropulse thumb.
- EPB
  - Lay hand flat and resist extension at the MCP.
- APL
  - Resist abduction at the metacarpal.
- APB
  - Resist abduction with thumbs up at P1.
- EDC
  - Assess the extension of the finger at the MCP.
  - May be masked by junctura (distal connections between EDC tendons).
- EDM
  - Assess independent extension of SF at MCP.
- EIP
  - Assess independent extension of IF at MCP.
- ECRB/ECU
  - Assess extension of the wrist; look for deviation with extension.
- Testing Intrinsics

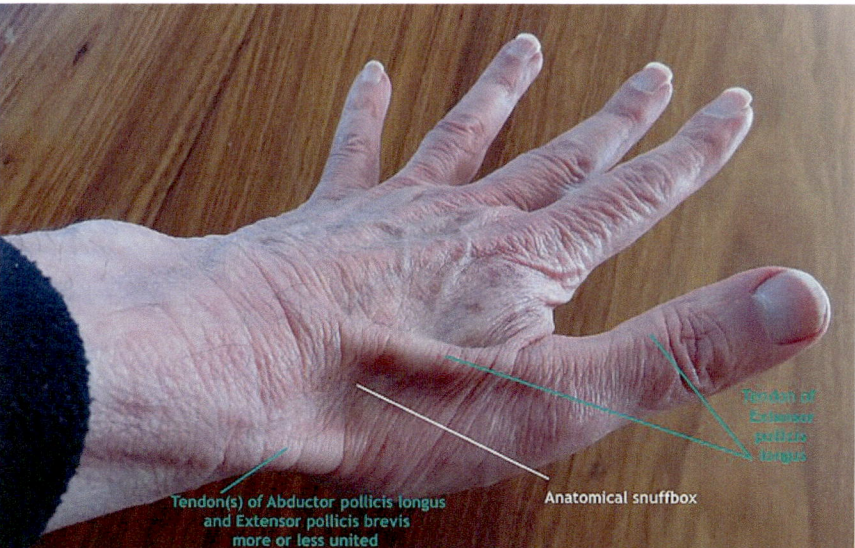

Fig. 46.5 Tendons of the anatomic snuffbox

- AdP
  - Test key pinch.
- FPB
  - Test flexion at P1.
- OP
  - Test the opponens of the thumb
- ADM
  - If the finger is held in abduction, then likely ADM is out (Wartenberg sign)
- Intrinsic vs extrinsic tightness
  - Intrinsic is tested by extending MCP to stress the intrinsic, then evaluating PIPJ.
  - Extrinsic is tested by flexing the MCP to stress the extrinsic, then evaluating PIPJ.
- Interossei test
  - Resisted abduction or adduction

- Testing vessels
  - Cap refill
    - Test fingernail, cap refill should be approx. 2 s.
  - Pulse ox
    - Cheap way to see if you have perfusion through the fingers
  - Allen test
    - Occlude both the radial and ulnar artery until the hand is white.
    - Release one, see if the entire hand perfuses, to see if the arch is complete.
- Testing nerves
  - Combine sensory and motor findings and figure out the nerves injured
  - Quick Test
    - Median
      - Inability to make the "OK" sign; suggests AIN injury and loss of FPL/FDP to the index
      - Sensation at tip of IF
    - Radial
      - Cannot give thumbs up (abductors and EPL)
      - Sensation in dorsal first webspace

- Ulnar
  - Cannot cross fingers (interossei)
  - Sensation at the tip of the SF

References

1. Huuman WW. Injuries to the hand and wrist. Adolesc Med. 1998;9:611–25.
2. Mastey RD, Weiss AP, Akelman E. Primary care of hand and wrist athletic injuries. Clin Sports Med. 1997;16:705–24.
3. Newton AW, Hawkes DH, Bhlaik V. Clinical examination of the wrist. Orthop Traumatol. 2017;31:237–47.
4. Newton AW, Tonge XN, Hawkes DH, Bhalaik V. Key aspects of anatomy, surgical approaches, and clinical examination of the hand. Orthop Trauma. 2019;33:1–13.
5. Panchal-Kildare S, Malone K. Skeletal anatomy of the hand. Hand Clin. 2013;20:459–71.

Chapter 47
Hand Infections

Nirbhay S. Jain

Evaluation of a Hand Infection [1, 2]

- Systemic signs of an infection.
- Local signs of infection (pain, rubor, calor, swelling).
- Elevated WBC count.
- Fever.
- Fluctuance: sign of an abscess, would need drainage.
- Labs such as CRP and ESR, though typically drawn, are nonspecific.
- Historical factors include immunocompromising states, exposures, injuries, and trauma.
- All patients require an XR at least.

Treatment Principles

- Surgical drainage and debridement should be done with as wide an incision as necessary.
- Excise all necrotic tissue for source control.
- Broad-spectrum antibiotics as needed.
- Culture as needed:

N. S. Jain (✉)
Division of Plastic Surgery, Department of Surgery, University of California, Los Angeles, Los Angeles, CA, USA
e-mail: nsjain@mednet.ucla.edu

- Most common organisms causing hand infections are the typical skin flora, including *Strep, Staph*, and *MRSA*; direct empiric therapy against these organisms, but may need to be broadened

Types of Acute Infection

- Acute paronychia
  - Most common infection in the hand.
  - Infection of the tissue around the fingernail, mainly by *Staph*.
  - Often due to manicures or nail biting.
  - Early infection treated by betadine soaks and antibiotics.
  - Abscesses need to be drained.
  - If extensive abscess, needs elevation of eponychial fold and drainage.
- Chronic paronychia
  - Chronically indurated tissue around the nail
  - Most commonly GPCs, *Candida*, and mycobacteria
  - May be related to diabetes, immunocompromise, or a foreign body
  - Often fail antibiotics and require marsupialization (incision proximal to nail fold to externalize nail matrix and allow drainage)
- Felon
  - Infection of the finger pad, walled off by septa from spreading down the hand.
    - Once the septa break down, it can cause osteomyelitis.
  - Most commonly staph after trauma to the fingertip.
  - Uncommon infections (20%), mainly in diabetics.
  - Requires drainage if an abscess is present.
- Pyogenic Flexor Tenosynovitis [3]
  - Hand surgical urgency
    - Failure of recognition can lead to destruction of the flexor tendons, which causes severe disability from lack of flexion.
    - Bacteria destroy the synovium, which feeds tendons.
  - Most commonly due to *Staph, Strep*, and *Pasteurella*
    - Gonorrhea can also cause this (disseminated gonococcal infection) but in the setting of other arthralgias.
  - Exam
    - Classically defined by the four Kanavel signs

- Finger held in passive flexion
- Fusiform swelling (sausage digit, Fig. 47.1)
- Pain with passive extension (diffuse)
- Tender to palpation down the flexor sheath proximally
- Can spread proximally down the flexor sheath into various spaces.
  - Flexor sheath communicates with ulnar bursa, which (through Parona space) communicates with radial bursa, leading to horseshoe abscess
- Treatment is almost always operative.
  - If early or due to gonorrhea, can trial nonoperative management
  - Otherwise, operate
    - Irrigate the tendon sheath; release the A1 pulley

- Mid Space Infections
  - Horseshoe abscess
    - Connection of radial and ulna bursae via the space of Parona
    - Involves the small finger and thumb
    - Needs operative decompression
- Deep Space Infection
  - Involves either the thenar, hypothenar, or midpalmar spaces.

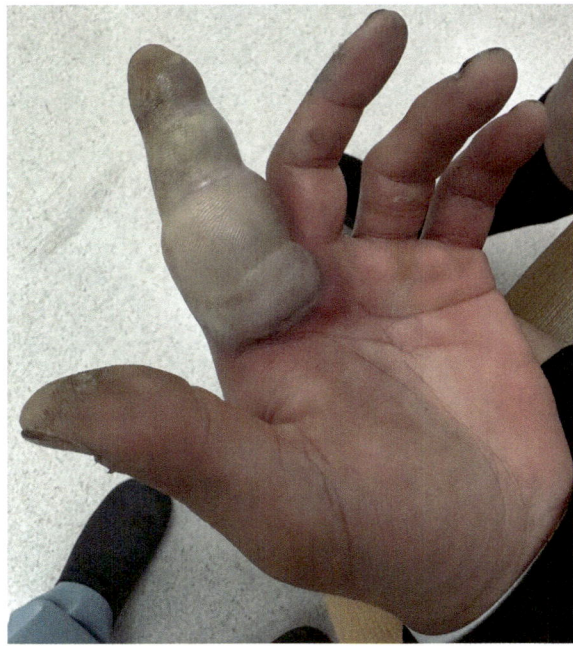

Fig. 47.1 Sausage digit. (Author's own work)

- All dorsal to the flexor tendons.
- Thenar most common.
  - Spreads to first dorsal interossei and AdP dorsally
- Hypothenar least common, not in continuity with the flexor tendon sheath.
- All need surgical drainage.

- Collar Button abscess (Fig. 47.2)
  - Abscess in the webspace
  - Often starts dorsally but spreads volarly
  - Needs surgical drainage with both volar and dorsal incisions, avoid incision on skin in actual web space to avoid contracture

- Septic Arthritis
  - Infection in the closed space of the joint.
  - Key physical exam sign is pain with axial loading of the joint.
  - Serum WBC may be normal; joint WBC will be elevated (high PMN also).
  - Needs emergent surgical drainage.
  - Can result in boutonniere deformity at the PIP and mallet at the DIP.

- Osteomyelitis
  - Infection in the bone, 1–6% of all hand infections.
  - Rarely due to seeding from the blood, usually due to direct trauma
    - Hematogenous is more common in children and in immunocompromised; *Salmonella* is a common offender.
  - Laboratory studies are typically normal, and symptoms are nonspecific.

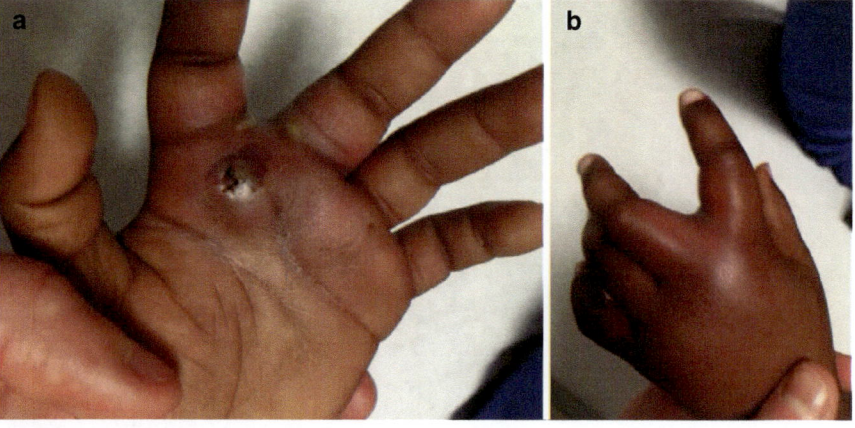

Fig. 47.2 Collar button abscess

- Acute changes on XR may not be present but are seen after chronic osteomyelitis sets in
- Requires long-term antibiotics and debridement of necrotic tissue.
- May need amputation.

Specific Vectors of Infection

- Animal bites
  - Mainly dog bites, along with normal skin flora, need to be covered by Pasteurella.
  - Augmentin, a typical first-line antibiotic.
  - Tularemia and *Bacteroides* are less common.
- Marine organisms
  - Main concerns are *Mycobacterium marinum* and *Vibrio cholera*.
    - Mycobacterium is an indolent infection; *Vibrio* is acute and deadly.
  - Aeromonas is associated with leeches, Cipro, and Bactrim, key drugs.
- Human bites
  - Main concern is *Eikenella*, along with bloodborne viruses.
  - Augmentin is typically the first-line antibiotic.
- Prosthetic infections
  - Often covered in biofilm, hard to eradicate
  - Often require removal of prosthetic, washout, and maybe an antibiotic spacer
- Herpetic whitlow
  - Caused by HSV 1 and 2.
  - Early stage is similar to other herpetic lesions, commonly the thumb and index finger.
  - These turn into bullae, which rupture.
  - Fades by day 10 after infection, and viral shedding occurs over the next 2 weeks.
  - Antivirals are only helpful in the early stage.
  - Treatment is otherwise observation.
- Injection Injuries
  - Paint gun and other injectors can lead to necrosis and infection in the hand.
    - If oil-based pain, 50% amputation rate

- Requires emergent surgical decompression, removal of injected material, and debridement of necrotic tissue
- Not commonly infected, but managed as such

Necrotizing Infections [4, 5]

- Similar principle to necrotizing fasciitis elsewhere
  - Crepitus
  - Gas on imaging
  - Dishwater fluid
- Needs urgent surgical debridement and broad-spectrum antibiotics

Chronic Infections

- Managed differently than acute infection, as often due to bacteria such as tuberculosis or fungi that require a separate approach
- Often seen in immunocompromised patients
- Often a nonspecific presentation
- Bacteria
  - Actinomycosis
    - Related to bites
    - Often presents as a nodule or abscess, spreads
    - Yellow sulfur granules on the drainage
    - Treated well with penicillin
  - Syphilis
    - Often can cause dactylitis if congenital
    - Treat with penicillin
- Neutrophilic dermatoses/pyoderma gangrenosum (Fig. 47.3)
  - Ulcerative dermal disease with neutrophilic infiltration
  - Synonymous with pyoderma gangrenosum
  - Does not have a true infection
  - Associated with systemic disease such as SLE or AML or UC
  - Presents as a large ulcer
  - Has poor response to biopsy

Fig. 47.3 Pyoderma gangrenosum

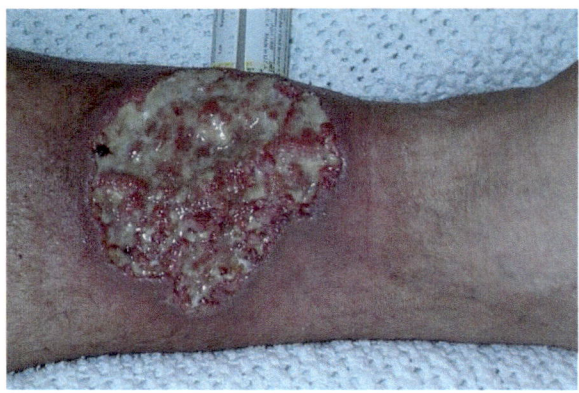

- Acute trauma from surgical procedure results in flare up
  - Manage with steroids, dapsone, azathioprine
- Fungi
  - Mainly in immunocompromised people.
  - Often due to *Candida* and *Aspergillus.*
  - Include tinea and ringworm and sporotrichosis.
  - Aspergillosis and blastomycosis are typically deeper.
  - Rhizopus and Mucor are much rarer and deadlier.
  - Manage with debridement and antifungals as needed.
- Other mycobacterial diseases
  - TB can cause infection in the hand, leading to rice bodies and osteomyelitis.
  - Leprosy can lead to neuropathy and sores.
- Scabies (Fig. 47.4)
  - Sores and itches that worsen at night, typically seen in web spaces between digits
  - Treat with permethrin and ivermectin.
- Non-herpetic viruses
  - AIDS can lead to lesions in the hand as well as Kaposiform disease.
  - Verruca vulgaris (warts), often due to HPV, can treat with salicylates or freezing.
  - Human orf virus infection looks like a tumor in an immunodeficient host.

Fig. 47.4 Scabies

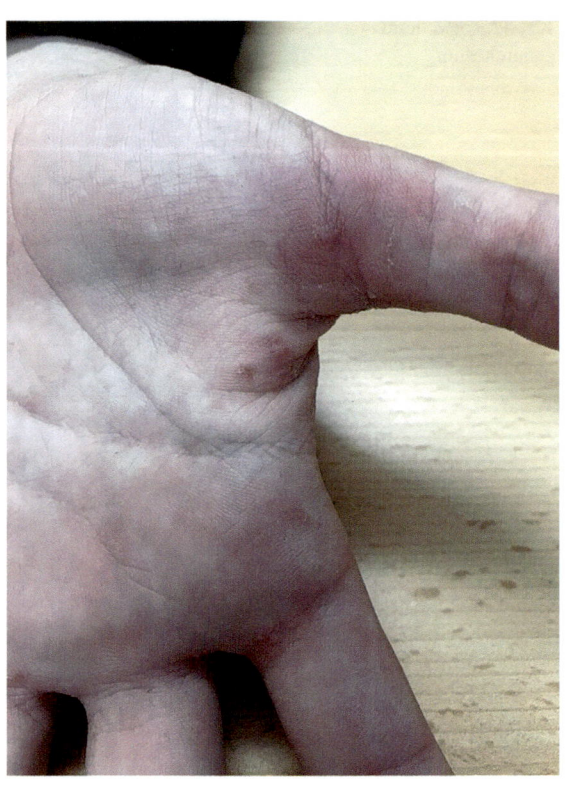

References

1. Abrahamian FM, Goldstein EJ. Microbiology of animal bite wound infections. Clin Microbiol Rev. 2011;24:231–46.
2. Barbieri RA, Freeland A. Osteomyelitis of the hand. Hand Clin. 1998;14:589–603.
3. Boles D, Schmidt C. Pyogenic flexor tenosynovitis. Hand Clin. 1998;14:567–78.
4. Calkins E. Nosocomial infections in hand surgery. Hand Clin. 1998;14:531–45.
5. Gonzalez M. Necrotizing fasciitis and gangrene of the upper extremity. Hand Clin. 1998;14:635–45.

Chapter 48
Compression Neuropathies

Nirbhay S. Jain

Nerve Compression Physiology [1, 2]

- As nerves get compressed, they essentially lose blood flow to the axon and Schwann cell, which starts to die and cause demyelination.
- These are not universally distributed and may depend on the anatomic branching of the nerve, which results in the symptoms.
- Double crush phenomenon—compression or injury at one point makes you more susceptible elsewhere.

Evaluation

- Systematic approach involving evaluation of all compression points.
- Provocative tests include Tinel's sign, Phalen's sign.
- Reproducing stressors can also trigger symptoms (cubital tunnel (elbow flexion) or radial tunnel (resisted supination)).
- Thoracic outlet syndrome/brachial plexus: narrowing of the aperture at the shoulder to compress.
- Other signs:
  - Froment's sign: loss of adductor pollicis in key pinch, patient will use flexor pollicis longus instead and flex the IP joint.

N. S. Jain (✉)
Division of Plastic Surgery, Department of Surgery, University of California, Los Angeles, Los Angeles, CA, USA
e-mail: nsjain@mednet.ucla.edu

- Wartenberg sign: deviation of the small finger at rest due to loss of palmar interossei adduction function being overpowered by extensors
  - Both signs of ulnar neuropathy
- Always do a sensory and motor test (evaluate two-point discrimination, gone before others).
- Scratch collapse test can also be important if done well.
  - Rub the nerve at the presumed compression point and then have the patient attempt to resist shoulder inward rotation with the shoulder adducted, elbows flexed, and forearms out.
- Electromyography (less reliable) and nerve conduction studies (more reliable) also give information and context.

Median Nerve Compression Points (Fig. 48.1) [3]

- Carpal Tunnel
  - Anatomy
    - Entryway of the median nerve at the wrist includes FDS, FDP, and FPL.
    - Roof is the flexor retinaculum; floor is the carpus.
    - Palmar cutaneous branch NOT in the carpal tunnel; the patient will have intact palmar sensation in carpal tunnel syndrome.
      - Loss of palmar sensation suggests more proximal injury or compression.
  - Presents with weakness in the thenar muscles and first two lumbricals and decreased sensation and paresthesias in the volar thumb, index finger, long finger, and radial side of the ring finger.
  - Initially managed nonoperatively with splinting, steroid injections, NSAIDs.
  - Operative treatment can be endoscopic or open, with similar results.
  - Can recur.
- Elbow/Forearm
  - Anatomy
    - Median nerve runs over the brachial artery on the medial side of the brachialis and passes through the antecubital fossa under lacertus.
    - Dives between heads of pronator and splits into the anterior interosseous nerve and the distal median nerve.
  - Pronator syndrome
    - Includes sensory branches, motor to FCR/FDS/PL, and AIN.

Fig. 48.1 Nerves of the upper extremity

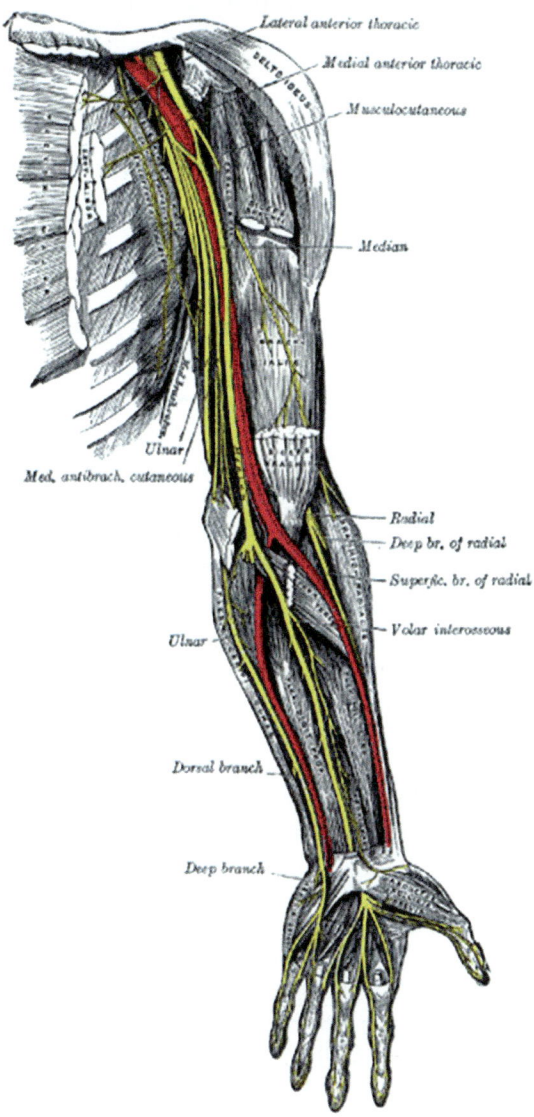

- Palmar sensation will be diminished, unlike in the carpal tunnel.
- Test with resisted pronation.
- Can also be compressed by the ligament of Struthers at the supracondylar process.

- AIN
  - Motor only
  - More distal in the pronator region

- Treat mainly with operative technique
  - Release ligament of Struthers, pronator arch, lacertus, and FDS

Ulnar Nerve Compression (Fig. 48.2) [4, 5]

- Cubital tunnel syndrome—at the elbow ("funny bone")
  - Anatomy
    - Nerve runs posteromedial to the brachial artery and anterior to the triceps in the upper arm.
    - Passes through the arcade of Struthers, then the intramuscular septum (where MABC is often).
    - Then, enters the cubital tunnel proper around the elbow, including the ligament of Osborne and FCU.
    - Then, travels under the flexor pronator mass in the forearm.
    - There may be an anconeus muscle as well.
  - Presents with weakness in intrinsic muscles of the hand, FCU, and decreased sensation and paresthesias in the small finger and ulnar side of the ring finger.
  - All these points need to be released.
  - Can trial elbow extension splinting for symptom relief, but often need surgery.
  - After release of the cubital tunnel and freeing the ulnar nerve, can transpose the nerve anterior to the olecranon if there is subluxation with elbow flexion and extension.
  - May also take out a portion of the medial epicondyle.
- Ulnar tunnel (Guyon canal)—at the wrist
  - Has three zones: I has motor/sensory, II is motor only, III is sensory only.
  - Runs by the hook of the hamate and pisiform.
  - Floor of the Guyon canal is the roof of the carpal tunnel (transverse carpal ligament), and the roof is the volar carpal ligament.
  - Can splint, but the main treatment is operative (release the pisohamate and volar carpal ligament).
  - Need to watch the ulnar artery as it dives deep.

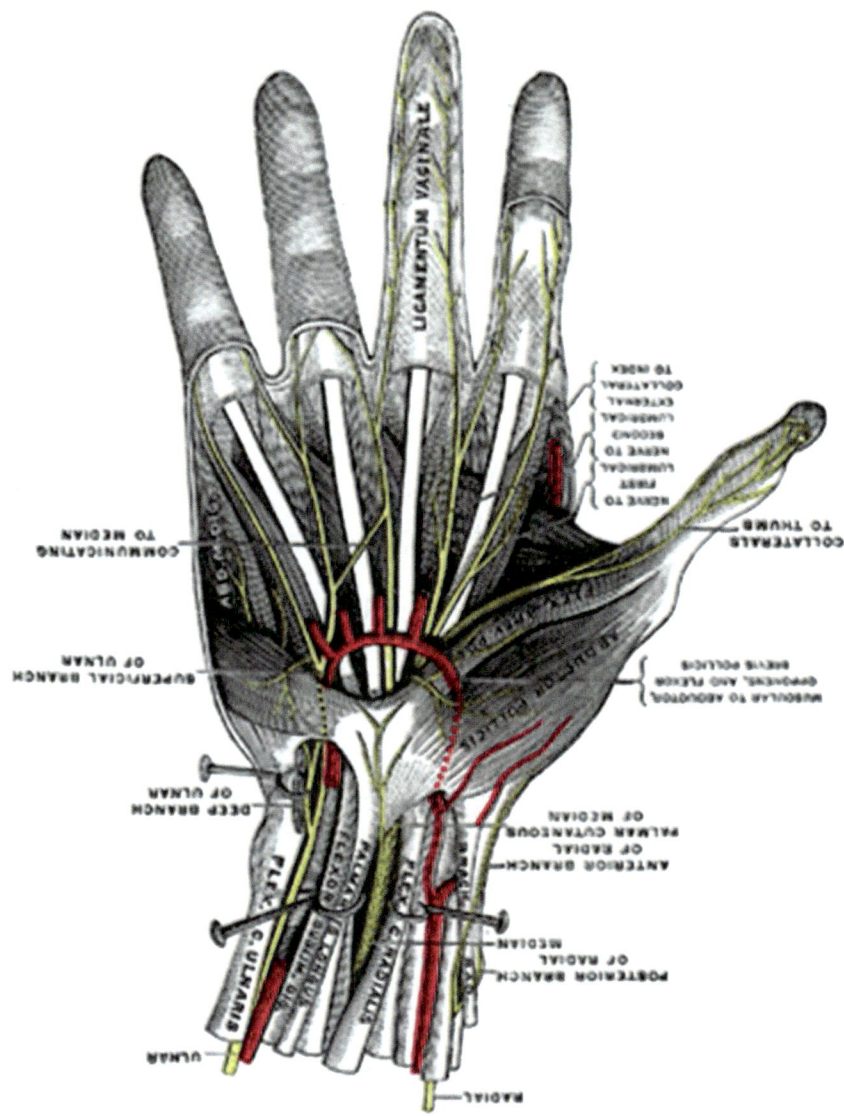

Fig. 48.2 Branching of the median nerve in the hand

Radial Nerve Compression (Fig. 48.3)

- Posterior interosseous nerve
  - Motor only
  - Compressed mainly at the arcade of Frohse (superior superficial part of the supinator)
  - Need to split BR and release the supinator

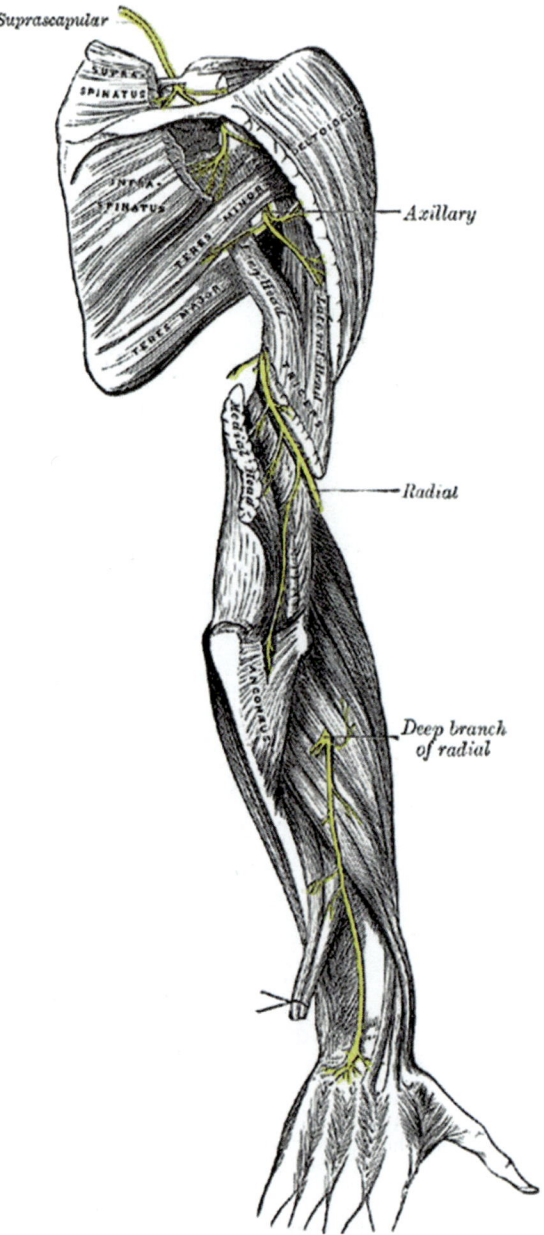

Fig. 48.3 Branching of the radial nerve

- Radial tunnel syndrome (full radial nerve)
  - Main symptom is pain, less frequently weakness
  - Presents like tennis elbow
  - In between BR and ECRL/B up to arcade of Frohse
  - Need to split BR and release the supinator
- Wartenberg syndrome (not sign)
  - Superficial radial nerve compression between BR and ECRL
  - Fascial release and BR tendon excision
- Can be compressed in triangular space as well, less common (axillary in quadrangular space)

Thoracic Outlet Syndrome (Fig. 48.4)

- Structures compressed as they leave the thoracic cavity, can be vascular or neurogenic
  - Vascular due to compression of subclavian artery, usually due to cervical rib
  - Most are electrically negative but symptomatic neurogenic.
  - Causes compression of C8–T1 mainly.
  - Usually activity or positional (nerve compression), not osseous.
- Plexus runs through the scalenes, can be compressed there or by cervical ribs.
- Costoclavicular triangle is a rare spot, as is the subcoracoid space.
- Evaluation shows loss of sensation and motor function in a dermatomal/myotomal pattern, not a peripheral nerve pattern.
- Worsens with limb abduction.

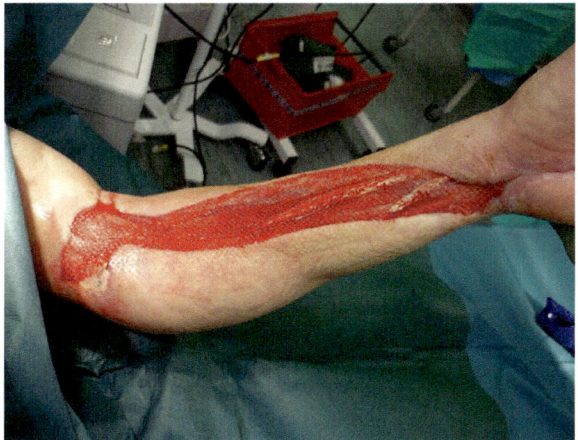

Fig. 48.4 Compartment syndrome after release

- Nonoperative treatment is first line, often with PT and strength training.
- If that fails, then it progresses to operative management, including rib resection and decompression.

Compartment Syndrome (Fig. 48.4)

- Essentially acute nerve compression
- Pathophysiology
    - High pressures (due to reperfusion, trauma, venous blockage) cause ischemia to muscles and nerve loss.
    - Affects deeper structures (AIN compartment volarly) first.
    - Then, more superficial.
    - Surgical emergency.
- Management (initial)
    - Decompression with fasciotomy incisions
    - Need to release all compartments
        - Hand
            - Thenar
            - Hypothenar
            - Four abductor, three adductor palmar
            - Adductor pollicis
            - Carpal tunnel
            - Guyon canal
        - Forearm
            - Deep and superficial volar
            - Deep and superficial dorsal
            - Mobile wad
- Management (sequelae)
    - If it fails, get Volkmann contracture of the muscles, severely limiting function.
    - Treat with tendon transfers, tendon lengthening procedures, or free flap as needed.

References

1. Apefelberg DB, Larson SJ. Dynamic anatomy of the ulnar nerve at the elbow. Plast Reconstr Surg. 1973;51:76–81.
2. Dellon AL, Mackinnon SE. Chronic nerve compression model for the double crush hypothesis. Ann Plast Surg. 1991;26:259–64.

3. Lanz U. Anatomic variations of the median nerve in the carpal tunnel. J Hand Surg Am. 1977;2:44–53.
4. Lowe JB, Mackinnon SE. Management of secondary cubital tunnel syndrome. Plast Reconstr Surg. 2004;113:1–16.
5. Novak CB, Mackinnon SE. Selection of operative procedures for cubital tunnel syndrome. Hand. 2009;4:50–4.

Chapter 49
Nerve Transfers, Repairs, and Complex Amputation

Nirbhay S. Jain

Nerve Anatomy and Physiology (Fig. 49.1) [1–3]

- Peripheral nerves contain axons, wrapped in endoneurium.
- Axons are bundled in fascicles surrounded by perineurium.
- Fascicles are bundled in nerves surrounded by epineurium.
- Nerves have topography (can identify which fascicle goes to which muscle throughout the course).
- Nerves receive blood through the vasa nervorum.
- Nerves preferentially run alongside fat and blood vessels.
- Responses to injury.
  - Wallerian degeneration occurs distal to the injury, driven by Schwann cells, which leave behind trophic factors.
  - Proximal axons develop growth cones that grow guided by these trophic factors until a target is reached.
    - That target can be a muscle, skin, the framework left behind by Wallerian degeneration, or itself (leading to a neuroma).
    - This is the process that allows repaired nerves to regrow and find the original (or new in the case of a transfer) target.
  - Similar pattern whether injury is sharp or traction.

N. S. Jain (✉)
Division of Plastic Surgery, Department of Surgery, University of California, Los Angeles, Los Angeles, CA, USA
e-mail: nsjain@mednet.ucla.edu

Fig. 49.1 Anatomy of a nerve

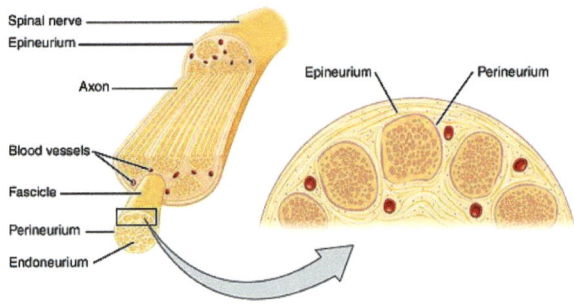

Clinical Exam

- Understanding anatomic relationships of nerves helps isolate injuries as peripheral or central
- Need to know timeframe from injury, sensory, motor, or both
- Need to know mechanism as well
- Performing a nerve exam is just performing a motor and sensory exam and analyzing the pattern of injury to identify the nerve

Electrodiagnostics (Fig. 49.2)

- Two forms: nerve conduction studies (NCS) and electromyography (EMG).
- NCS is a measure of the nerve itself.
    - More reliable.
    - Amplitude is the number of healthy axons.
    - Velocity/latency is a measure of healthy myelin.
        - Myelin provides insulation for saltatory conduction and allows faster conduction along the nerve.
- EMG is a measure of the muscle response.
    - Not as reliable.
    - Fibrillation—sign of denervation.
    - Motor unit potential (MUP)—if normal, then normal; if decreased, then denervated and if increased, then reinnervated.
    - Positive sharp waves (PSW)—another sign of denervation.
    - Nascent potential is another sign of reinnervation.

Fig. 49.2 Common EMG patterns

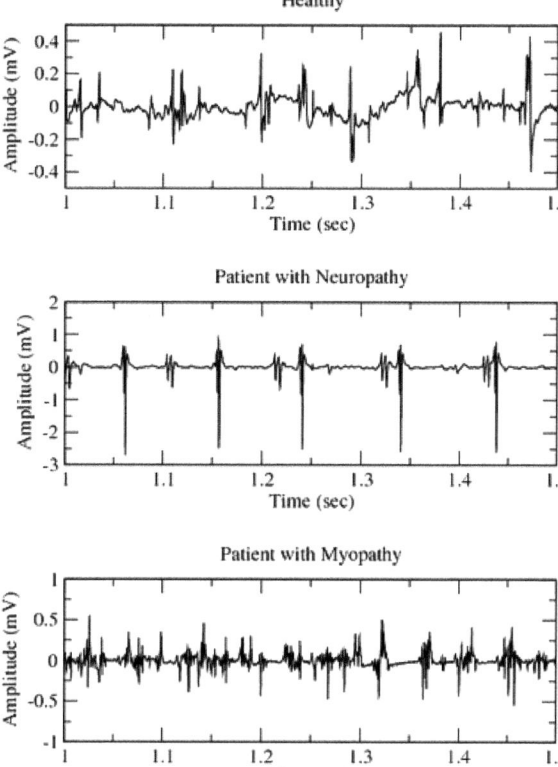

Classification of Nerve Injuries [4]

- Sunderland I (neuropraxia)
  - Conduction block
  - No actual axonal damage, only myelin sheath damage
  - No Tinel sign
  - No change on EMG
  - No need for surgery
- Sunderland II (axonotmesis)
  - Axon damage
  - Advancing Tinel sign
  - EMG with denervation and reinnervation
  - No need for surgery
- Sunderland III (axonotmesis)
  - Endoneurial damage

- Advancing Tinel sign
- EMG with denervation and reinnervation
- No need for surgery (usually)
- Sunderland IV (axonotmesis)
  - Perineural damage
  - Stationary Tinel sign
  - EMG with denervation alone
  - Need surgery
- Sunderland V (neurotmesis)
  - Epineural damage
  - Stationary Tinel sign
  - EMG with denervation alone
  - Needs surgery
- Sunderland VI (neuroma in continuity)
  - Mixed features

In summary, nerve repair is typically indicated to facilitate nerve regrowth if it does not occur spontaneously (advancing Tinel).

Nerve Repair Methods [5, 6]

- Timing
  - Ideally, repair nerves within a timeframe so that downstream function is not lost.
    - For motor nerves, repair is typically required within 1 year on average.
      - Rule of 18's—nerve should be able to regrow from injury to motor end plate within 18 months, by estimating 1 inch per month of regrowth.
      - Proximal injuries need earlier repair or may never reach their destination before end plate degeneration.
    - Affected by age.
  - For sharp injuries, explore ASAP if a nerve deficit is noted.
    - Motor nerves lose NT by 72 h, so they may not be able to stimulate distally.
  - Avulsive nerve may need to have delayed exploration to allow extent of damage to declare itself.
  - Closed injuries normally wait 3 months with serial exams and electrodiagnostic studies to evaluate if the nerve is healing.

- Primary repair
  - Preferred, if possible, without tension.
  - Epineural stitches and fascicular stitches have the same outcome.
    - Fascicular repairs are bulkier and may cause more scarring, though the nerves are better aligned.
- Grafting
  - Done if there is a gap and repair cannot be done primarily without tension.
  - Options include allograft (Axogen), although reliability at >5 cm is unclear.
  - Can also do a conduit or vein graft, but best for short distances.
  - Autograft is most reliable, typically the sural nerve or MABC.
  - Anterior interosseous nerve/posterior interosseous nerve are good donors for digital nerves.
- Nerve transfers
  - Take the principle of tendon transfer and use it for nerves.
  - Sacrifice one to augment another.
  - Common transfers:
    - Cranial nerve XI → suprascapular
    - Triceps → axillary
    - FCU → biceps, FCR → brachialis (single or double fascicular transfer)
    - FCR → PIN
    - FDS → ECRB
    - AIN to distal motor Ulnar (end-to-side "babysitter" transfer)
      - Allows maintenance of distal motor end plates while the ulnar nerve regrows from a high injury.
    - ECRB → AIN
  - Spinal cord transfers:
    - New developments are nerve transfers from unaffected myotomes to restore function to affected myotomes.
    - Brachialis to AIN, supinator to PIN, deltoid to triceps: most common.
  - Free functional muscle transfers are a last resort if no available muscles in the area (i.e., delayed reconstruction after motor end plate degeneration).
    - Gracilis is most commonly used on the obturator nerve.
- Repaired nerves are never the same.
  - Younger, earlier, better repair helps, but rarely get normal function.

Complex Amputations

- Nerve management during amputation of the upper or lower extremity may prevent painful neuroma growth and give the patient the ability to control "smart" myoelectric prostheses.
- Targeted muscle reinnervation
    - Main nerve branches that are truncated by amputation are coapted to motor branches in the residual extremity to give the nerves a "destination" rather than undergoing disorganized growth into a neuroma.
    - Primarily a pain operation, myoelectric integrated prostheses are secondary.
        - Decreases narcotics reliance, improves pain, and has higher rates of ambulation in lower extremity patients
    - Transhumeral amputation transfers
        - Long head of triceps → triceps
        - Lateral head of triceps → PIN
        - Median biceps → median
        - Brachialis → ulnar
        - Lateral biceps → MC
- Regenerative peripheral nerve interface
    - Small muscle graft wrapped around the distal truncated nerve, again to give a destination to prevent neuroma formation
    - Primarily used to prevent neuropathic and phantom limb pain
    - May be used for prosthetics down the line

References

1. Novak CB, Mackinnon SE. Distal anterior interosseous nerve transfer to the deep branch of the ulnar nerve for reconstruction of high ulnar nerve injuries. J Reconstr Microsurg. 2002;18:459–64.
2. Kim DH, Kam AC, Chandika P, et al. Surgical management and outcome in patients with radial nerve lesions. J Neurosurg. 2001;95:573–83.
3. Addas BM, Midha R. Nerve transfers for severe nerve injury. Neurosurg Clin N Am. 2009;20:27–38.
4. Gaul JS. Intrinsic motor recovery—a long-term study of ulnar nerve repair. J Hand Surg Am. 1982;7:502–8.
5. Sunderland S. A classification of peripheral nerve injuries producing loss of function. Brain. 1961;74:491–516.
6. Mackinnon SE, Novak CB. Nerve transfers. Hand Clin. 1999;15:643–66.

Chapter 50
Brachial Plexus

Nirbhay S. Jain

Anatomy (Fig. 50.1)

- The brachial plexus is formed from cervical roots from C5 to T1 and divided into roots, trunks, divisions, cords, and nerve branches (*Red Trucks Drive Cats Nuts*).
- The plexus itself lies on the scalene muscles and surrounds the axillary artery.
- Once the nerves reach the infraclavicular region, they have already branched.
- Nerves that come off the brachial plexus:
    - Phrenic (C3–5)
    - Long thoracic (C5–7)
    - Dorsal scapular (C5–6)
    - Subclavius (C5–6)
    - Suprascapular (C5–6)
    - Lateral pectoral (C5–6)
    - Upper subscapular (C5–6)
    - Lower subscapular (C5–6)
    - Thoracodorsal (C6–8)
    - Medial brachial cutaneous (MBC) (C5–6)
    - Medial antebrachial cutaneous (MABC) (C6–8)
    - Medial pectoral (C8–T1)
    - Median (C5–T1)
    - Ulnar (C8–T1)
    - Radial (C5–T1)
    - Axillary (C5–6)

N. S. Jain (✉)
Division of Plastic Surgery, Department of Surgery, University of California, Los Angeles, Los Angeles, CA, USA
e-mail: nsjain@mednet.ucla.edu

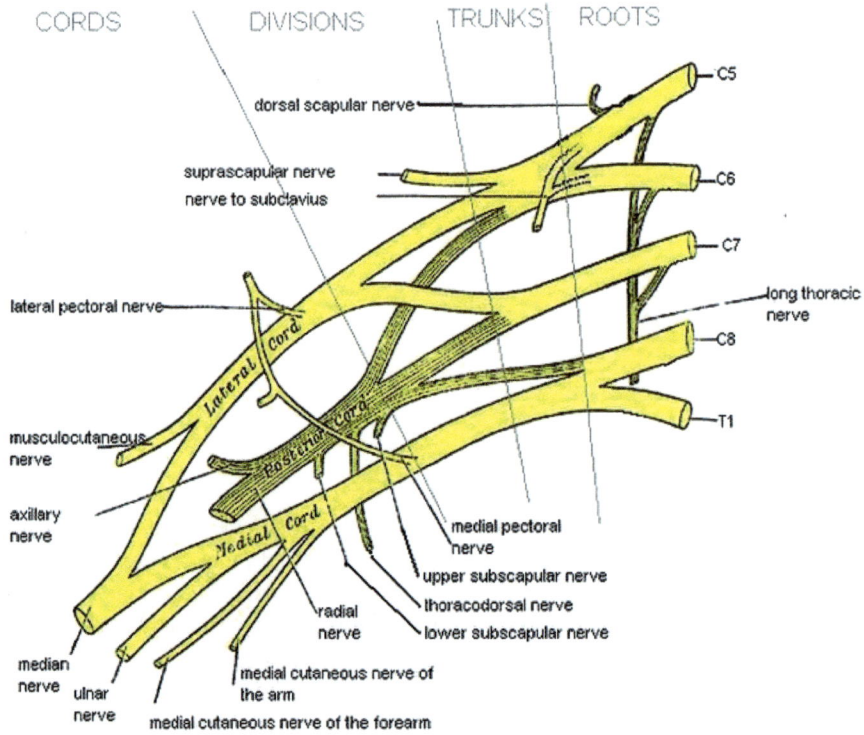

Fig. 50.1 Anatomy of the brachial plexus

- Musculocutaneous (MC) (C5–7)

Mechanisms of Injury [1–3]

- Most injuries are associated with other trauma (head, arm, thoracic).
- Traction injury:
  - Most common etiology of injury to the plexus; requires high velocity injury to cause true damage to the plexus, requiring surgical intervention.
  - If arm elevated (shoulder neck angle acute) during injury, then likely C8/T1 injury (Klumpke Palsy).
  - If arm is depressed (shoulder neck angle obtuse), then C5/6 injury (Erb palsy).
  - Most injuries are supraclavicular.
  - Klumpke is more likely to avulse from the cord; Erb's palsy is more likely to be in the nerve itself after it exits the foramina.
- Penetrating trauma

- Gunshot and knife
- Often associated with orthopedic and vascular injury

Common Injury Patterns

- Erb palsy
  - 15% of patients
  - Deficits in shoulder stability, abduction, internal/external rotation, sometimes elbow flexion, and supination
    - Waiter's tip deformity
  - Radial sensory deficit
- C5–7 injury
  - 1/3 of patients with Erb's palsy will also have loss of C7, with weakness in the wrist and sometimes finger extensors as well as sensation in the hand.
- Klumpke palsy
  - 10% of patients
  - Deficits in the motor function of the hand and ulnar sensation
  - Horner syndrome may be present because the T1 roots include the sympathetic ganglion and injury here can disrupt the path to the eye, causing ptosis, miosis, and anhidrosis
- Pan plexus
  - Most common form of palsy with a flail and insensate hand
- Parsonage-Turner syndrome
  - Variable patterns of injury, idiopathic in nature
  - Typically presents as abrupt, severe pain in the unilateral shoulder or arm, followed by variable nerve deficits
  - Often resolves with time

Preoperative Evaluation

- Physical examination is critical to evaluate the specific muscle and sensory patterns injured.
- Routine imaging for trauma evaluation is necessary for initial injury workup; further imaging is not strictly necessary.

- Electrodiagnostic testing is done at 1 month post-injury with follow-up at 3 months to evaluate recovery; if no recovery is present, then it likely requires surgical intervention.

Timing of Surgical Management

- Primary repair is indicated in sharp injuries or possibly if exploration is otherwise indicated.
- Blunt injury typically gets explored by 3 months.
    - Gunshot wounds often cause neuropraxia from burn; usually wait to see if there is recovery of function, and explore if not.
- Delayed presentation often requires tendon transfers due to the length of time for the nerve to regrow to the destination and loss of neuromuscular junctions.

Nerve-Based Surgical Options If Primary Repair/Grafting Is Not Possible [4]

- C5–6 roots
    - Goal is to restore shoulder abduction and elbow flexion for feeding.
    - Spinal accessory to suprascapular.
    - Medial branch of the triceps to the axillary.
    - Nerve to the FCU to the biceps.
    - Nerve to the FCR to the brachialis.
- C8–T1 roots
    - Mainly tendon transfers and free functional muscle transfers due to the distance from nerve roots to distal targets
- Pan-plexus Injury
    - Intercostal transfers for biceps and free functional transfers

Non-Nerve-Based Surgical Options [5]

- Based on a joint injury
- Shoulder
    - Tendon transfers to stabilize the shoulder

- Trapezius
        - Latissimus
        - Pectoralis
      - Arthrodesis
  - Elbow
    - Tendon transfers
      - Flexor advancement
      - Pectoralis
      - SCM
      - Triceps
      - Latissimus
  - Wrist
    - Arthrodesis
- For specific details on tendon transfers, see Chap. 54.

Pediatric Considerations

- Erb's palsy has a high rate of spontaneous recovery within 6 months.
  - Often due to shoulder dystocia
- If no return of function by 6 months, likely requires surgical intervention
- May require neurolysis and grafting, joint manipulation and release, and bone manipulation

References

1. Alnot JY. Traumatic brachial plexus in the adult: indications and results. Hand Clin. 1995;11:623–31.
2. Bertelli JA, Ghizoni MF. Reconstruction of C5 and C6 brachial plexus avulsion injury by multiple nerve transfers. J Hand Surg Am. 2004;29:131–9.
3. Birch R. Brachial plexus injury. Neurosurg Clin N Am. 2009;20:15–23.
4. Doi K. New reconstructive procedure for brachial plexus injury. Clin Plast Srug. 1997;24:75–85.
5. Sedel L. The results of surgical repair of brachial plexus injuries. J Bone Joint Surg Br. 1982;64:54–66.

Chapter 51
Hand Fractures

Nirbhay S. Jain

Relevant Anatomy

- There are five metacarpals, which articulate with the carpal bones of the distal row (trapezium, trapezoid, capitate, hamate).
- Metacarpals are numbered from 1 (thumb) to 5 (small finger).
- There are specific tendons that attach to the metacarpals in a reliable pattern.
  - First: APL
  - Second: ECRL, FCR
  - Third: ECRB
  - Fifth: ECU, FCU
  - The fourth metacarpal does not have any tendinous attachments and is thus narrower on imaging.
- The CMC joint at the fourth and fifth metacarpals is mobile, allowing for tolerance of greater angles of fractures.

General Principles of Treatment [1, 2]

- The goal of intervention is, as with fractures elsewhere in the body, to align the bones to allow them to heal in the best possible functional position.
- This involves reduction of all displaced fractures, and if the reduction is not able to be maintained in a splint or cast, operative intervention and fixation.

N. S. Jain (✉)
Division of Plastic Surgery, Department of Surgery, University of California, Los Angeles, Los Angeles, CA, USA
e-mail: nsjain@mednet.ucla.edu

- General indications for operative intervention include:
  - Irreducible fractures
  - Malrotation
  - Unstable articular fractures
  - Open fractures
  - Bone loss
  - Polytrauma
  - Extensor lag (inability to actively fully extend fingers) > 15°
- Methods of Fixation include:
  - Percutaneous pinning (K-wire) with or without open reduction
  - Internal fixation with plate, cerclage wire, or intramedullary nail

Specific Fracture Patterns and Considerations for Treatment [3]

- Metacarpal Fractures (non-thumb)
  - Metacarpal Head Fractures (Fig. 51.1)
    - More rare than other metacarpal fractures
    - Often intraarticular, mainly in the index finger
    - Typically require fixation
  - Metacarpal Neck Fractures
    - Called a "boxer's fracture" in the fifth neck.
    - Angle of displacement that can be tolerated after reduction changes based on the metacarpal involved, due to more mobility in the ulnar hand.
      - Second: 10°
      - Third: 20°
      - Fourth: 30°
      - Fifth: 40°
    - Can attempt reduction with the Jahss maneuver, but this is often unstable and requires surgery.
  - Metacarpal shaft fractures (Fig. 51.2)
    - Management is similar to neck fractures, except angles tolerated differ.
      - Second: 10°
      - Third: 20°
      - Fourth: 40°
      - Fifth: 60°

Fig. 51.1 Third metacarpal shaft fracture and second metacarpal head fracture

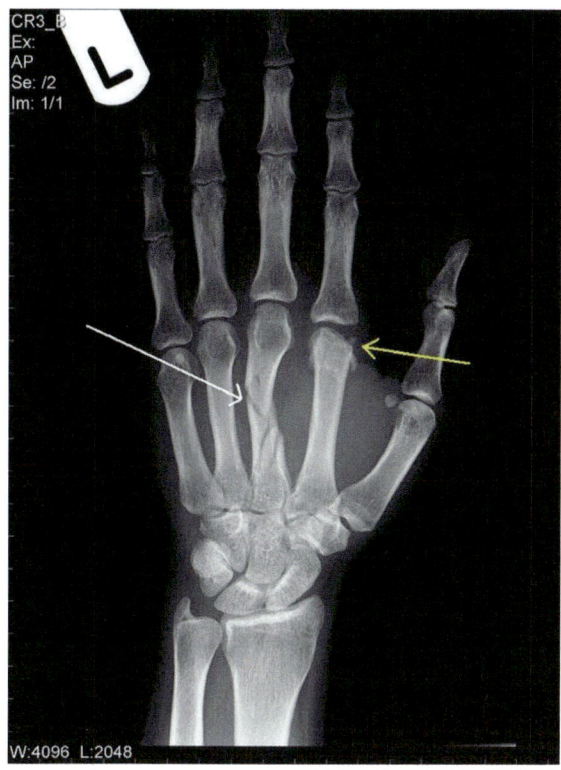

- If need fixation, good candidate for intramedullary screw.
- Segmental metacarpal loss
  - Stabilize fragments and graft
- Metacarpal base fractures and CMC fracture dislocations
  - Mainly in the fifth metacarpal (Baby Bennett).
  - FCU maintains the fifth metacarpal; the small fragments are dislocated.
  - Universally requires ORIF if displaced.
- Phalangeal Fractures [4–6]
  - Distal (Fig. 51.3)
    - Tuft fractures are usually due to crush injury and may have a subungual hematoma; require immobilization only.
    - Nondisplaced shaft fractures also require immobilization only, if displaced may need pinning.
    - Epiphyseal fractures result from hyperflexion of the joint.
      - If open, called Seymour fracture (through growth plate, Salter Harris II)

Fig. 51.2 Fourth and fifth metacarpal shaft fractures with angulation

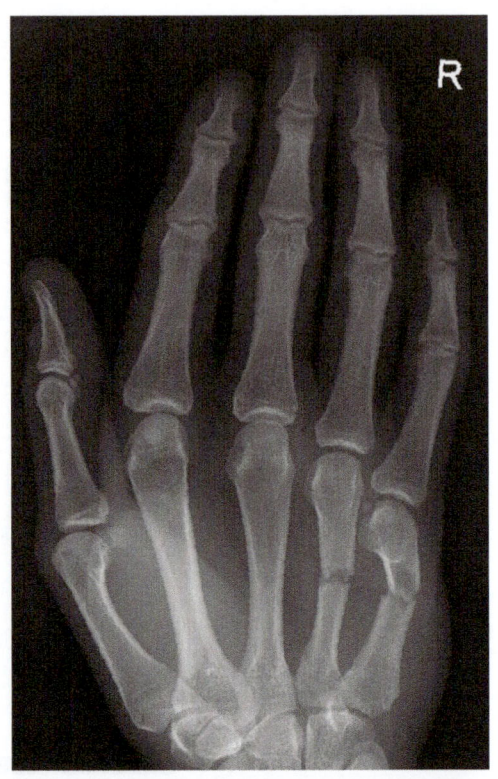

Fig. 51.3 Distal tuft fractures

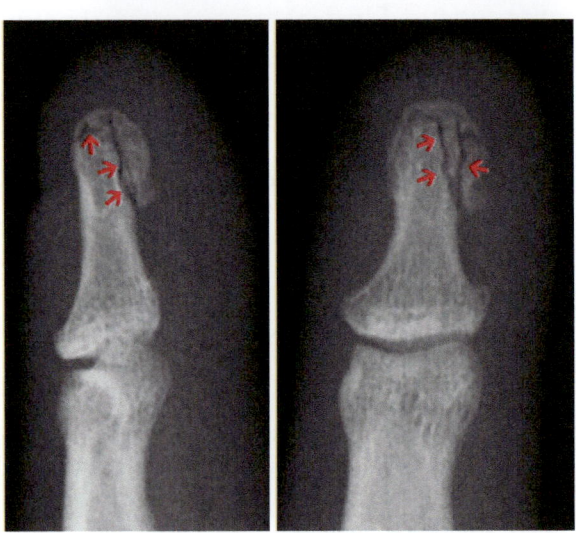

- Associated with mallet finger
- Need to repair nail plate and wash out relatively urgently
- Reduction usually held without fixation

- Middle and proximal

    - Buddy taping typically manages nondisplaced, stable fractures.
    - Condylar fractures:

        - Type I is stable
        - Type II is unicondylar and unstable.
        - Type III is bicondylar or comminuted.
        - Typically requires fixation for II or III.
        - Extensor lag can be managed with dynamic extension splinting.

    - Base fractures:

        - If stable up to 30°, dorsal extension block splint.
        - If more the 30°, then dynamic traction reduction or operation.
        - Hemihamate arthroplasty is a secondary surgery reserved for delayed resurfacing of the joint surface by using part of the hamate to remake the phalangeal base. Typically performed as a salvage operation.

    - Neck and shaft fractures:

        - If displaced, then operate
        - If nondisplaced, buddy tape

- Thumb Fractures

    - Phalangeal

        - Tufts rarely require fixation.
        - Proximal phalanx is managed similarly to the rest of the fingers.

    - Metacarpal (Fig. 51.4)

        - Bennett

            - Two-part articular fracture of the thumb base
            - Small fragment is held in place, large fragment displaced by APL.
            - Reduce with pronation, traction, and abduction

        - Rolando

            - Three-part or more Bennett-type fracture
            - Needs operative fixation

Fig. 51.4 Rolando fracture

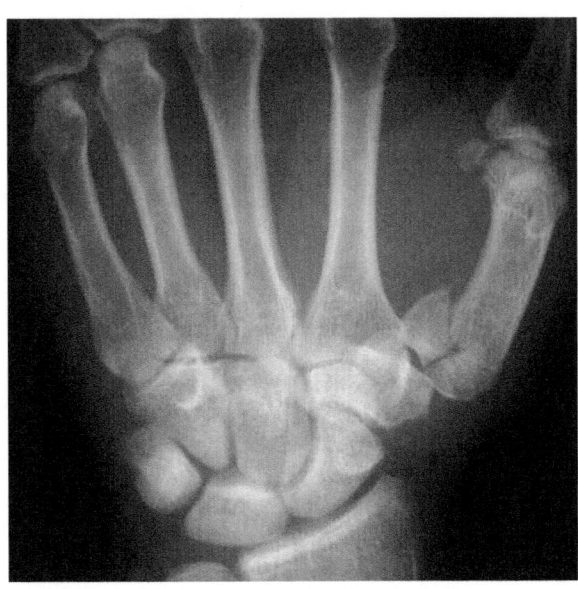

References

1. Al-Qattan MM. Metacarpal shaft fractures of the fingers. J Hand Surg Br. 2006;31:377–82.
2. Burkhalter WE. Closed treatment of hand fractures. J Hand Surg Am. 1989;14:390–3.
3. Cannon SR, Dowd GS, Williams DH, et al. A long-term study following Bennett's fracture. J Hand Surg Br. 1986;11:426–31.
4. Chung KC, Spilson SV. The frequency and epidemiology of hand and forearm fractures in the United States. J Hand Surg Am. 2001;26:908–15.
5. Duncan RW, Freeland AE, Jabaley ME, et al. Open hand fractures: an analysis of the recovery of active motion and of complications. J Hand Surg Am. 1993;18:387–94.
6. Stern PJ. Management of fractures of the hand over the last 25 years. J Hand Surg Am. 2000;25:817–23.

Chapter 52
Wrist Fractures

Nirbhay S. Jain

Function and Anatomy of the Wrist Articulation [1, 2]

- The wrist joint is made up of interactions between the radius, scaphoid and lunate, and separately the distal radioulnar joint, there is no true ulnocarpal joint.
- Distal radioulnar joint (DRUJ) is the key to pronation/supination, radius rotates around ulna.
- Sigmoid notch of the radius interacts with the head of the ulna.
- Ulna is typically shorter than the radius in this region.
- Distal tip of the ulna has a triangular fibrocartilage complex (TFCC) on it, which provides stability to DRUJ through its connections to the radius.
- Fovea is primary attachment for ligaments, at base of styloid of ulna.
  – Strongest portions of the TFCC attaches to base of ulna, weaker to styloid
- ECU runs over ulna, provides stabilizing forces (ECU subsheath).
- Intracarpal articulations and ligaments are beyond the scope of this book (fellow-level and beyond).

Physical Examination of the Wrist [3, 4]

- Range of motion: expect 90° of dorsiflexion to 90° of palmar flexion, full pronation and supination, and approximately 45° of ulnar deviation and radial deviation.

N. S. Jain (✉)
Division of Plastic Surgery, Department of Surgery, University of California, Los Angeles, Los Angeles, CA, USA
e-mail: nsjain@mednet.ucla.edu

© The Author(s), under exclusive license to Springer Nature Switzerland AG 2025
J. Roostaeian et al. (eds.), *Plastic Surgery Clerkship*, Contemporary Surgical Clerkships, https://doi.org/10.1007/978-3-031-99098-4_52

- Watson test: tells if the scaphoid is out of place.
- Snuffbox tenderness for scaphoid fracture (palpate between the first and third compartment tendons over the dorsal hand).
- Four-view XR, CT for acute trauma, and MRI for ligaments.
    - The four-view XR includes the A–P, oblique, lateral, and navicular views; a clenched fist view can be added on for further evaluation of the scaphoid.
- Piano key sign: used for the DRUJ—relative movement and laxity between radius and ulna
- Foveal tenderness: used for TFCC.

Specific Injury Patterns and Management

- DRUJ/TFCC Injuries
    - Can be traumatic or degenerative.
    - Oftentimes can manage with splints.
    - DRUJ typically dislocates dorsally.
    - If fail, then need to do an open repair, especially of the foveal portion, and address the cause (ulnar impaction syndrome).
    - Can be associated with ulnar styloid fragments, which do not normally need to be fixed unless the TFCC is involved.
- Radius
    - Distal radius fractures are the most common fractures seen in the ER.
    - Indications for treatment.
        - Loss of height < 11 mm (Fig. 52.1)
        - Dorsal tilt >10° (Fig. 52.2)
        - Inclination <15° (Fig. 52.3)
        - Both bone fractures
    - Types of fractures
        - Colles: apex dorsal
        - Smith: apex volar
        - Barton: sliding off the articular surface
        - Chauffer: styloid
    - Treatment
        - Casting
        - Fixation
            - Volar approach is more common (between the FCR and radial artery, the volar plate has less irritation to tendon).

Fig. 52.1 Radial inclination

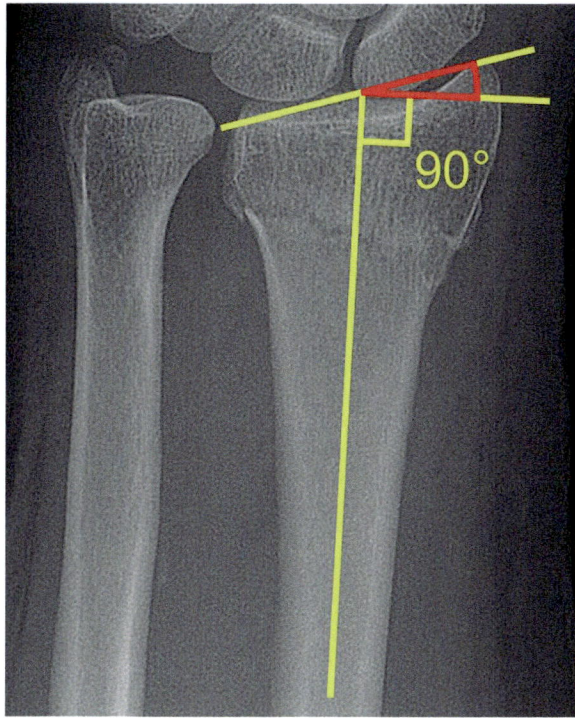

- Dorsal approach is easier but worse long term.
- Dorsal spanning plate can be placed temporarily but prevents motion at the wrist and must be removed after bony healing.

- Ulna
  - Ulnar impaction syndrome—where the ulna repeatedly hits the carpus, needs to shorten the ulna
  - Ulnar shaft fracture indications for surgery
    - 10-degree angulation
    - displaced
    - 50% shift
- Scaphoid [5–7]
  - Most commonly fractured carpal bone.
  - 90% heal well.
  - Anatomy is special (Fig. 52.4).
    - Proximal pole fed by retrograde flow, so a proximal pole fx has a risk of avascular necrosis, which can lead to scaphoid nonunion advanced collapse (SNAC) wrist, which can progress to debilitating arthritis (Fig. 52.4).
    - Waist is the most common place for fracture.

Fig. 52.2 Volar (or dorsal) tilt

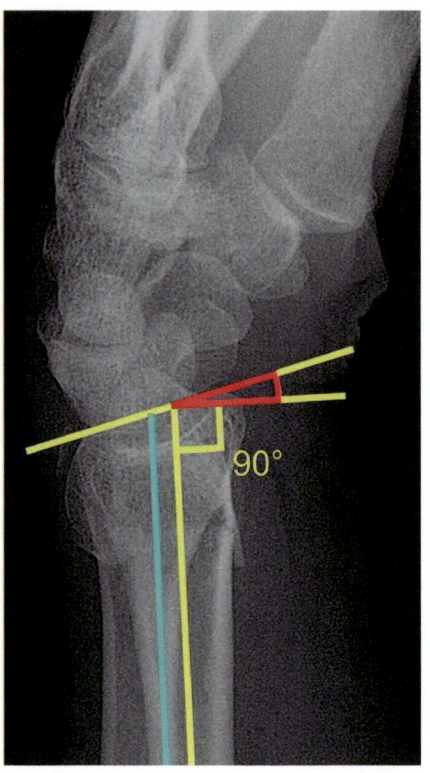

- Evaluation requires a navicular view exam on XR and/or MRI to evaluate for perfusion (CT also reasonable).
- If stable fracture, can put lag screw across.
- Indication for fixation typically if displaced or proximal pole, if nondisplaced often thumb spica for 10–12 weeks
  - Longer time period of casting due to poor vascularity and slow healing.
  - Some patients request fixation to avoid 3 months of casting.
- If proximal, the pole undergoes avascular necrosis:
  - Nonvascular bone graft; may not heal
  - Vascular bone graft—medial femoral condyle (MFC) free flap or 1,2 SRA
- Long-term complication: SNAC wrist
- Salvage
  - Four-corner fusion (4CF) or proximal row carpectomy (PRC)
- Other Carpal Bones
  - All other fractures are quite rare
  - Triquetral

Fig. 52.3 Distal radius fracture with radial impaction and dorsal tilt

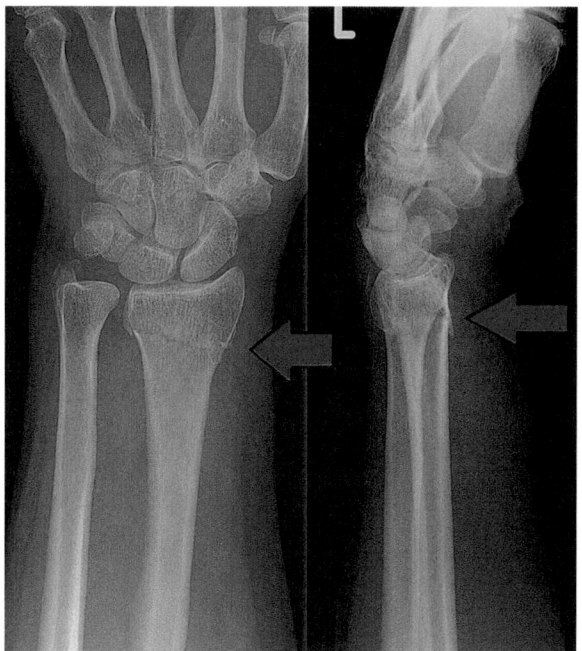

- Next most common
- Universally heal with casting

– Trapezium

- Third most common
- Again, cast unless majorly displaced

– Capitate

- Fourth most common
- Cast unless majorly displaced

– Hamate

- Fifth most common.
- Ball and stick injury.
- May lead to Guyon canal compression.
- Hook may need to be removed.

– Pisiform

- Sixth most common
- Cast

– Trapezoid

- Rarest carpal fracture

Fig. 52.4 Vasculature of a scaphoid

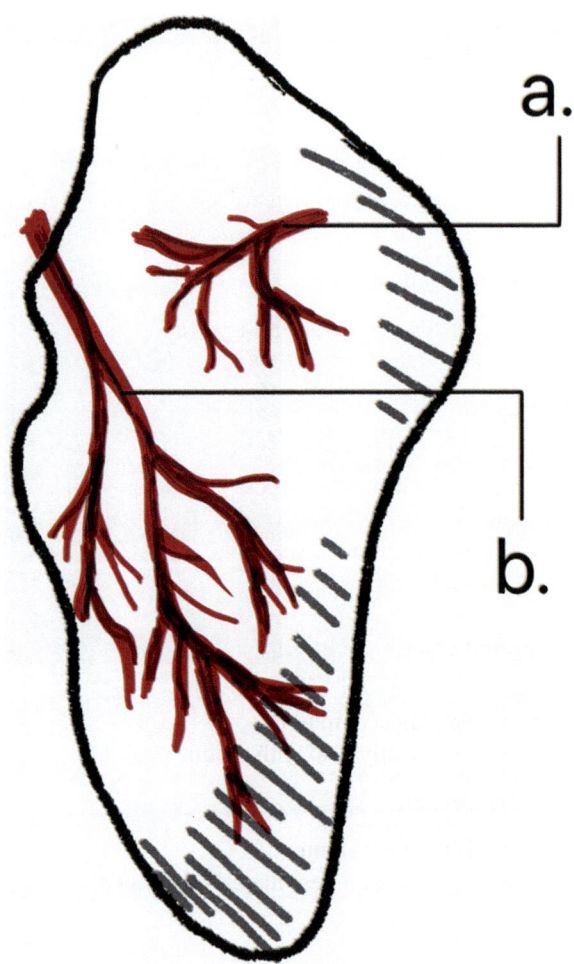

- Cast
- Lunate [8]
    - Seventh most common.
    - May need to repair the ligaments as well.
    - May need fixation.
    - Kienbock disease—avascular necrosis of the lunate, idiopathic.
        - Can bone graft to fix, or just leave it, unless it causes pain
    - Lunate collapse may not have long-term issues.

References

1. Chung KC, Kotsis SV, Kim HM. Predictors of functional outcomes after surgical treatment of distal radius fractures. J Hand Surg Am. 2007;31:76–83.
2. Cole DW, Elsaidi GA, Kuzma KR, et al. Distal radioulnar joint instability in distal radius fractures: the role of sigmoid notch and triangular fibrocartilage complex revisited. Injury. 2006;37:252–8.
3. Cooney WP III, Dobyns JH, Linscheid RL. Complications of Colles' fractures. J Bone Joint Surg. 1980;62:613–39.
4. Adler JB, Shaftan GW. Fractures of the capitate. J Bone Joint Surg Am. 1962;44:1536–47.
5. Alshryda S, Shah A, Odak S, et al. Acute fractures of the scaphoid bone: systematic review and meta-analysis. Surgeon. 2012;10:218–29.
6. Amadio PC, Berquist TH, Smith DK, et al. Scaphoid malunion. J Hand Surg Am. 1989;14:679–87.
7. Berger RA. The anatomy of the scahpoid. Hand Clin. 2001;17:525–32.
8. Bochud RC, Buchler U. Kienbock's disease, early stage 3: height reconstruction and core revascularization of the lunate. J Hand Surg Br. 1994;19:466–78.

Chapter 53
Hand Tendon Injuries

Nirbhay S. Jain

Detailed Anatomy of Tendons [1, 2]

- Flexors (Pulleys) (Fig. 53.1)
  - A1: over MCP, A2: over P1, A3: over PIP, A4 over P2, A5: over DIP
  - C1 between A2/3, C2 between 3/4, C3 between 4/5
  - A2/4 are most important to prevent bowstringing, need to maintain
- Extensors at the Wrist (Fig. 53.2)
  - Dorsal compartments
    - 1: APL/EPB
    - 2: ECRL/ECRB
    - 3: EPL
    - 4: EDC/EIP
    - 5: EDM
    - 6: ECU
      - Needs subsheath for stability
  - Juncturae tendinum.
    - Interconnections between extensor tendons distally
    - Allows EDC to transmit forces to other fingers if cut PROXIMAL to the juncturae
    - Prevent MF/RF from extending on its own

N. S. Jain (✉)
Division of Plastic Surgery, Department of Surgery, University of California, Los Angeles, Los Angeles, CA, USA
e-mail: nsjain@mednet.ucla.edu

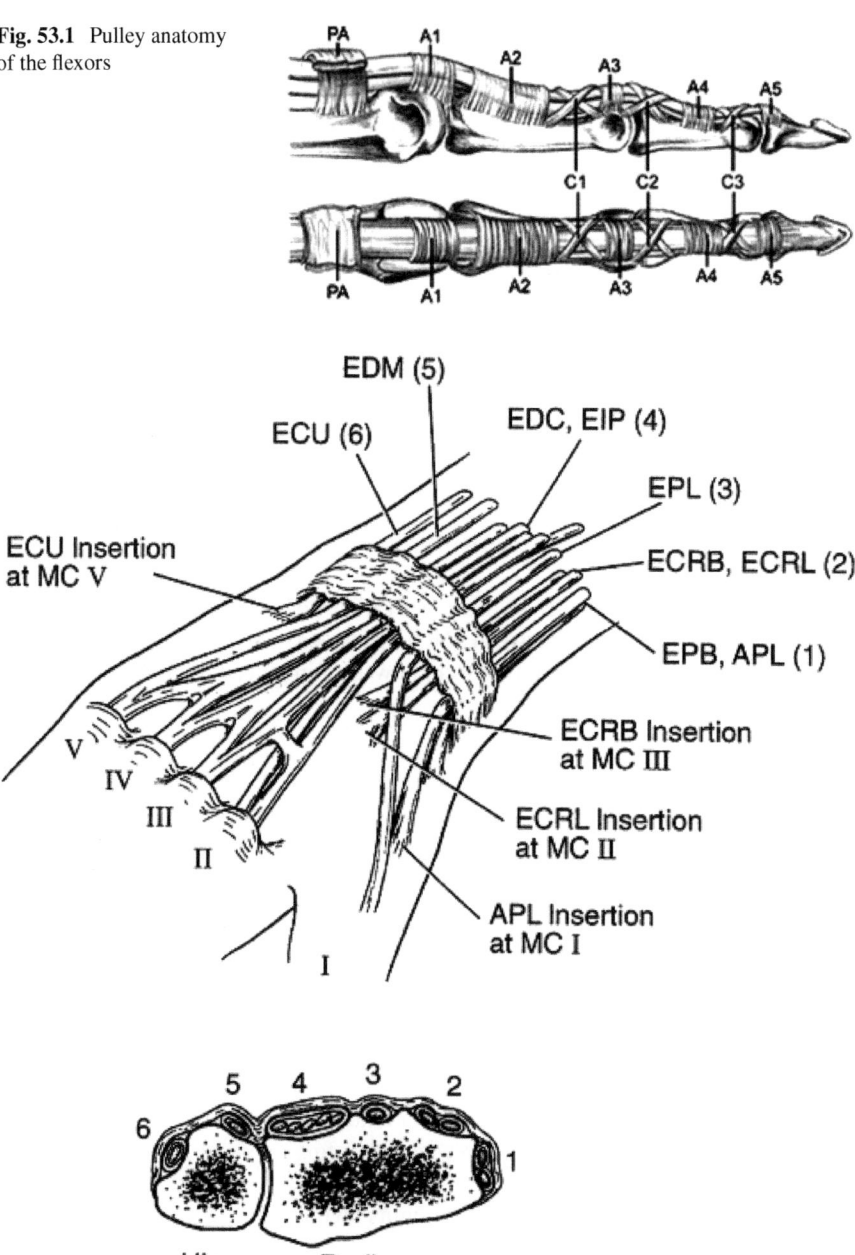

Fig. 53.1 Pulley anatomy of the flexors

Fig. 53.2 Extensor compartments

- EIP and EDM give an independent function to IF and SF.
- Sagittal bands maintain the MP EDC position.
- Extensor mechanisms at the finger.
  - EDC does NOT insert on the proximal phalanx; force is transmitted by the sagittal bands.
  - EDC trifurcates at P1 to form lateral slips and the central slip.
  - Lateral slip joins with lumbricals and interossei, as does the central.
  - Central inserts on P2, lateral on P3 in terminal tendon.
- Transverse retinacular ligament and the oblique retinacular ligament maintain the palmar position of the lateral slips over P2.
  - ORL may not be real, helps organize PIP and DIP functions (transfers power from one to the other, keeps them in sync).
- TL maintains dorsal position over DIP.
- MP function driven by EDC, IP by intrinsics.

Principles of Repair [3]

- Repair timing
  - Generally, primary repair should be done within 2 weeks; otherwise, muscles contract and proximal tendons will no longer reach.
- Repair methods (graft, primary, transfer)
  - Primary repair is preferred.
    - Repair if >50% is injured.
    - Flexor tendons retract more than extensors, so need to fix sooner.
  - Grafting and transfer are salvage options:
    - Grafting is often used if no appropriate donor is available.
    - Need to have an intact tendon sheath to graft in one stage with good soft tissue coverage.
    - If not, need to develop the sheath by placing a temporary silicone rod (Hunter Rod) and then graft at the second stage.
  - Suture options
    - Core sutures give strength (~80%), and the epitendinous provide the rest.
    - Want 4–6 strand repair on average.
- Postoperative considerations and complications
  - Splinting and early active motion are ideal.

- Careful balance because early forces risk rupturing the repair, but if fingers don't move, then the tendons will scar to surrounding tissues and will not move.
- Duran protocol for flexor tendons.
- Also need to watch out for rupture.

Flexor Tendon Injuries [4, 5]

- Based on flexor zones (Fig. 53.3)
  - I (between insertion of FDS and FDP)
    - FDP only injury.
    - Jersey.
    - Quadriga effect causes inability to completely flex remaining digits if FDP is over-advanced during a repair, because FDP shares a common muscle belly and excursion is limited by the shortest tendon.
  - II between the A1 pulley and the insertion of FDS
    - Includes camper's chiasm.
    - "No man's land."

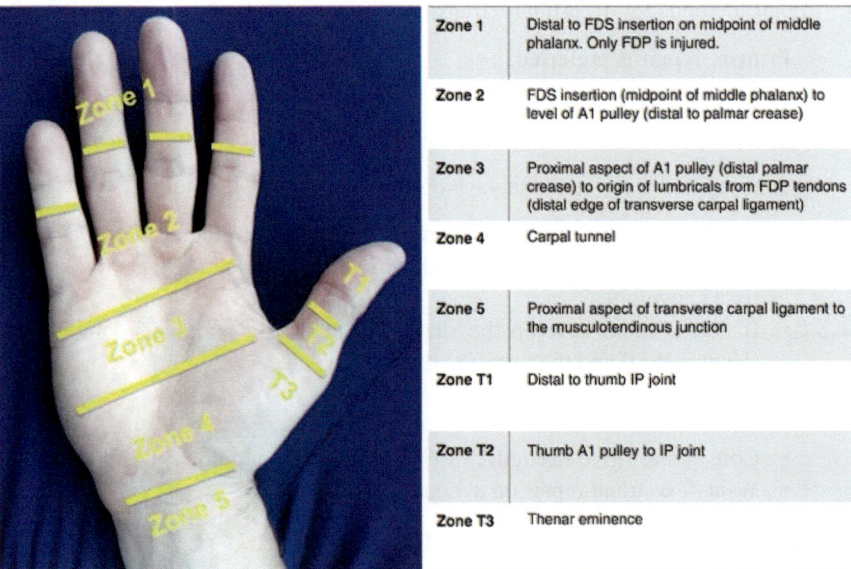

Zone 1	Distal to FDS insertion on midpoint of middle phalanx. Only FDP is injured.
Zone 2	FDS insertion (midpoint of middle phalanx) to level of A1 pulley (distal to palmar crease)
Zone 3	Proximal aspect of A1 pulley (distal palmar crease) to origin of lumbricals from FDP tendons (distal edge of transverse carpal ligament)
Zone 4	Carpal tunnel
Zone 5	Proximal aspect of transverse carpal ligament to the musculotendinous junction
Zone T1	Distal to thumb IP joint
Zone T2	Thumb A1 pulley to IP joint
Zone T3	Thenar eminence

Fig. 53.3 Flexor zones

- Most difficult place to repair given the potential injury to A2 and the need to fix FDS and FDP.
- FDP is more important to repair than FDS.
- III between the A1 pulley and the carpal tunnel
- IV within the carpal tunnel
- V proximal to the carpal tunnel

Extensor Tendon Injuries

- Based on extensor zones (Fig. 53.4)
  - I: mallet, swan neck
    - DIPJ.
    - Often get away with splinting or K-wire for 6 weeks continuously
    - May need repair if chronic or fusion.
    - Fowler tenotomy is also an option, releasing the central slip, which takes up the slack of the mallet.
    - Can progress to a swan neck deformity if left untreated.
  - II
    - Dorsal middle phalanx distal to the central slip
    - Does pretty well with repair

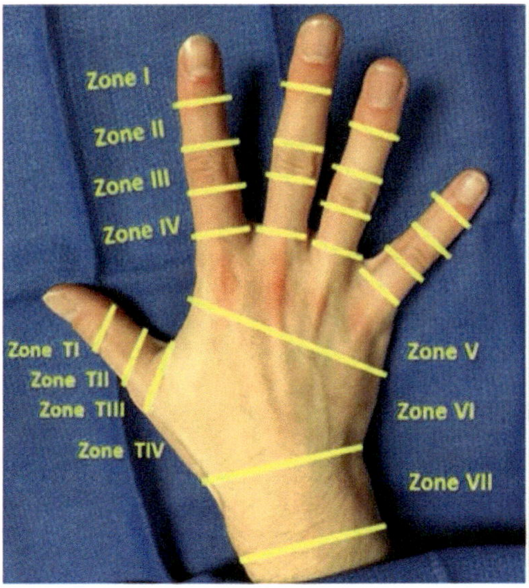

Zone I	Injury is distal to the DIP joint
Zone II	Injury is overlying the middle phalanx
Zone III	Injury is over the PIP joint
Zone IV	Injury is overlying the proximal phalanx
Zone V	Injury is over the MCP joint
Zone VI	Injury is over the metacarpal Most common zone of injury
Zone VII	Injury to the tendon and retinaculum over the wrist joint
Zone VIII	Injury to the muscle belly in the distal forearm
Zone TI	Injury is distal to the IP joint of the thumb
Zone TII	Injury is overlying the proximal phalanx of the thumb
Zone TIII	Injury is over the MCP joint of the thumb
Zone TIV	Injury is over the CMC joint of the thumb

Fig. 53.4 Extensor zones

- III: central slip (boutonniere)
    - Main injury is a central slip.
    - Treat with splinting (like a mallet), though operative repair may be needed.
    - Chronic may need release of the terminal tendon or TRL
    - Elson test
        - If the central slip is lacerated, it can extend the DIP with a flexed PIP.
        - When PIP is flexed, DIP cannot usually extend because of slack on the lateral bands.
        - This slack is released when the central slip is disrupted.
- IV
    - Over the proximal phalanx, just repair.
- V (sagittal band exam)
    - Sagittal bands over the MCP.
    - Cannot raise finger, but can maintain finger in extension if placed there.
    - Splint first, then repair.
- VI
    - Over the metacarpal, relatively favorable injury.
    - Easy to repair if you can find ends.
    - May not always have extension deficit on exam because of juncturae.
- VII
    - Over the wrist
    - May be in the extensor retinaculum
    - Need to find and repair, may have retracted
- VIII
    - Distal forearm, MT junction
- IX
    - Proximal forearm, again, repair if you find ends. Often muscle bellies in this area.

Other Tendon-Based Injuries

- Trigger Finger
    - Tendonitis of the FDS or FDP as they pass through the A1 pulley
    - Swollen FDP or FDS gets caught in A1 pulled, resulting in a fixed flexion that pops into extension.

- Steroids and NSAIDS at first; may need to be released.
- De Quervain's
  - Extensor compartment I tenosynovitis (APL, EPB)
  - Steroids, brace, NSAIDs, or release
  - Have to check for and release separate subcompartments for each tendon; otherwise, may recur
- Intersection
  - Intersection of compartments I/II
  - Splint, rest, NSAIDs
- Tennis elbow
  - Lateral epicondylitis
  - Primarily pathology of ECRB origin
  - Rest, NSAIDs

References

1. Blue AI, Spira M, Hardy SB. Repair of extensor tendon injuries of the hand. Am J Surg. 1976;132:128–32.
2. Mason ML. Rupture of the tendons of the hand. Surg Gynecol Obstet. 1930;50:611–24.
3. Wehbe MA. Junctura anatomy. J Hand Surg Am. 1992;17:1124–9.
4. Doyle JR. Anatomy of the finger flexor tendon sheath and pulley system. J Hand Surg Am. 1988;13:473–84.
5. Tang JB. Indications, methods, postoperative motion and outcome evaluation of primary flexor tendon repairs in zone 2. J Hand Surg Eur. 2007;32:118–29.

Chapter 54
Tendon Transfers

Nirbhay S. Jain

Indications for Tendon Transfers [1]

- Used to recreate the functions of paralyzed muscles from nerve palsy.
- Does not restore sensation or normal strength, but does give motion to lost actions.
- Can be done at any time after an injury, but often done after nerve transfers failed or no longer are possible.
  - Nerve transfers are feasible for up to 1 year after injury; afterwards, tendon transfers are typically the only options that are feasible due to loss of neuromuscular junctions.
- Can also be done if primary tendon repair is not possible or if grafting is not reasonable.
  - This can occur after 1–2 months after injury.

Principles of Tendon Transfers (What Is Needed for a Successful Tendon Transfer) [2]

- Supple Joints:
  - Tendon transfers are only useful if joints are still mobile—rerouted tendons cannot move frozen joints.

N. S. Jain (✉)
Division of Plastic Surgery, Department of Surgery, University of California, Los Angeles, Los Angeles, CA, USA
e-mail: nsjain@mednet.ucla.edu

- Postoperative joints cannot move more as preoperative joints.
- Stiff joints are a contraindication to tendon transfers.
- Tissue equilibrium.
  - Local tissue is healed with minimal scarring/present planes for tendon gliding.
- Donor with adequate strength as the recipient.
- Approximate amplitude of motion.
  - Amplitudes of motion should be nearly the same in tendon donors and recipients.
  - Can be augmented using the tenodesis effect.
- Straight line of pull.
- One tendon, one function.
- Synergy of function—donor tendon should generally have a synergistic function (like wrist extension to finger flexion because those movements typically occur concurrently).
- Expendable donors.
- Patient will often require some cortical retraining postoperatively through rehab.

Transfers for Specific Injury Patterns [3]

- Finger and wrist extension
  - Standard Trio
    - PT → ECRB
    - PL → EPL
    - FCR → EDC
      - FCR is preferred because FCU is a more important wrist stabilizer.
      - FCU also gives a power grip.
      - Does require tenodesis for most effect (maximal finger extension with wrist flexion).
  - Boyes transfers
    - PT to ECRL/ECRB
    - FCR to APL/EPB
    - FDS-III (to ring finger) to EDC
    - FDS-IV (to small finger) to EPL/EIP
  - Thumb extension
    - EIP to EPL

- Finger and Wrist Flexion
  - Transfers to restore thumb opposition
    - FDS-III
    - EIP
      - Pulley around the ulna to allow for opposition
    - ADM (Huber), mainly in pediatric patients
    - PL (Camitz), mainly in carpal tunnel syndrome
  - Transfers for thumb flexion
    - BR to FPL
  - Transfers for finger flexion
    - ECRL to FDP
  - Thumb adduction
    - ECRB to AdP
    - FDS to AdP
  - SF adduction
    - EDC to ADM
  - FDP loss
    - Side to side tenorrhaphy
  - Key Pinch
    - ECRB
  - ADM
    - EDM

References

1. Adams J, Wood VE. Tendon transfers for irreparable nerve damage in the hand. Orthop Clin North Am. 1981;12:403–32.
2. Beasley RW. Principles of tendon transfer. Orthop Clin North Am. 1970;1:433–8.
3. Lieber RL, Jacobson MD, Fazeli BM, et al. Architecture of selected muscles of the arm and forearm: anatomy and implications for tendon transfer. J Hand Surg Am. 1992;21:612–8.

Chapter 55
Ligament Injuries

Nirbhay S. Jain

Distal and Proximal Interphalangeal Joint Injuries [1, 2]

- Anatomy
    - Collateral ligaments (proper and volar components) for the ulnar and radial aspects of the joint.
    - Volar plate forms the floor.
        - Checkrein ligaments are the proximal lateral portion, preventing hyperextension of the joint.
- Evaluation
    - XR as always.
        - Look for the V sign to evaluate incongruent joints.
    - Stability under digital block:
        - Active: able to voluntarily range the digit through motion
        - Passive: test in flexion for collaterals, extension for volar plate
- Types of injury
    - Dorsal dislocation
        - Involves injury to the volar plate
        - If stable through the full range of motion, then buddy tape
        - If unstable, then extension block splint and progressively extend

---

N. S. Jain (✉)
Division of Plastic Surgery, Department of Surgery, University of California, Los Angeles, Los Angeles, CA, USA
e-mail: nsjain@mednet.ucla.edu

- If the volar plate interposed, then needs open reduction
- Lateral dislocation
  - Typically manage with buddy taping
- Volar dislocation
  - Rare injury
  - Due to rupture of extensor mechanism/central slip
  - If not reducible, then need to operate

Metacarpophalangeal Joints of the Fingers (Excluding the Thumb) [3]

- Anatomy
  - Dorsally supported by a loose extensor tendon.
  - Volar side has the volar plate and collaterals laterally.
  - Sagittal bands and intrinsic tendons provide secondary support.
  - Collaterals taut in flexion.
- Dorsal dislocations
  - Irreducible due to interposed volar structures
    - Forms a noose around MC neck
  - Keeps finger in hyperextension
  - Reduce by flexing the wrist and volarly displacing the proximal phalanx
- Volar
  - Rare, typically reducible
- RCL rupture of MCPJ
  - Can splint or repair depending on degree of injury
- Locked MCPJ
  - Flexion deformity of the MCPJ with normal PIP/DIP
  - Usually due to restriction of the collateral ligament by a prominent osteophyte
  - Mainly in long fingers
  - Radially deviate and externally rotate the joint to displace the ligament to free it
  - If fails, may need operative exploration

MCPJ (Thumb) (Fig. 55.1)

- Anatomy
    - Proper and accessory collateral ligaments on both sides
    - Volar plate and intrinsics form the floor
    - AdP inserts ulnarly at the joint, AbP radially
    - Ligaments are 1/3 volar
- UCL injuries
    - Acute—skier's thumb, if 10–20° can be splinted; if greater, then repair.
    - Test in extension for accessory, flexion for proper.
    - Stener lesion occurs when the adductor interposes between the ruptured ends of the UCL, requires operative exploration.
    - Chronic—gamekeeper thumb, direct repair unlikely, needs reconstruction or a tightrope.
- RCL lesion
    - Associated with abductor injury but rarely interposition

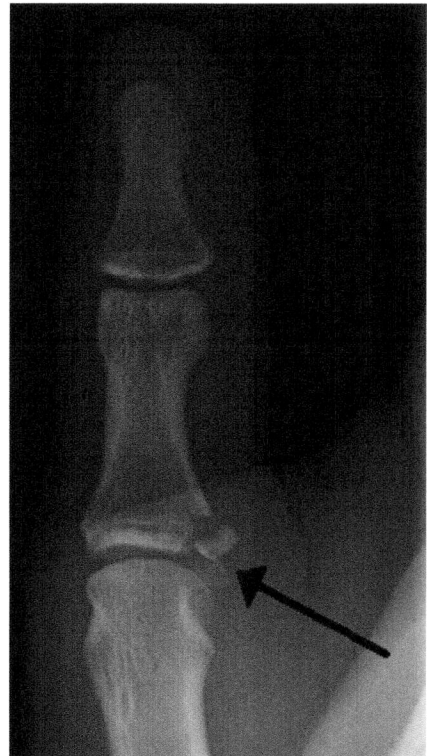

Fig. 55.1 UCL tear with associated fracture

- Common finding is the dorsoradial prominence of the metacarpal head
- Indication for management similar to UCL

CMC (Thumb)

- Four key ligaments: volar beak, intermetacarpal, dorsal oblique/APL, and dorsoradial
- Dislocation almost always dorsal with a volar beak tear
- Reduce and splint if stable, otherwise reduce and repair the volar beak

Wrist [4, 5]

- Perilunate
  - Complex carpal derangements involving injury to the ligaments surrounding the lunate bone
  - Evaluation
    - Watson test for scaphoid
    - Gilula's arcs on XR
    - Stress views
  - Stage I
    - Scapholunate injury
    - Associated with a Dorsal Intercalated segment Instability (DISI) deformity, Terry Thomas sign
    - Can be dynamic (only with clenched first) or static (always)
    - Clenched fist view
    - Needs to be repaired, risk of scaphoid lunate advanced collapse (SLAC) wrist, which progresses to debilitating arthritis of the wrist (Fig. 55.2)
  - Stage II
    - Lunocapitate ligamentous injury
    - Capitate dislocates dorsally from lunate (lesser arc)
    - Fenton syndrome—scaphoid and capitate fracture (greater arc)
  - Stage III
    - Lunotriquetral ligamentous injury
    - Volar intercalated segment instability (VISI) deformity
  - Stage IV
    - True lunate dislocation

Fig. 55.2 SLAC wrist with severe radiocarpal erosion

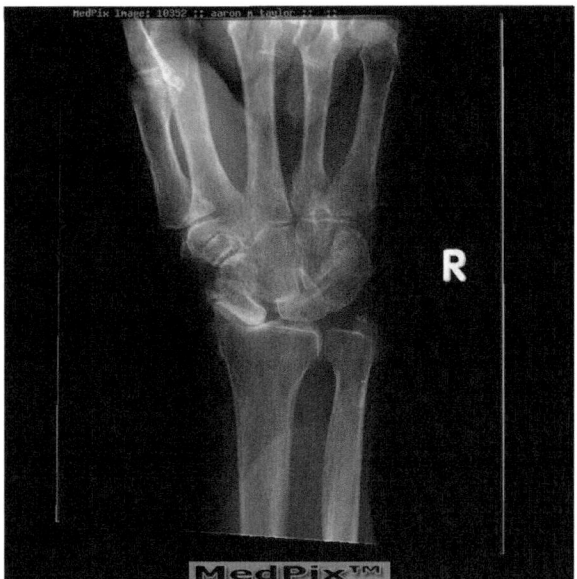

- Short radiolunate ligament all that is left
- Lunate goes volar
- Needs operative intervention
- Acute carpal tunnel risk
- Dislocates into the space of Poirier

– Initial goal of surgery is to reconstruct ligaments.

- If it fails, go to salvage procedures like fusion and proximal row carpectomy (PRC).

References

1. Bohart PG, Gelberman RH, Vandell RF, et al. Complex dislocations of the metacarpophalangeal joint. Clin Orthop Relat Res. 1982;164:208–10.
2. Campbell CS. Gamekeeper's thumb. J Bone Joint Surg Br. 1955;37:148–9.
3. Diao E, Eaton RG. Total collateral ligament excision for contractures of the proximal interphalangeal joint. J Hand Surg Am. 1993;18:393–402.
4. Kaplan SJ. The Stener lesion revisited. J Hand Surg Am. 1998;23:833–6.
5. Rettig ME, Dassa G, Raskin KB. Volar plate arthroplasty of the distal interphalangeal joint. J Hand Surg Am. 2001;26:940–4.

Chapter 56
Digital Replantation and Revascularization

Corbin Muetterties

Pathophysiology

Ischemic Injury

- Ischemia leads to tissue hypoxia, which increases anaerobic metabolism and ultimately leads to the buildup of lactic acid, activation of cellular enzymes, and eventually cell necrosis [1].
- In general, more proximal amputation injuries require more urgent replantation due to the increased presence of muscle tissue, which is much less tolerant of ischemia compared to skin or adipose tissue.
- Replantation should proceed. as soon as possible; however, successful digital replantation has been reported in cases with up to 33 h of warm and 96 h of cold ischemia [2].

Reperfusion Injury

- Reperfusion of ischemic tissue leads to the release of reactive oxygen species (ROS), which in turn lead to the release of inflammatory mediators, complement activation, leukocyte adhesion, and direct cell damage, ultimately leading to increased vascular permeability and cell death [1].
- Methods used to mitigate these factors and improve replantation success include cooling of the amputated digit, timely revascularization of affected tissue, and postoperative use of antithrombotic agents.

C. Muetterties (✉)
UCLA Medical Center, Los Angeles, CA, USA
e-mail: CMuetterties@mednet.ucla.edu

© The Author(s), under exclusive license to Springer Nature Switzerland AG 2025
J. Roostaeian et al. (eds.), *Plastic Surgery Clerkship*, Contemporary Surgical Clerkships, https://doi.org/10.1007/978-3-031-99098-4_56

Indications for Replantation

- Thumb amputations (40% of hand function)
- Multi-finger amputations (with a focus to allow for the restoration of pinch or grasp)
- Proximal hand, wrist, or forearm amputations
- Single-digit amputation distal to FDS insertion
- Any amputation in a child
- Dominant hand, particularly in patients with occupational needs (ex musician)

Relative Contraindications to Replantation

- Severe crush or avulsion injuries
- Segmental injuries
- Extreme tissue contamination
- Single digit proximal to FDS insertion (poor prognosis)
- Index finger amputations
- Uncontrolled mental illness or inability to participate in a rehabilitation program after surgery
- Prolonged warm ischemia time
- Ribbon sign (indicates avulsion injury to digital vessels)

Absolute Contraindications

- Concomitant, life-threatening injuries or significant medical comorbidities precluding the ability to undergo a replantation procedure

History and Physical Exam

- ATLS (Advanced Trauma Life Support) protocol should be used to assess for concomitant life-threatening or other traumatic injuries.
  - ABCDE of Trauma
    - Airway
    - Breathing
    - Circulation
    - Disability/Deficit
    - Exposure

- Obtain history of medical comorbidities, including occupation, handedness, smoking history, diabetes, and prior surgeries.
- Obtain plain film X-rays of the hand and amputated digit.
- Assess amputated part and stump site to determine mechanism of injury (sharp, crush, avulsion), location, and viability of involved tissue.

Preoperative Care

- Amputated part should be gently cleaned, wrapped in a saline-soaked gauze, and placed into a sealed plastic bag, which in turn is placed into a saline/ice bath.
- Avoid direct exposure of ice to the amputated part, as this can lead to frostbite injuries.
- Bleeding should be controlled with hand elevation and pressure with gauze (avoid clipping vessels and tourniquet before entering the operating room).
- Consent should be obtained for the planned procedure, including discussion of the possible need for vein grafting, nerve grafting, skin grafts, local flap coverage, and revision amputation if the digit is unable to be salvaged.
- Typically, both regional and general anesthesia are used, with regional anesthesia providing the additional benefit of sympathetic blockade and vasodilation.

Intraoperative Sequence of Events

Back Table Evaluation of the Amputated Part

- Wound irrigation and debridement of devitalized tissue.
- An operating microscope or loupes should be used to identify and tag all structures, including digital arteries and nerves, dorsal skin veins, and tendons.

Bony Fixation

- Generally, bony fixation is performed first after identification of structures.
- Bony shortening should be considered if it allows for secure fixation and lessens the need for nerve or vessel grafting.
- Intraosseous 90-90 wiring allows for both compression across the fracture and stabilization of rotational forces without requiring extensive periosteal stripping.
- Plate fixation is useful for more proximal amputations. The smallest possible plates should be used to minimize periosteal stripping.

- Crossed K-wires allow for quick bony stabilization and can be placed retrograde into the amputated digit on the back table and then driven into the proximal bone for fixation.

Tendon Repair

- Technique varies by surgeon; however, the most commonly used technique is a 4-0 modified Kessler core stitch with a 6-0 epitendinous suture.
- Pulleys should be preserved during tendon repair to prevent bowstringing.
- Distal core suture can be placed on the back table of the amputated digit.
- Proximal tendon is identified and secured in place with a 25-gauge wire in proximity to the distal tendon.
- Most important factor in tendon repair is early return to motion, which has been shown to improve both active and passive range of motion without significantly increasing the risk of tendon rupture [3].

Artery Repair

- The arteries should be examined and trimmed back until a healthy vessel is identified.
- The lumen should be inspected for intimal flaps or other signs of endothelial damage, which can increase the risk of thrombosis.
- The lumen is then flushed with dilute heparinized saline and examined for pulsatile flow.
- Vascular clamps are applied, and the repair is then completed with 9-0 or 10-0 nylon sutures.
- If a vessel gap exists following trimming, vein grafts can be harvested from the volar palm, volar forearm, or dorsal foot to bridge the defect.
- In all cases, attempts should be made to repair both digital arteries if possible.

Vein Repair

- Successful vein repair is critical to improving replant survival in cases of complete amputation.
- In partial amputations, a small skin bridge can allow for sufficient venous drainage to allow for survival of the revascularized digit.
- Dorsal skin veins can be identified by looking for areas of bruising along the dorsal skin.

- Often, partial amputations with intact dorsal skin have adequate venous drainage.
- Veins should be repaired with vein grafts as required
  - Typically taken from the proximal volar wrist
- Multiple vein repairs have been shown to increase the success rate of digital replantations, with two veins having the highest success rate when compared to single or no veins repaired [4].
- Vein repair should be performed prior to release of arterial clamps to prevent congestion of the replanted digit.
- In cases where no vein can be identified for repair, digital salvage with temporary alternative methods for venous drainage, including leeches, arteriovenous anastomoses, nail plate removal, and heparin injections, has been reported [1].

Nerve Repair

- Nerve repair is essential to allow for protective sensation and sensibility of the replanted digit.
- Sharp injuries can often be performed primarily, particularly if bone shortening techniques are used.
- The nerve ends should be carefully inspected under an operating microscope and trimmed back to healthy fascicles. Evidenced by pinpoint bleeding and normal fascicular architecture.
- In cases where a nerve gap exists, conduits or nerve grafts can be utilized to bridge the defect.
- A careful epineural repair should be completed using a meticulous technique to ensure a tension-free nerve repair.
- Nerve allograft or autologous nerve grafts can be used with the most common autologous donor sites, including the posterior interosseous nerve, median antebrachial cutaneous nerve, or sural nerve.

Soft Tissue Coverage

- Following repair of all structures, skin closure and soft tissue coverage are performed.
- Skin grafts should be used liberally to avoid tight skin closure, which may compromise the repair.
- In cases of extensive soft tissue injury, placement of a wound matrix or delayed soft tissue coverage with local flaps or free tissue transfer may be required.
- In cases of volar digital wounds with both arterial and skin defects, venous flow through flaps harvested from the volar wrist can be used.

Postoperative Care (Fig. 56.1)

- Following replantation, patients are typically admitted to allow for postoperative monitoring of the replanted digit.
- Digital vascularity can be monitored with pulse oximetry, bedside arterial doppler exams, and physical exam to monitor for signs of ischemia or congestion.
- In order to prevent thrombosis, some providers use anticoagulation protocols in the immediate postoperative period, with many different agents utilized, including heparin, aspirin, or dextran
- 80% of vascular occlusions occur within the first 48 h after surgery [1].
- If recognized immediately, salvage rates following revision of microvascular anastomoses range anywhere from 60% to 80% [1].
- Rehab is initiated 5–7 days after surgery with initial gentle active and passive range of motion, taking care to protect the vessel and nerve repairs.
- Sensory reeducation and desensitization protocols are also followed in patients who undergo nerve repairs.

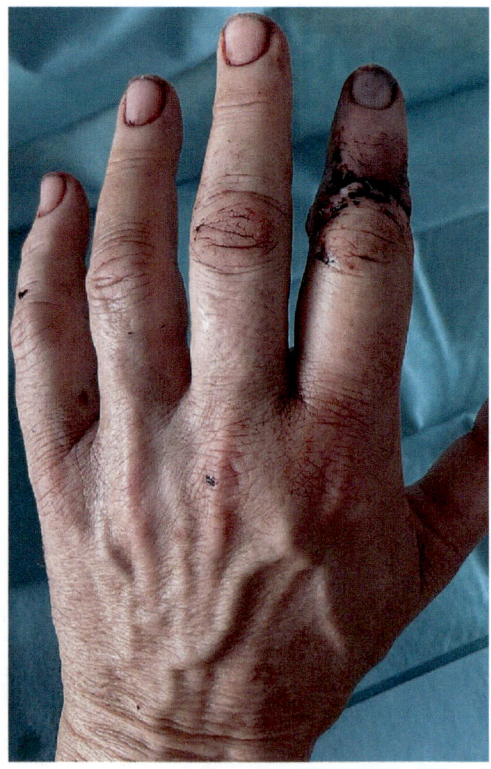

Fig. 56.1 Index finger after replantation

Key Points

- General sequence of events: back table identification of structures > bone fixation > tendon repair > arterial repair > venous repair > nerve repair > skin closure.
- Candidates for replantation should have the amputated digit wrapped in a saline-soaked gauze, placed into a plastic bag, which is then placed on ice before transfer to a replantation center.

References

1. Dzwierzynski W. Replantation and revascularization. In: Nelligan P, editor. Plastic surgery. 3rd ed. London: Elsevier; 2013. p. 228–49.
2. Prucz RB, Friedrich JB. Upper extremity replantation: current concepts. Plast Reconstr Surg. 2014;133:333–42.
3. Starr HM, Snoddy M, Hammond KE, Seiler JG 3rd. Flexor tendon repair rehabilitation protocols: a systematic review. J Hand Surg Am. 2013;38(9):1712-7.e1–14.
4. Yamano Y. Replantation of the amputated distal part of the fingers. J Hand Surg. 1985;10A:211–8.

Chapter 57
Thumb Reconstruction

Udayan Betarbet

Overview/General Considerations [1–6]

- After functional tissue loss of the thumb, always assess viability of surrounding skin, determine integrity of the neurovascular bundle, and determine extent of bony loss.
- Always ask about the patient's smoking history of any tobacco or nicotine products in addition to preexisting comorbidities.
- At presentation, obtain standard three view hand radiographs and at least one view of any amputated parts.
- Reconstructive goals are to restore protective sensation and opposition of the thumb according to the patient's occupational needs.
- To restore thumb opposition, sufficient length must be preserved for pinch and grasping motions. Amputation of the thumb at or proximal to the shaft of the proximal phalanx can cause serious difficulties for thumb pinch. In comparison to the thumb interphalangeal joints (IP) and metacarpophalangeal joints (MP), the carpometacarpal joint (CMCJ) is most important for active thumb function.
- Discuss reconstructive goals and rehabilitation demands with each patient after considering occupation, patient's age, and hand dominance.
- Revision amputation should only be performed if other options for stability and sensate tissue coverage are not available.
- Reconstruction can be divided into thumb defects as described by Dr. Lister:

1. Acceptable length with soft tissue deficit
2. Subtotal amputation with possible adequate length
3. Total amputation with preservation of CMCJ
4. Total amputation with destruction of CMCJ

Acceptable Length with Soft Tissue Defect [1, 2, 4, 5, 7, 8]

- Amputation above or at the level of the interphalangeal joint can provide adequate bony length and function, provided a sensate thumb tip is reconstructed.
- If the soft tissue defect is less than 1 cm^2 at the distal phalanx, then the recommended treatment is to let the wound heal by secondary intention.
- Local flaps, such as local advancements and free skin grafts, are possible for small defects as well. The V-Y volar advancement, also known as the Atasoy flap, is used for defects just distal to the midpoint of the nail bed, with the base of the flap at the volar IP joint crease. Similar lateral or oblique V-Y flaps can be performed in a unilateral or bilateral fashion.
- If greater than 50% of the thumb distal phalanx soft tissue is disrupted with exposure of bone, then soft tissue coverage with the Moberg advancement flap, cross-finger flaps, or neurovascular island flaps is necessary to preserve length and sensation to the remaining thumb. Free toe pulp transfers have also been described.
- Moberg Advancement Flap (Fig. 57.1):
  - This flap resurfaces distal thumb pulp defects that are less than 50% of the volar surface by advancing proximal volar tissue with neurovascular structures.
  - Is viable in the thumb because the thumb has robust dorsal vasculature.
  - This flap advances sensate tissue into the defect. This flap can be advanced to cover defects up to 1.5 cm or less, though this can be increased to 2.5 cm if a proximal releasing incision is made or a V-Y extension is made at the base.
  - Summary of Procedure: After nonviable tissue is debrided, radial and ulnar mid-axial incisions are made from the defect to the proximal thumb crease. The flap is elevated from the flexor tendon sheath with care to include the neurovascular bundles. Next, the IP and MP joints are flexed to allow for sufficient advancement of the flap to cover the defect. The IP joint is commonly flexed 45° while the MP joint is flexed 30°.
  - Flexion of the MP and IP joints may cause a long-term flexion deformity. To avoid significant flexion of the distal thumb joints and gain additional advancement, proximal releasing incisions can be used. In this procedure, the mid-axial incisions are made to the proximal third of the proximal phalanx and

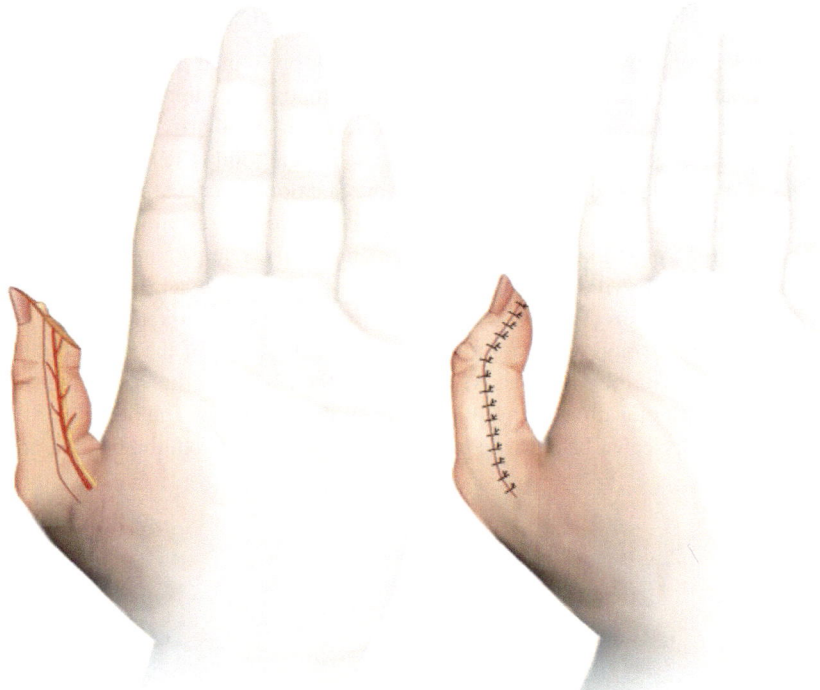

Fig. 57.1 Moberg flap with advancement

then transversely connected. The flap is then advanced and the proximal defect is covered with a full-thickness skin graft.

- Cross-Finger Flap (Heterodigital Flap):
  - This flap is designed to provide sensate skin coverage for significant soft tissue defects of the thumb distal phalanx.
  - Summary of Procedure: After the nonviable tissue has been debrided, a sterile piece of paper is used to create a template of the defect that is then outlined on the dorsal radial aspect of the proximal phalanx of the index finger. The incisions are then made, leaving the radial aspect intact as a pivot point of the flap. The flap is raised in an ulnar to radial dissection above the extensor paratenon with incision of Cleland ligaments. The flap is rotated on its radial border and inset onto the thumb defect. The donor site is then covered with a full-thickness skin graft. The flap is divided after 2–3 weeks.
  - Return of flap protective sensation is best in patients younger than 20 years old.
  - Modifications of this flap can include incorporation of the dorsal sensory branch of the radial nerve.

- First Dorsal Metacarpal Artery (FDMA) Island Flap (Fig. 57.2):
    - This is a versatile flap that reduces the need for prolonged immobilization.
    - Summary of Procedure: Similar to the cross-finger flap, a template is made of the thumb defect and then outlined on the dorsum of the proximal phalanx of the index finger from the proximal interphalangeal joint (PIP) and index MP joint. A Doppler is then used to identify the first dorsal metacarpal artery from the radial aspect of the index MP joint distally to the proximal pivot point between the proximal first and second metacarpals. The proximal portion of the flap near the MP joint is extended further proximally in a lazy-S pattern to the level of the pivot point. The flap is raised in the ulnar to radial and distal to proximal fashion with care to preserve the entry point of the FDMA at the radial border of the MP joint. After reaching the MP joint, the lazy-S incision is made with elevation of the skin in a deep dermal plane. The pedicle of the FDMA is dissected back to the level of the pivot point. Next, the flap is trans-

Fig. 57.2 FDMA flap

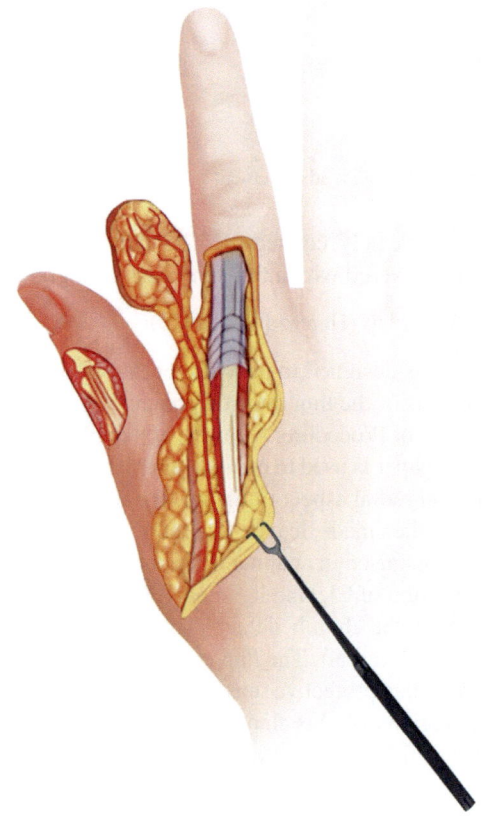

ferred through a subcutaneous tunnel to the defect. The donor site is covered with a full-thickness skin graft.
  - This flap can be modified to incorporate the sensory branch of the radial nerve.
- Neurovascular Island Pedicle Flap:
  - A local flap that allows for reconstruction of sensate tissue, though with notable donor site morbidity.
  - The neurovascular island pedicle flap utilizes the ulnar palmar skin of the long finger if the median nerve is intact and the ring finger if the median nerve is not intact.
  - Summary of Procedure: Similar to other flaps in this section, a paper template is used to outline the thumb defect onto the ulnar long or ring finger. The flap is marked out from the ulnar distal aspect of the donor digit from the distal phalanx proximal to the volar MP joint crease. First, the neurovascular bundle is identified in the webspace, and the digital artery and nerve to the donor digit are isolated. This neurovascular bundle is dissected distally to the edge of the flap. The flap is then elevated distally to proximally and transferred to the defect under a skin bridge. The flap is secured to the recipient defect and the donor site is covered with a full-thickness skin graft. The palmar defect is closed primarily.
  - This flap sacrifices the ulnar sensation of the long or ring finger as well as the radial blood supply to the adjacent digit.
- Dorsal-ulnar and dorsal-radial reverse flow homodigital island flaps, innervated by the superficial radial nerve, have also been described.

Subtotal Amputation with Possible Adequate Length [1, 2, 4, 5]

- Loss of bony length proximal to the mid-point of the proximal phalanx is at increased risk for impaired pinch and grasping function. With preservation of the CMC joint arc of rotation, improved function can be achieved by deepening the first webspace with either a simple or four-flap Z-plasty procedure. These procedures can be performed if at least half the proximal phalanx is present, adequate mobility of the first metacarpal, and minimal scarring of skin and muscle. The simple Z-plasty is designed with the vertical limb along the distal ridge of the first webspace, with 60° limbs of the same length as shown in Fig. 57.3. The flaps are then incised and raised at the level of the muscle fascia. The thumb is then abducted to allow for transposition of the flaps that are then sutured in place. A modification of this is the four-flap Z-plasty.
- If there is scarring of the first webspace or contracture of the first metacarpal, phalangization or relative lengthening of the first metacarpal with a dorsal rotation flap is needed to restore the first webspace.

Fig. 57.3 Standard Z-plasty

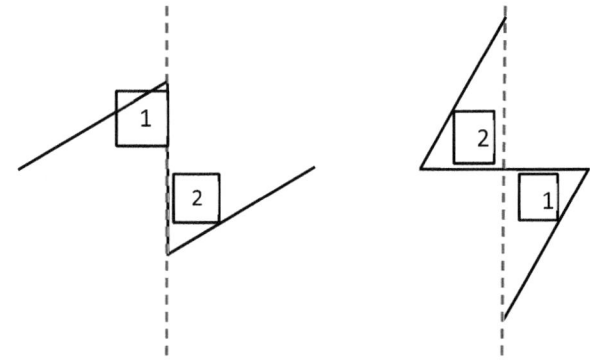

Total Amputation with Preservation of CMCJ [1, 2, 4, 5]

- At this level of amputation, the goal is to restore adequate length for thumb functionality. Toe-to-thumb transfer is a reliable option for patients to address this level of defect, which will be discussed in a separate section. Osteoplastic reconstruction and composite radial forearm island flap are other potential reconstructive options that will be briefly discussed as well.
- Osteoplastic reconstruction is performed as a two-stage procedure to reconstruct the thumb length with a bone graft and a pedicle flap. In the first stage, a tricortical bone graft from the iliac crest is fashioned to have a proximal 2 cm stem or peg. This bone graft peg is then inserted into a hole previously carved into the medullary canal of the remaining first metacarpal. The combined first metacarpal bone graft construct is then inserted into a tubed groin flap. In the second stage, the groin flap is divided, and a neurovascular island flap is raised from the ulnar long finger to cover the volar aspect of the neo-thumb.
- Composite Radial Forearm Island Flap: This is a single-stage procedure that involves raising a radial forearm flap with a 2–3 cm bone flap from the lateral radius vascularized by perforators of the radial artery. The skin and bone flap is mobilized under a skin bridge of the first webspace to the thumb defect. The volar aspect of the skin-bone graft is covered with a neurovascular island flap from the ulnar long finger. The radial forearm donor site is covered with split-thickness skin graft.
- Metacarpal distraction osteogenesis with secondary iliac bone crest grafting can be performed to increase length up to 3.0 cm if two-thirds of the first metacarpal is still intact with adequate soft tissue coverage.

Toe-to-Thumb Reconstruction [2, 5, 8]

- Important considerations in performing a toe-to-thumb reconstruction include better outcomes for younger patients and donor site morbidity as it relates to cosmesis and decreased ability to perform certain foot movements.

- This procedure can be performed at the time of initial injury or as a secondary reconstruction after wound closure has been performed with an effort to maintain bony length, tendons, nerves, and arteries. If performed as secondary reconstruction, a groin flap is a viable option for immediate reconstruction of the thumb defect, and local flaps should be avoided. Delayed toe-to-thumb transfer also allows time for the patient to understand the risks and benefits of the procedure.
- Great toe-to-thumb reconstruction can be performed in patients with thumb amputations as distal as the IP joint. The functional success of the great toe-to-thumb transfer decreases the more proximal the amputation due to the greater degree of thenar musculature damage. Amputations below the level of the MCP joint will have a critical loss of opposition function. Indications for great toe-to-thumb transfer include thumb amputation at the level of the proximal phalanx or metacarpal.
- Second toe transfer can also be performed, particularly if the thumb amputation is proximal to the CMC joint, since additional bony length can be achieved, since there are multiple phalanges compared to the great toe. An additional advantage to using the second toe transfer is that the toe is not involved in gait, unlike the great toe.
- Vasospasm is the most common complication within the first 24–72 h. Early management includes warming the transplanted thumb, lowering the level of the operated hand below the level of the heart, and releasing a few skin sutures. Operative reexploration is indicated if circulation has not returned within 1 h (Fig. 57.4).

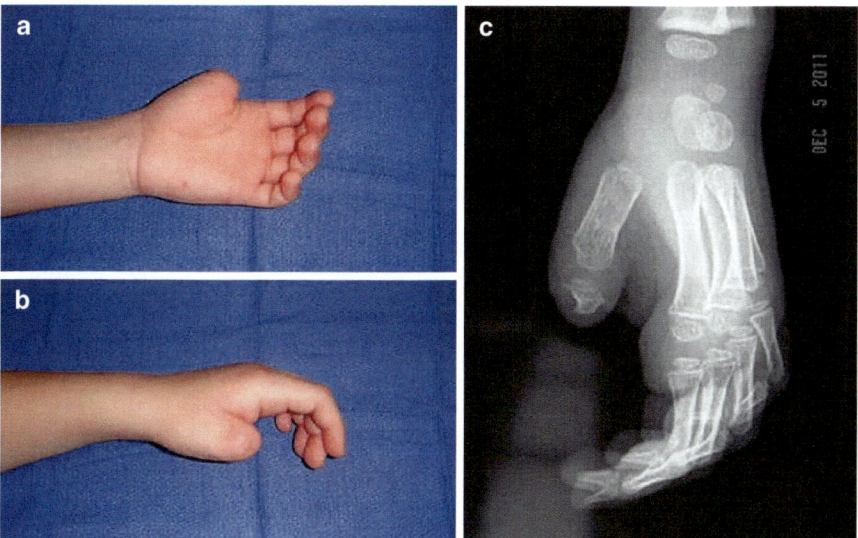

Fig. 57.4 Thumb amputation (**a**) AP view, (**b**) lateral view (**c**) X Ray demonstrating bony defect

Total Amputation with Destruction of CMCJ [1, 2, 4, 5]

- Loss of the basal thumb joint results in the absence of critical movement of the thumb leaving only arthrodesis of a reconstructed digit to perform opposition as an option. A reconstructed digit can be crafted via the pollicization of an intact index or ring finger, osteoplastic reconstruction (as previously described), or free transfer of an injured digit. Pollicization will allow for reconstruction of a basal joint
  - Methods for pollicization
  - Take ipsilateral index finger
  - Tendon transfers
    - ABP → 1DO
    - ADP → 1PO
    - APL → EDC
    - EPL → EIP
    - FDP → FPL
    - FDS → FPL
- Prosthetics can be used when reconstructive options are limited. Osseous-integrated prosthetics used dental implant hardware to improve stable fixation for opposition.

References

1. Azari K. Thumb reconstruction. In: Wolfe SW, Hotchkiss RN, Pederson WC, Kozin SH, Cohen MS, editors. Green's operative hand surgery. 7th ed. Philadelphia: Elsevier; 2017.
2. Graham DJ, Venkatramani H, Sabapathy SR. Current reconstruction options for traumatic thumb loss. J Hand Surg Am. 2016;41(12):1159–69.
3. Lister G. The choice of procedure following thumb amputation. Clin Orthop Relat Res. 1985;195:45–51.
4. Parker WL, Mathes DW. Thumb reconstruction. In: Janis J, editor. Essentials of plastic surgery. 2nd ed. Boca Raton: CRC Press; 2014.
5. Pet MA, Ko JH, Vedder NB. Reconstruction of the traumatized thumb. Plast Reconstr Surg. 2014;134(6):1235–45.
6. Waljee JF. Thumb reconstruction. In: Brown DL, Borschel GH, Levi B, editors. Michigan manual of plastic surgery. 2nd ed. Philadelphia: Lippincott Williams & Wilkins, A Wolters Kluwer Business; 2014.
7. Germann G, Rudolf KD, Levin SL, Hrabowski M. Fingertip and thumb tip wounds: changing algorithms for sensation, aesthetics, and function. J Hand Surg Am. 2017;42(4):274–84.
8. Wei F-C, AlDeek NF. Toe-to-hand transplantation. In: Wolfe SW, Hotchkiss RN, Pederson WC, Kozin SH, Cohen MS, editors. Green's operative hand surgery. 7th ed. Philadelphia: Elsevier; 2017.

Chapter 58
Dupuytren's Disease

Meaghan L. Barr

Background [1, 2]

- Dupuytren's disease most frequently affects middle-aged men of Northern European descent.
- Men are more likely than women to be afflicted (M:F is approximately 6:1).
- Dupuytren's disease is heritable. Although previously considered autosomal dominant with variable penetrance, newer studies suggest polygenetic inheritance.
- Disease prevalence varies by geographic location, with rates reported from 2% to 42%
- Associations have been demonstrated between Dupuytren's disease and manual labor, alcohol consumption, tobacco, diabetes, and epilepsy. However, whether any of these associations are causal remains controversial.

Pathophysiology [1–5]

- In Dupuytren's disease, normal hand anatomy becomes distorted when anatomic bands become pathologic "cords" due to an increase in type III collagen and proliferation of contractile myofibroblasts.
- In the non-diseased hand, there is a strong yet supple fascial system. Named components include:

M. L. Barr (✉)
Division of Plastic Surgery, Department of Surgery, University of California, Los Angeles, Los Angeles, CA, USA
e-mail: meaghanbarr@mednet.ucla.edu

© The Author(s), under exclusive license to Springer Nature Switzerland AG 2025
J. Roostaeian et al. (eds.), *Plastic Surgery Clerkship*, Contemporary Surgical Clerkships, https://doi.org/10.1007/978-3-031-99098-4_58

- Palmar aponeurosis—distal extension of the palmaris longus, located at the proximal palm.
    - Pretendinous bands—distal, longitudinal extensions of the palmar aponeurosis, extend towards the fingers.
    - Transverse ligament—runs transversely at the distal palmar crease, proximal and parallel to the natatory ligament but deep to the pretendinous bands.
    - Spiral bands—connection between the palmar and digital fascial structures.
    - Natatory ligament—travel transversely at the base of the fingers.
    - Lateral digital sheath receives contributions from the spiral band and natatory ligament.
- Soft-tissue nodules in the palms and fingers are typically the first signs of disease
- Nodules undergo three sequential phases: a proliferative stage, followed by an involution stage, followed by a residual phase
- Nodules typically precede cords, which is simply the term for a diseased fascial band.
- Cords mature into rigid, fixed structures that cause contractures, preventing finger extension. These typically begin in the volar hand and progress distally to the fingers.
- Named cords include:
    - Pretendinous cord (Fig. 58.1)—arises from a pretendinous band. Most common cord, responsible for flexion deformity at the metacarpophalangeal (MCP) joint.
    - Central cord—midline extension of a pretendinous cord.
    - Spiral cord—comprised of contributions from the pretendinous band, the spiral band, the lateral digital sheath, and Greyson's ligament. The spiral cord is of great surgical significance, as it causes volar and medial displacement of the neurovascular bundle.

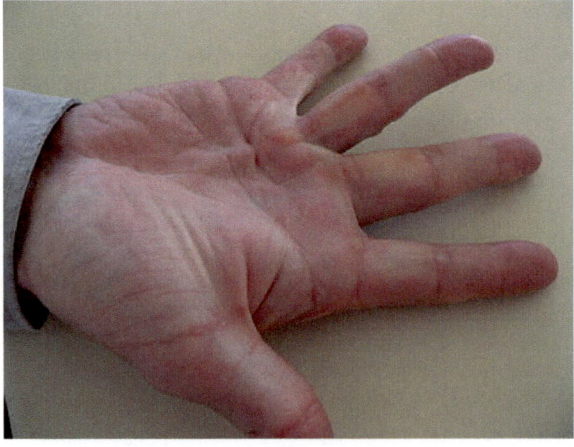

Fig. 58.1 Pretendinous cord to the ring finger

- Natatory cords—arise from natatory ligaments, causing webspace contracture.
- Lateral cord—arises from the lateral digital sheath, may cause proximal interphalangeal (PIP) and distal interphalangeal (DIP) contractures with medial displacement of the neurovascular bundle.
- Retrovascular cord—deep to the neurovascular bundle, can cause DIP joint contracture.
- Abductor digiti minimi cord—from the abductor digiti minimi tendon, causes flexion contracture of the PIP joint.
- Proximal commissural cord—from the proximal commissural ligament, causes the first webspace contracture.
- Distal commissural cord—from the distal commissural ligament, causes the first webspace contracture.

- Other manifestations of Dupuytren's disease include
  - Garrod's nodes (or knuckle pads)—ectopic lesions on the dorsal hand over the PIP joint
  - Peyronie's disease—ectopic lesions of the penis
  - Ledderhose disease—ectopic lesions of the plantar feet

Dupuytren's Diathesis [1]

- Describes more aggressive, refractory disease with early age of onset
- Characterized by bilateral hand disease, positive family history, lesions on the plantar feet (Ledderhose disease) and/or penis (Peyronie's disease)

Treatment [2, 4–6]

- Dupuytren's disease is benign but progressive; morbidity arises from contractures that limit hand function. The goal of treatment is to disrupt these diseased cords. Not all patients will require treatment, as not all disease results in severe contractures. Furthermore, despite treatment, Dupuytren's has a predilection for recurrence and progression. As such, the modality and timing of treatment should be individually tailored.
- Treatment is generally indicated for ≥30° of MCP contracture and/or any degree of PIP contracture.
  - PIP contracture is much more difficult to correct.
- The "tabletop test" is an easy way for both clinicians and patients to monitor symptoms; the patient is asked to lay their hand flat on a table. If the patient cannot lay their hand flat, intervention is usually warranted.

- There are three major treatment modalities: needle aponeurotomy, collagenase injection, and limited fasciectomy.
- In needle aponeurotomy (NA), a needle is introduced through the skin and into the underlying cord repeatedly in order to transect the cord. The digit is then passively extended to fully disrupt the cord. NA is safer for certain cords; the risk of neurovascular bundle injury is elevated when treating spiral cords. NA may be performed in the office or in the operating room.
- The collagenase *Clostridium histolyticum* (brand name Xiaflex) can be injected directly into a diseased cord in the office setting. The patient returns 1–7 days later and undergoes manipulation under local anesthesia to fully rupture the cords. The most common complications include skin tears, bruising, and edema; the risk of major complications such as tendon or neurovascular injury is <1%.
- Limited fasciectomy involves surgical removal of diseased tissue in the operating room. While studies demonstrate favorable long-term results without recurrence compared to collagenase injections and NA, the recovery process is significantly longer.

References

1. Hindocha S. Risk factors, disease associations, and Dupuytren diathesis. Hand Clin. 2018;34(3):307–14. https://doi.org/10.1016/j.hcl.2018.03.002.
2. Shaw RB, Chong AKS, Zhang A, Hentz VR, Chang J. Dupuytren's disease: history, diagnosis, and treatment. Plast Reconstr Surg. 2007;120(3):44e–54e. https://doi.org/10.1097/01.prs.0000278455.63546.03.
3. Leibovic SJ. Normal and pathologic anatomy of Dupuytren disease. Hand Clin. 2018;34(3):315–29. https://doi.org/10.1016/j.hcl.2018.04.001.
4. Wolfe SW, Pederson WC, Hotchkiss RN, Kozin SH. Green's operative hand surgery: 2-volume set. 6th ed. New York: Churchill Livingstone; 2010.
5. Beasley RW. Beasley's surgery of the hand. New York: Thieme Publishing Group; 2003.
6. Boe C, Blazar P, Iannuzzi N. Dupuytren contractures: an update of recent literature. J Hand Surg Am. 2021;46(10):896–906. https://doi.org/10.1016/j.jhsa.2021.07.005.

Chapter 59
Hand Tumors

Udayan Betarbet

General History and Physical Examination of Soft Tissue and Bony Tumors

- History should include prior history of similar tumor, current or prior history of malignancy, prior history of radiation, detailed timeline of changes in the size and skin characteristics of the tumor, and any functional or sensory changes caused by the tumor.
- Visual inspection of dorsal and volar surfaces of hand for skin changes such as ulceration, changes in skin color, presence of a punctum, or bleeding.
- A complete physical examination should include the presence of regional lymphadenopathy, complete neurologic exam, and assessment of joints, tendons, and bones.
- Examination should include if the tumor is firm or soft, fixed or mobile, or painful. Additionally, the description should include the location of the suspected tumor with respect to joint spaces and vasculature.
- Malignant tissue tumors are more commonly fixed to surrounding tissues, firm, and painful.
- Common imaging modalities include plain radiographs, ultrasound, computerized tomography (CT), or magnetic resonance imaging (MRI).

U. Betarbet (✉)
University of Texas Medical Branch, Galveston, TX, USA
e-mail: udbetarb@UTMB.EDU

Benign Soft Tissue, Nerve, and Vascular Tumors

Name: Ganglion Cysts and Mucous Cyst [2, 4, 15, 26, 32, 33] (Fig. 59.1)

- *Incidence*: Most common mass of the hand. Ganglion cysts are more commonly found in women between the second and fourth decades of life.
- *Pathogenesis/Anatomy*:
    - Mucin filled cysts that are possibly caused by synovial herniation with mucoid degeneration or have traumatic origins.
    - Most commonly found on dorsal wrist over the scapholunate ligament between the third and fourth extensor compartments. However, ganglion cysts can arise at any joint in the hand and wrist.
    - The second most common site is the volar wrist arising from the radiocarpal joint between the first extensor compartment and the flexor carpi radialis tendon sheath.
    - Flexor tendon sheaths ganglions typically arise from the A1 or A2 pulley and do not move with flexor tendon motion.
    - A ganglion cyst of the dorsal distal interphalangeal joint (DIPJ) between the joint crease and the eponychium is called a mucous cyst.
- *Diagnosis/Imaging*: Ganglion cysts are commonly soft and mobile and will transilluminate. They are frequently located adjacent to a joint space, tendon, or tendon sheath. Examination should include maneuvers assessing medial and ulnar nerve compression if in close proximity to the cyst. An Allen's test should be performed if the cyst is close proximity to the radial artery. Radiographs are not routinely completed if clinical examination is consistent with a ganglion cyst though may be performed if an interosseous component is suspected. Diagnostic ultrasound can be useful if the clinical examination is not revealing.
- *Treatment*:
    - If the ganglion cyst is not symptomatic, the cyst can be observed.

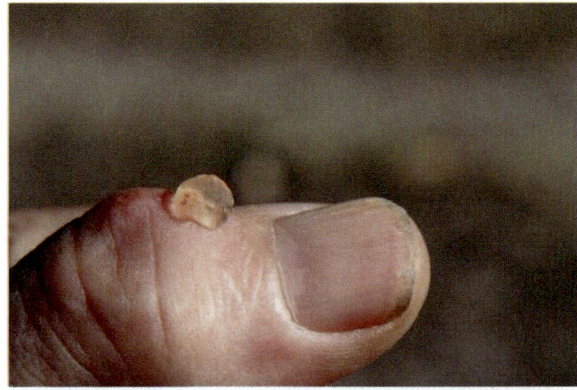

Fig. 59.1 Ganglion cyst

- Aspiration is a temporizing symptomatic treatment with a high recurrence rate. Injection of the cyst capsule or surrounding tendon sheath with lidocaine and betamethasone have been described for symptom relief as well.
- For symptomatic ganglion cysts, surgical excision of the ganglion cyst and stalk with coagulation of the stalk base is the preferred treatment with careful dissection of adjacent joint capsule or vasculature. Volar wrist ganglion cysts are frequently near the radial artery. Resection of osteophytes during excision of DIPJ ganglion cysts is required to reduce rates of recurrence.
- Pediatric ganglion cysts may be managed with observation.

Name: Giant Cell Tumors of the Tendon Sheath (GCTTS) [2, 4, 15, 16, 27, 29]

- *Incidence*: GCTTS are the second most common hand mass after ganglion cysts.
- *Pathogenesis/Anatomy*: These masses occur frequently on the volar surfaces of the thumb, index, and middle fingers in close proximity to the interphalangeal joints, predominantly the DIPJ. GCTTS are well-circumscribed, painless, and slow-growing tumors. Patients may describe numbness and paresthesias depending on the proximity of the mass to the neurovascular bundle.
- *Diagnosis/Imaging*: Biopsy is indicated for definitive diagnosis. GCTTS do not transilluminate. Radiographs can reveal bony erosion and/or invasion due to pressure from the mass on the bone.
- *Treatment*: Marginal surgical excision with meticulous dissection is the preferred treatment for GCTTS with characteristics of satellite lesions, poor encapsulation, intraosseous involvement, and involvement of adjacent joints and tendons, indicating higher rate of recurrence. Arthrodesis (fusion) of an interphalangeal joint may be indicated if there is extensive joint involvement. Radiation therapy after surgical excision is associated with lower recurrence rates. Systemic therapy with colony-stimulating factor-1 inhibitor have been studied for patients with diffuse and recurrent disease with involvement of neurovascular structures.

Name: Epidermal Inclusion Cyst (EIC) [4, 15, 27, 34]

- *Incidence*: Most commonly occur in men in the third and fourth decades in the thumb and distal phalanx of the long finger.
- *Pathogenesis/Anatomy*: EICs develop from the traumatic implantation of keratinized epithelium into the subcutaneous tissue.
- *Diagnosis/Imaging*: These cysts are filled with keratin and present as painless well circumscribed masses on the volar palm and digits. Radiographs may be obtained if high index of suspicion of bony erosion around the cyst.
- *Treatment*: Marginal surgical excision is the preferred treatment with curettage and bone grafting of osteolytic lesions. Biopsy is recommended prior to surgical excision if a lytic lesion of the distal phalanx is observed.

Name: Lipoma [4, 15, 27]

- *Incidence*: No known gender, age, or other demographic predominance.
- *Pathogenesis/Anatomy*: Lipomas are slow growing benign fatty tumors that may occur anywhere on the hand subcutaneously or intramuscularly. Lipomas may

occur in the deep palmar space, carpal tunnel, or Guyon canal, causing nerve compression.
- *Diagnosis/Imaging*: Lipomas commonly present as soft, mobile, and painless masses. MRI can be used to further delineate deeper anatomy structures surrounding the lipoma and aid in operative planning. Patients may present with numbness and paresthesia if compressing the median, radial, or ulnar nerves.
- *Treatment*: Marginal surgical excision is the preferred treatment for symptomatic masses with low recurrence rates.

Name: Schwannomas (Neurilemomas) [4, 15, 24, 33] (Fig. 59.2)

- *Incidence*: Most common nerve tumor in the upper extremity. This tumor is common in the fourth, fifth, and sixth decades of life.
- *Pathogenesis/Anatomy*: Benign peripheral nerve tumors derived from Schwann cells that arise over flexor surfaces of the forearm or hand. Schwannomas are well-encapsulated and slow growing tumors around a nerve.
- *Diagnosis/Imaging*: Schwannomas presents as soft and mobile (in the transverse direction) masses that may be associated with paresthesias and radiating pain upon palpation. CT and MRI may be used to evaluate the location. These patients typically have positive Tinel's signs but no deficit in function.
- *Treatment*: Surgical enucleation from the nerve sheath and separation from the nerve is the preferred treatment. Postoperative neurologic deficit may occur in up to 15% of patients.

Name: Neurofibromas [2, 4, 15, 27, 33]

- *Incidence*: Second most common benign nerve tumor in the hand. The fusiform subtype of neurofibromas is more common in young females, and plexiform subtype is commonly seen in patients with neurofibromatosis.
- *Pathogenesis/Anatomy*: Neurofibromas develop and proliferate within nerve fascicles. Solitary lesions can arise spontaneously whereas multiple lesions are associated with neurofibromatosis. There is higher risk for malignant degeneration in patients with neurofibromatosis.

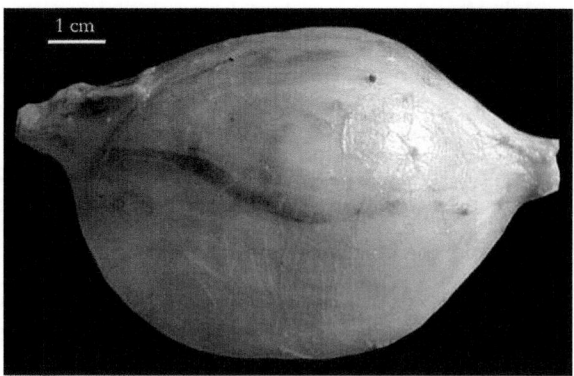

Fig. 59.2 Schwannoma ex vivo

- *Diagnosis/Imaging*: Neurofibromas are similar to schwannomas in clinical presentation and appear as slow growing soft masses causing variable neurologic deficit. MRI may be useful in further delineating surrounding anatomy. These patients have positive Tinel's signs and often deficits in function.
- *Treatment*: Marginal excision of symptomatic neurofibromas with division of the proximal and distal nerve fascicles associated with the mass is the standard treatment. Nerve fascicular repair or nerve grafting may be required after excision. Neurologic deficit is more common after excision of a neurofibroma than a schwannoma.

Name: Glomus Tumor [1, 15, 22, 23]

- *Incidence*: 1%–5% of hand tumors.
- *Pathogenesis/Anatomy*: A glomus tumor is a benign hamartoma that evolves from the glomus body of the distal phalanx. The glomus apparatus is arteriovenous anastomosis involved with temperature regulation.
- *Diagnosis/Imaging*: Glomus tumors present as dark red or purple masses in the subungual area that may cause changes to the nail plate. Common symptoms are tenderness and cold-sensitivity. Ultrasound and MRI are common imaging modalities for diagnosis,
- *Treatment*: The preferred treatment is surgical excision through the sterile nail matrix that often requires removal of the nail. There is low recurrence after complete excision.

Name: Vascular Malformations (VMs) [1, 15, 22, 23]

- *Incidence*: VMs are uncommon in the hand and upper extremity. Hemangiomas of the upper extremity are more common in children and on the palm. Venous malformations are the most common vascular malformation in the hand. Ulnar artery aneurysms are common in laborers who use hammers.
- *Pathogenesis/Anatomy*: VMs are errors of vascular development that can be venous, arterial, or arteriovenous in nature. They present *at birth* and are further characterized by slow-flow and high flow lesions. Hemangiomas are dermal-epidermal lesions that arise from vascular endothelial cells *after birth*. Hemangiomas progress through two stages of proliferation (0–12 months) and involution (12 months to 10 years). Minimal change in a hemangioma is expected after 12 years of age. Ulnar artery aneurysms are caused by repetitive motion near the ulnar artery.
- *Diagnosis/Imaging*: Slow-flow venous lesions present with dependent swelling and overlying skin changes. Slow-flow capillary lesions present as small pink nodules that become nodular over time. High-flow arterial lesions present as pulsatile masses with digital ischemic changes. Diagnosis commonly requires Doppler ultrasonography and MRI angiography, and venography to assess surrounding structures and flow velocities. Arteriography may be used if embolization is planned.

- *Treatment*:
    - Hemangiomas are typically observed as most lesions involute. If hemangiomas become ulcerative or cause destruction to surrounding structures, treatment options include laser therapy with pulsed dye laser, systemic or intralesional corticosteroids, or beta-blockers such as propranolol (dose 2 mg/kg/day). If a symptomatic hemangioma is unresponsive to non-surgical therapies, surgical excision is indicated.
    - Capillary malformations may be treated with a pulse dye laser over multiple treatments.
    - Small venous malformations may be treated with compression therapy and/or sclerotherapy, while larger venous malformations can be excised.
    - Arterial and arteriovenous malformations can be treated by embolization followed by resection. Ulnar artery aneurysms are treated with surgical resection, with ligation of the artery or interposition graft if poor circulation is seen.
    - Sclerotherapy or embolization in the hand is at high risk for nerve injury and ischemic changes in the digits and surgical excision is the preferred treatment for preservation of surrounding structures.
- More details can be found in the vascular malformations chapter.

Malignant Skin and Soft Tissue Tumors

Name: Basal Cell Carcinoma (BCC) [15, 17, 19, 27, 34]

- *Incidence*: Second most common malignant skin tumor of the hand. Risk factors include sun exposure, old age, immunosuppression, and prior history of skin cancer.
- *Description/Anatomy*: BCCs arise from the basal keratinocytes in the basal layer of the epidermis and pilosebaceous adnexa. Subtypes include nodular, pigmented, morpheaform (sclerosing), and superficial spreading. BCCs have a low rate of metastasis due to reticular dermis.
- *Diagnosis/Imaging*: BCCs present as raised lesions with possible ulceration, skin discoloration, telangiectasias, and raised borders. No imaging routinely indicated. Punch biopsy (incisional or excisional) can be used for initial pathology diagnosis.
- *Treatment*:
    - Wide Local Excision: 7–10 mm margins for morpheaform subtype and lesions greater than 2 cm. Wide local excision with 3–5 mm margins is indicated for other BCC subtypes up to 2 cm in size.
    - Mohs Micrographic Surgery is indicated for widespread lesions with unclear margins or recurrent BCC to aid with tissue preservation and confirmation of clear tissue margins.

- Electrodessication and curettage (EDC) or cryotherapy can be used for small lesions (<1 cm non-recurrent lesions).
- Radiation therapy can be used as primary requiring multiple treatments or as adjuvant therapy for invasive BCC.
- Topical therapies include Imiquimod and 5-fluorouracil for superficial BCCs.

Name: Squamous Cell Carcinoma (SCC) [15, 17, 19, 27, 34]

- *Incidence*: Most common malignant skin tumor of the hand and of the nail bed. Risk factors include fair skin, blue eyes, red hair, immunosuppression, history of chronic wound (Marjolin's ulcer) and history of prior sunburns. SCCs have a high rate of metastasis compared to BCC.
- *Description/Anatomy*: SCCs arise from the superficial keratinocytes of the epidermis. The most common location for SCC on the hand is the dorsum. SCC precursor lesions include actinic keratosis, keratoacanthoma, and Bowen's disease (SCC in-situ). Subtypes include verrucous, ulcerative, Marjolin's ulcer, or subungual.
- *Diagnosis/Imaging*: Punch biopsy (incisional or excisional) can be used for initial pathology diagnosis for SCC. Factors for prognostication include degree of undifferentiation, tumor size, tumor depth, and perineural invasion. High-risk lesions include size greater than 2 cm, greater than 2 mm of invasion depth, low ratio of differentiation to undifferentiation, and perineural invasion.
- *Treatment*:
  - Wide Local Excision: 4 mm margin for low-risk lesions and 6 mm margins for high-risk lesions. Consider sentinel lymph node biopsy for high-risk lesions.
  - Mohs micrographic surgery is indicated for high-risk lesions, penetrating tumors, or recurrent SCC to aid with tissue preservation and confirmation of clear tissue margins.
  - Radiation therapy can be used as primary or adjuvant therapy after excision. Radiation therapy is typically used for poor operative candidates or inoperable lesions.
  - EDC, cryotherapy, phototherapy, 5-fluorouracil, and topical imiquimod have been studied for treatment, however surgical excision is more recommended.

Name: Melanoma [9, 12, 15, 17, 19, 25, 28, 34]

- *Incidence*: Melanoma accounts for 3% of all hand tumors. Risk factors include Fitzpatrick types I and II, history of UV radiation exposure, prior melanoma, and family history of melanoma.
- *Description/Anatomy*: Suspicious lesion characteristics can be remembered by the ABCDE acronym: Asymmetric, Border Irregularity, Color variation, Diameter greater than 6 mm, and evolving. Precursor lesions include congenital nevi, acquired melanocytic nevi, lentigo maligna (in situ melanoma), and dysplastic nevi. Melanoma subtypes include superficial spreading, lentigo maligna

melanoma, acral lentiginous melanoma, nodular melanoma, and amelanotic melanoma.
- *Diagnosis/Imaging*: Staging is done after determining TMN staging with Breslow depth as the most important indicator of lymph node metastasis and survival. Refer to AJCC 8th Edition Melanoma Staging for full TMN staging. Narrow excisional or complete biopsy with 1–3 mm margins around the entire lesion is preferred.
- *Treatment*:
    - Surgical excision is the primary treatment for melanoma, with possible digit amputation of joint proximal to the lesion. Other therapies that have been studied include topical interferon-alfa, topical imiquimod, cryotherapy, and laser therapy.
    - Indications for sentinel lymph node biopsy include cutaneous melanoma with >1 mm thickness, patients with stage T1b with of <0.8 mm thickness with ulceration or 0.8–1 mm regardless of ulceration, or stage T1a if adverse features are present including high mitotic rate, lymphovascular invasion, positive deep biopsy margin, and young age.
    - Lymph node dissection is performed if positive sentinel lymph nodes are identified.

Name: Merkel Cell Carcinoma (MCC) [5, 15, 19, 34]

- *Incidence*: Rare malignant neuroendocrine tumor. The primary risk factor for MCC is immunosuppression.
- *Description/Anatomy*: MCCs arise from cells in the basal epidermal layer. MCC presents as rapidly growing, painless blue-red nodules.
- *Diagnosis/Imaging*: Skin biopsy is required for diagnosis, with excisional biopsy preferred.
- *Treatment*:
    - Wide Local Surgical Excision with 1–2 cm margins down to investing muscle fascia is the preferred treatment. Sentinel lymph node biopsy is recommended, and fine needle aspiration or core biopsy should be performed if regional lymphadenopathy is present on clinical exam. Adjuvant radiation should be considered for local or locoregional disease.

Name: Soft Tissue Sarcomas [4, 7, 8, 10, 27, 30, 31, 33, 34]

- *Incidence*: 15% of all soft tissue sarcomas diagnosed yearly are in the upper extremity. Only 4% of these malignant tumors occur in the hand.
- *Pathogenesis/Anatomy*: Soft tissue sarcomas share an early mesenchymal origin but vary according to a specific cell type. Of the histological subtypes, epithelioid, synovial, and clear-cell sarcomas are the most common in the hand. Radiation exposure and exposure to herbicides may increase the risk of having a soft tissue sarcoma. Patients with neurofibromatosis and Li-Fraumeni syndrome are at higher risk for occurrence.
- *Diagnosis/Imaging*: Patients typically present with a long-term painless mass that has grown more recently. Full examination should include palpation of the

epitrochlear and axillary lymph nodes. Plain radiographs may be helpful initially to determine bony involvement, but an MRI will be needed to fully examine the local invasion and size of the mass needed for operative planning. A carefully planned incisional biopsy is recommended to identify the soft tissue sarcoma type and histologic grade. The histologic grade will help determine the aggressive features of the soft tissue sarcoma. Further staging of the mass is done after CT scans of the chest and axilla to identify metastasis to the lung or regional lymph nodes. Position emission tomography (PET)-CT scans may be used to evaluate regional lymph node metastasis. Staging of soft tissue sarcomas is based on grade, size, and presence of metastasis. For full staging, see AJCC 8th edition for Soft Tissue Sarcoma of the Extremities or Trunk.
- *Treatment*:
  - Wide local excision of the soft tissue sarcoma with a cuff of normal tissue of about 2–3 cm is recommended, though it is frequently difficult to perform on the hand.
  - Ray amputation may be required for distal tumors.
  - Radiation therapy is useful to reduce local recurrence for large (>5 cm) high- and low-grade lesions.
  - Neoadjuvant or adjuvant chemotherapy with doxorubicin and ifosfamide may be useful in certain large (>5 cm) high-grade lesions, notably if lung metastases are present. Chemotherapy based on doxorubicin may be indicated for unresectable lesions as well, due to proximity to neurovascular structures.

Benign Bone/Cartilage Tumors

Name: Enchondroma [4, 14, 21, 24, 27] (Fig. 59.3)

- *Incidence*: Enchondromas are the most common bony tumor of the hand, accounting for 90% of primary bony tumors of the hand. Patients with Ollier's disease and Maffucci syndrome typically present with multiple enchondromas with increased risk for malignant transformation to osteosarcoma or chondrosarcoma. Ollier's disease is associated with malignant degeneration, and Maffucci's with hemangioma.
- *Pathogenesis/Anatomy*: Enchondromas are typically found in the proximal phalanx, primarily followed by the middle phalanx, and metacarpals of ulnar digits.
- *Diagnosis/Imaging*: Patients may present with a pathologic fracture due to the locally destructive nature of the bony tumor. On plain radiographs, enchondromas appear as radiolucent, lytic, and well-circumscribed lesions with increased calcifications, causing a popcorn-like appearance. Biopsy is needed to confirm the diagnosis.
- *Treatment*: For symptomatic lesions, curettage excision or intralesional excision is recommended with or without placement of autogenous or allogenous bone graft. If a pathologic fracture is present, it may be beneficial to allow the fracture

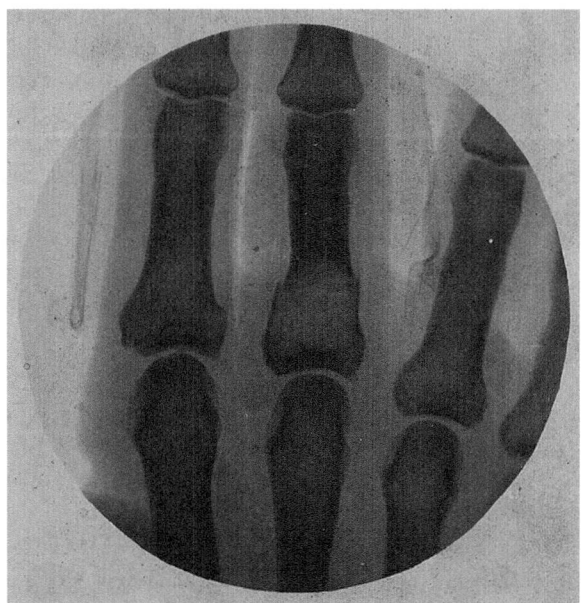

Fig. 59.3 Enchondroma at the base of P1

to heal prior to tumor excision, though single-stage treatments with injection of calcium sulfate cement have promising results.

Name: Osteoid Osteoma [4, 14, 27]

- *Incidence*: Five to fifteen percent of osteoid osteomas occur in the hand in patients in the second and third decades of life.
- *Pathogenesis/Anatomy*: Osteoid osteomas are non-progressive osteoblastic tumors that present with nighttime swelling relieved by nonsteroidal anti-inflammatory (NSAID) medications. These tumors are most commonly found in the proximal phalanges, metacarpals, and carpal bones.
- *Diagnosis/Imaging*: On plain radiographs, the osteoid osteomas have lytic lesions with a possible central radiolucent nidus less than 1 cm surrounded by sclerosis.
- *Treatment*: For persistent symptomatic osteoid osteomas, curettage excision with bone grafting is recommended, with low recurrence rates. Patients may alternatively continue NSAIDs if surgical removal may be harmful. Radiofrequency ablation for osteoid osteomas has not been well studied in the hand.

Name: Periosteal Chondromas [4, 14]

- *Incidence*: Periosteal chondromas are rare cartilaginous tumors that occur in males in the second or third decade.

- *Pathogenesis/Anatomy*: Periosteal chondromas can be found in phalanges at the metaphyseal-diaphyseal junction.
- *Diagnosis/Imaging*: Plain radiographs of periosteal chondromas demonstrate a subperiosteal, unilobular lytic lesion with "scalloping" of the cortex very similar to an enchondroma.
- *Treatment*: These tumors are treated with marginal excision, including the periosteum, to reduce recurrence.

Name: Osteochondromas (Exostoses) [4, 14, 27]

- *Incidence*: These tumors are rare in the hand, except in cases of multiple hereditary exostoses.
- *Pathogenesis/Anatomy*: Osteochondromas have a predilection for the distal proximal phalanx, but cases have been reported in carpal bones.
- *Diagnosis/Imaging*: Patients with this tumor may present with numbness, limited range of motion, and/or tendon rupture due to compression of local superficial nerves and tendons. Plain radiographs demonstrate a protuberant bony growth extending beyond the cortex on a narrow stalk.
- *Treatment*: For symptomatic lesions, marginal excision is recommended.

Name: Giant Cell Tumors of the Bone (GCTB) [3, 4, 6, 14, 27] (Fig. 59.4)

- *Incidence*: Two to five percent of giant cell tumors of the bone occur in the hand and present in patients typically in the third and fourth decades of life. GCTBs of the distal upper extremity have higher rates of recurrence and metastasis compared to other bony regions.
- *Pathogenesis/Anatomy*: GCTBs occur predominantly in all the bones of the hand and less commonly in the distal radius. GCTBs in the hand and distal radius have the potential for pulmonary metastasis.
- *Diagnosis/Imaging*: Plain radiographs and CT scans demonstrate lytic lesions classified by the Campanacci Grading System as follows: Grade 1 is well-marginated with intact cortex, Grade 2 is well-marginated with expanded cortex, and Grade 3 is an ill-defined lesion with soft tissue extension and cortical destruction. A CT of the chest should be conducted to evaluate for pulmonary metastasis.
- *Treatment*: For Campanacci Grade 1 or 2, curettage excision with bone or cement grafting with adjuvant hydrogen peroxide, phenol, or liquid nitrogen is recommended to decrease recurrence rates. The efficacy of adjuvant therapies is not consistent in the literature. For Campanacci Grade 3, en bloc resection with bony reconstruction with non-vascularized iliac bone graft for smaller defects and vascularized fibular bone graft for defects larger than 10 cm. When performing any resection procedure, it is recommended to always plan for a possible amputation and to protect soft tissues from the tumor to avoid seeding. Close postoperative surveillance is recommended due to high recurrence rates. External beam radiation therapy should be avoided due to risk of malignant transformation of the tumor, leading to death.

Fig. 59.4 Giant cell tumor of bone

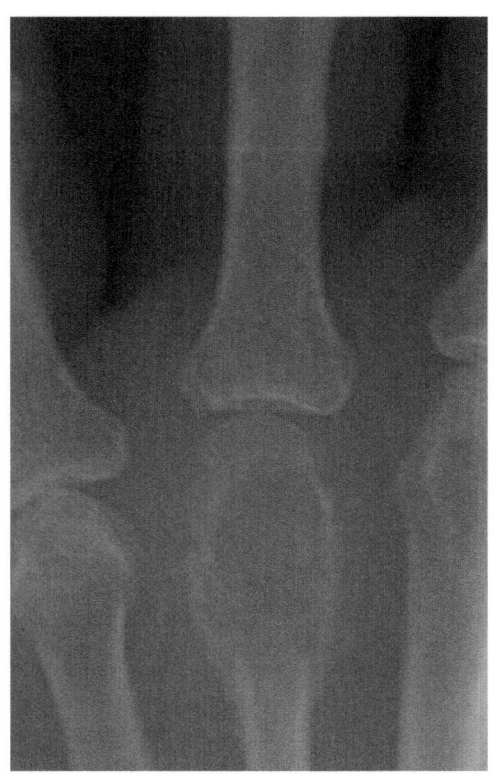

Name: Aneurysmal Bone Cysts (ABCs) [4, 14, 18]

- *Incidence*: These tumors are rare in the hand that can arise from other benign bony lesions or de novo. These tumors are more common in patients younger than 20 years old.
- *Pathogenesis/Anatomy*: ABCs are more common in metacarpals than phalanges.
- *Diagnosis/Imaging*: Plain radiographs demonstrate an expansile lytic lesion typically without soft tissue extension. Plain radiographs are necessary for the first evaluation of the bony tumor, but MRI is performed to adequately evaluate fluid levels in the lesion for diagnosis.
- *Treatment*: To decrease recurrence rates, curettage excision, bone grafting, and adjuvant therapies of liquid nitrogen, cement, and argon laser. For aggressive lesions, amputation or wide local excision is recommended.

Malignant Bone Tumors

Name: Chondrosarcoma [4, 8, 22, 27]

- *Incidence*: Chondrosarcomas are the most common malignant bony tumor in the hand, accounting for up to 8% of all chondrosarcomas in the body. These tumors primarily occur in elderly patients.

- *Pathogenesis/Anatomy*: Enchondromas or osteochondromas can evolve to become chondrosarcomas, though some lesions appear de novo. Pulmonary metastases are more likely to be present from high-grade lesions or from local recurrence after intralesional excision. Most chondrosarcomas of the hand are low grade.
- *Diagnosis/Imaging*: Patient will present with long-standing, slowly evolving pain in the metacarpals or proximal phalanges. Plain radiographs will demonstrate an aggressive lytic bony lesion with cortical expansion with ill-defined borders, endosteal scalloping, and soft tissue extension. MRI is indicated to identify the extent of bony and soft tissue disruption for surgical planning. CT of the chest should be conducted to evaluate for pulmonary metastases in high-grade chondrosarcomas.
- *Treatment*: For low-grade lesions confined to the bone, intralesional excision followed by cryoablation and bone cement with close follow-up is recommended. For high-grade aggressive lesions, wide local excision or amputation is indicated to prevent recurrence. Chemotherapy and radiation are minimally effective for chondrosarcomas.

Name: Osteosarcomas [4, 8, 11, 22, 27]

- *Incidence*: The incidence of osteosarcoma in the hand is reported to be 0.2%–0.9% and typically occurs in middle-aged individuals. Risk factors for osteosarcoma include the history of chronic radiation exposure and Paget's disease of the bone.
- *Pathogenesis/Anatomy*: These tumors originate from osteoblastic cells that produce immature bone. Osteosarcomas in the hand are commonly low-grade lesions.
- *Diagnosis/Imaging*: Patients will present with the acute onset of pain and swelling to a metacarpophalangeal joint, proximal phalanx, or distal radius in contrast to the slow-growing nature of chondrosarcomas. Plain radiographs reveal a sclerotic lesion within or outside the cortex with soft tissue extension. MRI is indicated to identify the extent of bony and soft tissue disruption for surgical planning. CT of the chest and a bone scan may be useful to identify potential bony metastases.
- *Treatment*: For high-grade lesions, neoadjuvant chemotherapy followed by en bloc excision and adjuvant chemotherapy is recommended. Ray amputation may be indicated to ensure negative margins.

Name: Ewing Sarcoma [4, 8, 13, 14, 20, 27]

- *Incidence*: 1.4% of Ewing sarcomas occur in the upper extremity, predominantly in males in the second decade.
- *Pathogenesis/Anatomy*: When occurring in the hand, Ewing's sarcoma occurs in the metacarpals or phalanges. Metastases occur in up to 25% of patients.
- *Diagnosis/Imaging*: Patients may present with slow onset malaise, fever, swelling, and pain in the hand. Plain radiographs will demonstrate mixed sclerotic and lytic bony destruction with periosteal reaction with soft tissue extension. A CT of

the chest and total bone scan can be conducted for systemic staging. Incisional biopsy avoiding soft tissue contamination is recommended prior to administration of systemic antibiotics since the differential diagnosis often includes an infectious etiology.
- *Treatment*: Surgical treatment with wide local excision or amputation with combination of neoadjuvant or adjuvant chemotherapy. Radiation therapy may additionally aid in reduction of recurrence rates for inoperable tumors or inability to obtain wide margins though complications include contractures and stiffness.

References

1. Abouzeid S, Derderian CA, Burns JL. Vascular anomalies. In: Janis J, editor. Essentials of plastic surgery. 2nd ed. Boca Raton: CRC Press; 2014.
2. Aliu O. Hand tumors. In: Brown DL, Borschel GH, Levi B, editors. Michigan manual of plastic surgery. 2nd ed. Philadelphia: Lippincott Williams & Wilkins, A Wolters Kluwer Business; 2014.
3. Athanasian EA. Aneurysmal bone cyst and giant cell tumor of bone of the hand and distal radius. Hand Clin. 2004;20(3):269–81, vi.
4. Athanasian EA. Bone and soft tissue tumors. In: Wolfe SW, Hotchkiss RN, Pederson WC, Kozin SH, Cohen MS, editors. Green's operative hand surgery. 7th ed. Philadelphia: Elsevier, Inc.; 2017.
5. Brady M, Spiker AM. Merkel cell carcinoma of the skin. Treasure Island: StatPearls Publishing; 2022. Available from: https://www.ncbi.nlm.nih.gov/books/NBK482329/.
6. Campanacci M, Baldini N, Boriani S, Sudanese A. Giant-cell tumor of bone. J Bone Joint Surg Am. 1987;69(1):106–14.
7. Cates JMM. The AJCC 8th edition staging system for soft tissue sarcoma of the extremities or trunk: a cohort study of the SEER database. J Natl Compr Cancer Netw. 2018;16(2):144–52.
8. Chapman T, Athanasian E. Malignant tumors of the hand. J Am Acad Orthop Surg. 2020;28(23):953–62.
9. Crowson AN, Magro CM, Mihm MC. Prognosticators of melanoma, the melanoma report, and the sentinel lymph node. Mod Pathol. 2006;19(Suppl 2):S71–87.
10. Dick HM. Synovial sarcoma of the hand. Hand Clin. 1987;3(2):241–5.
11. Fowble VA, Pae R, Vitale A, Bryk E, Vigorita VJ. Case reports: osteosarcoma of the hand: one case and a literature review. Clin Orthop Relat Res. 2005;440:255–61.
12. Gershenwald JE, Scolyer RA, Hess KR, Amin M, Edge SB, Greene FL. Melanoma of the skin. Switzerland: Springer; 2017.
13. Gorlick R, Janeway K, Lessnick S, Randall RL, Marina N. Children's Oncology Group's 2013 blueprint for research: bone tumors. Pediatr Blood Cancer. 2013;60(6):1009–15.
14. Henderson M, Neumeister MW, Bueno RA Jr. Hand tumors: II. Benign and malignant bone tumors of the hand. Plast Reconstr Surg. 2014;133(6):814e–21e.
15. Henderson MM, Neumeister MW, Bueno RA Jr. Hand tumors: I. Skin and soft-tissue tumors of the hand. Plast Reconstr Surg. 2014;133(2):154e–64e.
16. Kotwal PP, Gupta V, Malhotra R. Giant-cell tumour of the tendon sheath. Is radiotherapy indicated to prevent recurrence after surgery? J Bone Joint Surg. 2000;82(4):571–3.
17. LeBlanc DM, Ramanadham SR, Wells DD. Basal cell carcinoma, squamous cell carcinoma, and melanoma. In: Janis J, editor. Essentials of plastic surgery. 2nd ed. Boca Raton: CRC Press; 2014.
18. Mascard E, Gomez-Brouchet A, Lambot K. Bone cysts: unicameral and aneurysmal bone cyst. Orthop Traumatol Surg Res. 2015;101(1 Suppl):S119–27.

19. Netscher DT. Skin tumors of the hand and upper extremity. In: Wolfe SW, Hotchkiss RN, Pederson WC, Kozin SH, Cohen MS, editors. Green's operative hand surgery. 7th ed. Philadelphia: Elsevier, Inc.; 2017.
20. Parida L, Fernandez-Pineda I, Uffman J, Navid F, Davidoff AM, Neel M, et al. Clinical management of Ewing sarcoma of the bones of the hands and feet: a retrospective single-institution review. J Pediatr Surg. 2012;47(10):1806–10.
21. Payne WT, Merrell G. Benign bony and soft tissue tumors of the hand. J Hand Surg Am. 2010;35(11):1901–10.
22. Pederson WC. Vascular disorders of the hand. In: Wolfe SW, Hotchkiss RN, Pederson WC, Kozin SH, Cohen MS, editors. Green's operative hand surgery. 7th ed. Philadelphia: Elsevier, Inc.; 2017.
23. Ranganathan K. Vascular anomalies, lymphedema, and tattoos. In: Brown DL, Borschel GH, Levi B, editors. Michigan manual of plastic surgery. 2nd ed. Philadelphia: Lippincott Williams & Wilkins, A Wolters Kluwer Business; 2014.
24. Siqueira MG, Socolovsky M, Martins RS, Robla-Costales J, Di Masi G, Heise CO, et al. Surgical treatment of typical peripheral schwannomas: the risk of new postoperative deficits. Acta Neurochir. 2013;155(9):1745–9.
25. Sobanko JF, Dagum AB, Davis IC, Kriegel DA. Soft tissue tumors of the hand. 2. Malignant. Dermatol Surg. 2007;33(7):771–85.
26. Stephen AB, Lyons AR, Davis TR. A prospective study of two conservative treatments for ganglia of the wrist. J Hand Surg. 1999;24(1):104–5.
27. Strike SA, Puhaindran ME. Tumors of the hand and the wrist. JBJS Rev. 2020;8(6):e0141.
28. Swetter SM, Tsao H, Bichakjian CK, Curiel-Lewandrowski C, Elder DE, Gershenwald JE, et al. Guidelines of care for the management of primary cutaneous melanoma. J Am Acad Dermatol. 2019;80(1):208–50.
29. Tap WD, Gelderblom H, Palmerini E, Desai J, Bauer S, Blay JY, et al. Pexidartinib versus placebo for advanced tenosynovial giant cell tumour (ENLIVEN): a randomised phase 3 trial. Lancet (London, England). 2019;394(10197):478–87.
30. Terek RM, Brien EW. Soft-tissue sarcomas of the hand and wrist. Hand Clin. 1995;11(2):287–305.
31. Ugurel S, Mentzel T, Utikal J, Helmbold P, Mohr P, Pföhler C, et al. Neoadjuvant imatinib in advanced primary or locally recurrent dermatofibrosarcoma protuberans: a multicenter phase II DeCOG trial with long-term follow-up. Clin Cancer Res. 2014;20(2):499–510.
32. Wang AA, Hutchinson DT. Longitudinal observation of pediatric hand and wrist ganglia. J Hand Surg Am. 2001;26(4):599–602.
33. Ward RA, Crosby MA. Benign and malignant masses of the hand. In: Janis J, editor. Essentials of plastic surgery. 2nd ed. Boca Raton: CRC Press; 2014.
34. Wolter KG. Malignant skin and soft tissue lesions. In: Brown DL, Borschel GH, Levi B, editors. Michigan manual of plastic surgery. 2nd ed. Philadelphia: Lippincott Williams & Wilkins, A Wolters Kluwer Business; 2014.

Chapter 60
Vascular Injuries of the Hand

Nirbhay S. Jain

Vasculature of the Hand (Fig. 60.1) [1, 2]

- The brachial artery is the source of blood the forearm and hand.
  - It divides into the radial and ulnar arteries in the antecubital fossa at the elbow, with both traveling in the volar space.
- Radial and ulnar form the deep and superficial arch in the hand.
  - They are also connected through the anterior interosseous artery (AIA) and posterior interosseous artery (PIA), which cannot supply enough blood in case of an injury.
  - Radial main supply to deep arch, ulnar to superficial.
    - Radial also gives off the princeps pollicis to the thumb.
- Venous drainage is mainly dorsal through the superficial system, though the deep system does have venae comitans (VC).
  - Damage to volar structures does NOT typically compromise venous drainage.
  - VCs of the radial and ulnar arteries form the deep drainage system.
  - Cephalic vein drains the superficial system radially, and the basilic vein drains ulnarly.

N. S. Jain (✉)
Division of Plastic Surgery, Department of Surgery, University of California, Los Angeles, Los Angeles, CA, USA
e-mail: nsjain@mednet.ucla.edu

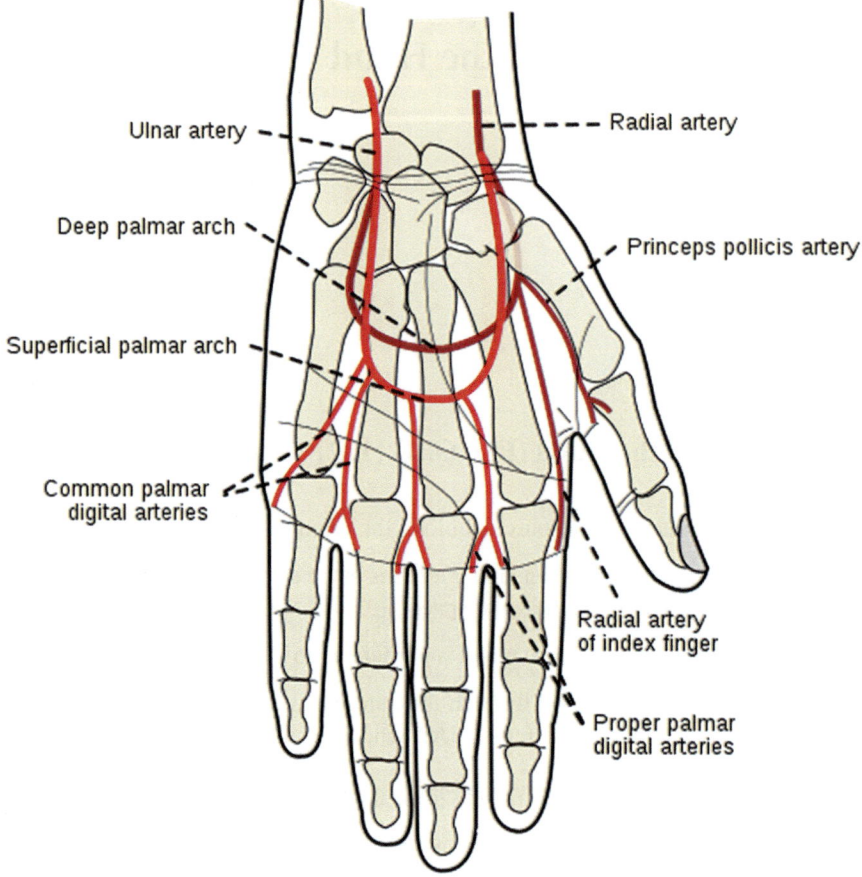

Fig. 60.1 Vasculature of the hand

Etiology of Ischemia

- Can be traumatic (rarely from A line) or embolic, typically, though vascular disease and vasopressor medications can cause this.
- Injury to one of the main vessels does not typically cause ischemia to the whole hand.

Evaluation

- After a history and key physical examination, maneuvers include
    - Allen's test

- Pulse palpation
- Doppler exam
  - Can replace with a pulse ox on fingers
  - Adequate pulse does not necessarily mean adequate flow
- Digital brachial index can be performed as well to assess the degree of flow loss
- Imaging
  - CTA
  - Direct angiogram

Types of Ischemia [3–5]

- Traumatic Injury
  - Often managed with ligation if only one vessel is injured (or reconstruction if the hand is ischemic, see chapter on replantation).
  - Can be a Surgical emergency if ischemia is present.
  - Supracondylar fracture can lead to brachial artery injury.
  - Special case: hypothenar hammer syndrome
    - Closed repetitive trauma to the ulnar artery in Guyon's canal
    - Can lead to rupture, aneurysm, thrombosis, and development of tortuosity
    - Presents with pain, ischemia in ulnar digits
    - Treat with ASA, nifedipine if ABI > 0.6
    - If ABI < 0.6, then needs resection and reconstruction with vein grafting v bypass
- Vascular disease
  - Typically, in the setting of systemic disease, such as ESRD, DM, and HLD.
  - Can also be related to an arteriovenous fistula for dialysis (steal syndrome).
    - If this is the case, symptoms improve with compression of the fistula, may need banding or ligation and distal revascularization (DRIL procedure).
  - Buerger disease is a rare form associated with smoking (also known as thromboangiitis obliterans) that causes swelling of blood vessels, leading to stasis and clots
    - Can be driven by sympathetic stimulation as well
- Vasospastic Disorders (Fig. 60.2)
  - Sympathetic disorders leading to vasospasm and symptomatology

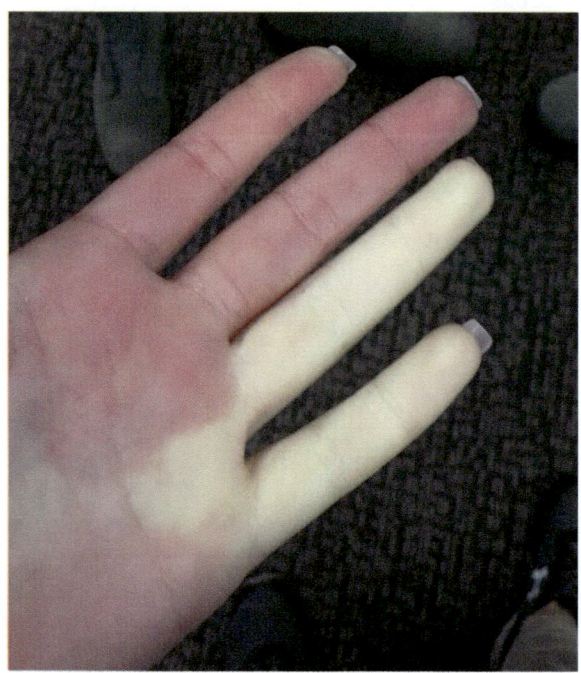

Fig. 60.2 Raynaud phenomenon

- Cold sensitivity is the most common (10% of the population), which can lead to ischemic changes if severe enough (Raynaud's disease).
- Associated with other connective tissue disorders like scleroderma or CREST.
- Can initially manage with calcium channel blockers, trigger avoidance (i.e., cold avoidance), sildenafil, and Botox (perivascular at the palm) to alleviate sympathetic symptoms.
- Sympathectomy is the main surgical approach.

- Other Conditions
  - Aneurysms
    - Rare in the hand, often false (does not involve all three layers of the arterial wall) due to arterial puncture for access
    - Typically, can be compressed or thrombosed by IR, may need excision and reconstruction
  - Deep venous thromboses
    - Extremely rare
    - Often present with compartment syndrome
  - Vascular malformations (see Chap. 17)
  - Glomus tumors (see Chap. 59)

- Compartment Syndromes
  - Rare, but can occur in either the hand or the forearm upper extremity
  - Requires fascial release

References

1. Chim H, Bakri K, Moran SL. Complications related to radial artery occlusion, radial artery harvest, and arterial lines. Hand Clin. 2015;31:93–100.
2. Coleman SS, Anson BJ. Arterial patterns in the hand based upon a study of 650 specimens. Surg Gynecol Obstet. 1961;113:409–24.
3. Dargon PT, Landry GJ. Buerger's disease. Ann Vasc Surg. 2012;26:871–80.
4. De Martino RR, Moran SL. The role of thrombolytics in acute and chronic occlusion of the hand. Hand Clin. 2015;31:*13–21*.
5. Marques E. Ulnar artery thrombosis: hypothenar hammer syndrome. J Am Coll Surg. 2008;206:188–9.

Chapter 61
Congenital Hand

Nirbhay S. Jain

Embryologic Development [1]

- Limb development is driven by mesenchyme and ectoderm and has reliable time points for the formation of specific structures.
  - Week 4: formation of the limb bud.
  - Week 5: formation of the brachial plexus and hand plate.
  - Week 6: formation of digits with webbing, muscles, and chondrogenesis.
  - Week 7: apoptosis for digital separation.
  - Week 8: formation of fingers from proximal to distal, ossification of forearm, and phalanges from distal to proximal.
  - Carpal ossification occurs after birth.
    - 1st year: Capitate
    - 2nd year: Hamate
    - 3rd year: Triquetrum
    - 4th year: Lunate
    - 5th year: Scaphoid
    - 6th year: Trapezium
    - 7th year: Trapezoid
    - 12th year: Pisiform
- Limb development occurs along three axes of development (Fig. 61.1) [2].
  - Proximal distal

N. S. Jain (✉)
Division of Plastic Surgery, Department of Surgery, University of California, Los Angeles, Los Angeles, CA, USA
e-mail: nsjain@mednet.ucla.edu

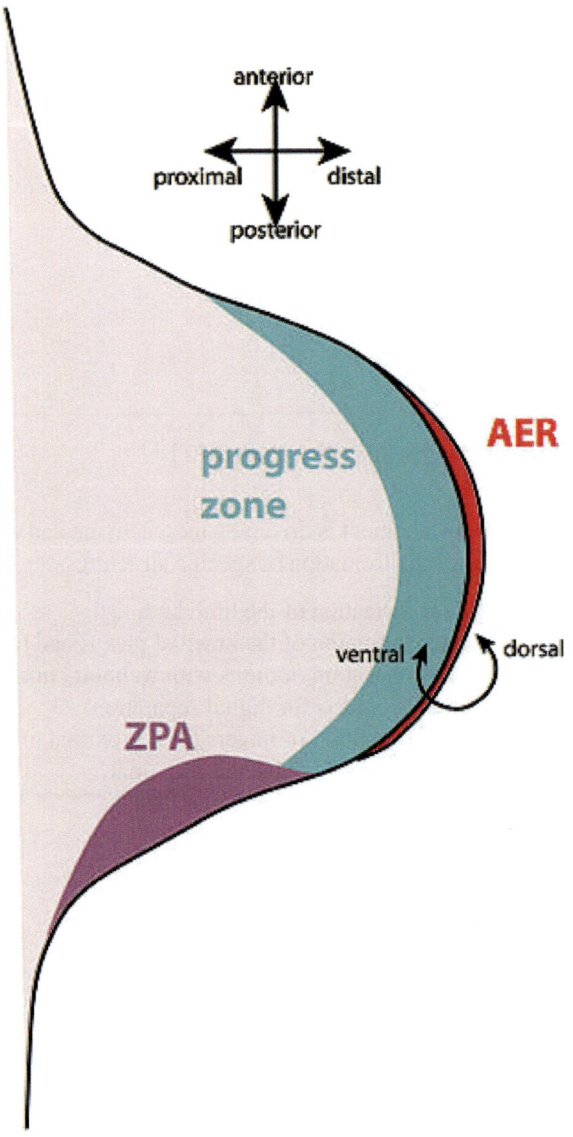

Fig. 61.1 Axes of development of the upper extremity

- Drives upper extremity length through the apical epidermal ridge (AER), main growth factor is FGF
- Radioulnar (lateral-medial)
  - Drives differentiation of radial and ulnar structures via the zone of polarizing activity and the sonic hedgehog (Shh) growth factor
- Dorsal-ventral (palmar)

- Differentiates dorsal and volar structures via the Wnt7 pathway

Classification Systems [3, 4]

- Two main classification systems
  - Swanson
    - Failure of Formation
    - Failure of Differentiation
    - Duplication
    - Overgrowth
    - Undergrowth
    - Constriction Band
    - Generalized/Other
  - Oberg, Manske, Tonkin (OMT)
    - Malformation
    - Deformation
    - Dysplasia

Key Patterns

- There are many patterns of congenital hand deformity [5].
- Syndactyly (Fig. 61.2)
  - Fusion of the soft tissue and possibly bony elements of the fingers due to failure of apoptosis driven by FGF/AER.
  - Can be classified as simple or complex based on if the bone is involved or not, and incomplete or complete based on how much of the finger is involved.
  - Incidence is approximately 1 in 2000 and is often bilateral and has a family history.
  - Most common is between LF/RF, then RF/SF.
  - Most patients require surgery unless there is no functional impairment.
    - Surgical release is typically done around 1 year of age.
    - Reconstruction of the commissure is typically with a dorsal rectangular flap with Z-plasty or a full-thickness skin graft.
    - May need to divide a digital artery, so should only operate on one side of a finger at a time.
    - May also need to split the digital nerve.
  - Acrosyndactyly

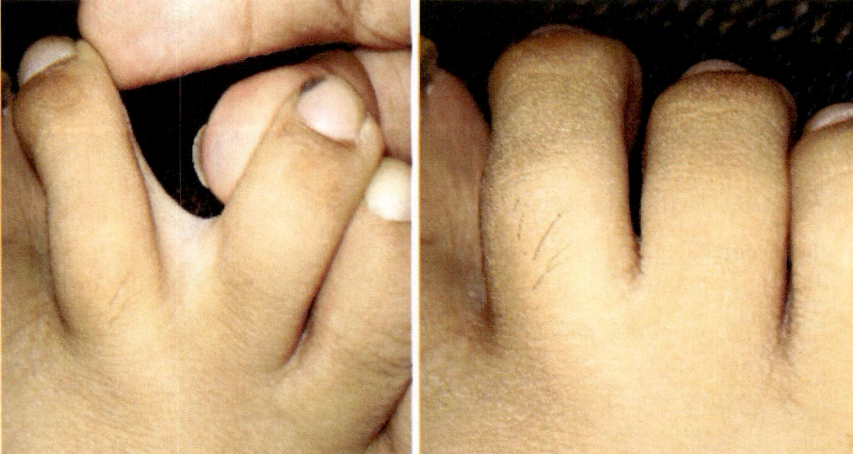

Fig. 61.2 Incomplete simple syndactyly

Fig. 61.3 Bilateral postaxial finger duplication

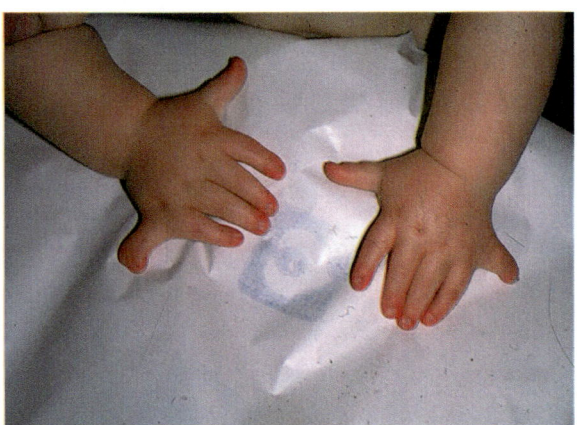

- Fingers are fused distally and fenestrated proximally.
- Often bilateral, associated with absent digits and syndromes such as Apert and amniotic band syndrome.

- Polydactyly
  - Can be preaxial (radial), postaxial (ulnar), or central
  - Postaxial polydactyly (Fig. 61.3)
    - Often inherited, more common in African Americans (1/143) than Caucasians (1/1339)
    - Classified as well developed (type A) or rudimentary (type B)
    - Type A more likely to be associated with syndrome
    - Type B often ligated in the nursery or office until it falls off (remove ulnar)

- Type A removed in operating room with ligation of vessels and nerves
- Risk of neuroma formation
- Central polydactyly
  - Most uncommon, if occurs likely part of a syndrome
  - Ring finger most affected
  - May be hidden in a syndactyly (synpolydactyly)
  - Often not managed surgically
- Preaxial Polydactyly
  - Thumb duplication, more common in Caucasian than others.
  - Most are sporadic cases.
  - Classified by the Wassel classification, which drives treatment.
  - Wassel IV is most common; VI is least common.
  - Surgery involves maintenance of the ulnar thumb and excision of the radial (or fusion) to spare the native UCL.
  - Need to make sure to centralize tendons and maintain UCL.

- Mirror Hand
  - Rare form of polydactyly where the thumb is replaced by a duplicated small, ring, and sometimes middle finger.
  - Can extend up into forearm with a duplicated ulna without radius.
  - Can also include vessels and even nerve and muscle duplication.
  - Due to a mutation in ZPA/Shh.
  - Treatment involves excision of abnormal digits and pollicization to form a thumb.

- Brachydactyly
  - Short fingers, may be isolated or part of a variety of syndromes.
  - One of the more common types of congenital hand deformities.
  - Middle phalanx is most commonly affected.
  - Severity of shorting can be great or minor, depending on the condition.
  - May be inherited but often sporadic.
  - Management depends on the severity of shortening; most need nothing, but if impacting function, then can do distraction osteogenesis or bone grafting.

- Cleft Hand
  - Central deficiency results in a V-shaped hand with ulnar fingers more likely to be preserved.
  - Autosomal dominant genes are typical.
  - Atypical cleft hands are found in symbrachydactyly (U-shaped), which often have finger nubbins, cleft hands have absent fingers, but the remaining ones are normal.
  - Most cleft hands function well; surgery is often for cosmetic reasons or to prevent worsening of the deformity.

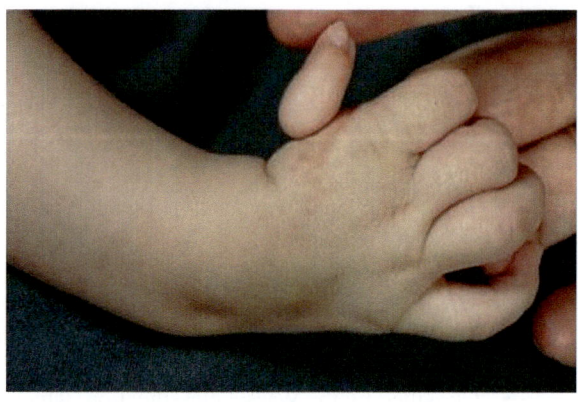

Fig. 61.4 Hypoplastic thumb, grade IV

- Absent Thumb (Fig. 61.4)
    - Considered part of the radial deficiency spectrum and associated syndromes (Holt Oram, TAR, VACTERL, Fanconi, CHARGE).
    - Classified based on the Blauth classification, which drives treatment (nothing, opponensplasty, pollicization).
    - Key structures to maintain include the UCL and the FDB.
- Amniotic Band Syndrome
    - Amniotic disruption constricts the distal parts of the upper extremity.
    - Distal to the constriction, there is edema or amputation.
    - If there is edema or swelling, may need immediate release with a Z-plasty to prevent ischemia.
- Symbrachydactyly
    - Spectrum of deformity from digit hypoplasia to loss of forearm, has features of undergrowth, differentiation, and formation.
    - Can be short finger, cleft hand, monodactylous, or peromelic.
    - Associated with Poland syndrome (hypoplasia of pectoralis and chest).
    - Central rays are typically the most commonly affected.
    - Management is based on addressing specific deformities (short fingers, absent fingers) as needed for functional benefit
- Clinodactyly (Fig. 61.5)
    - Angulation of digits in the radioulnar plane, often associated with a delta phalanx.
    - Considered pathologic at 10° of angulation or more.
    - True incidence has been estimated at 1%–20%, depending on the study.
    - Due to malformation of the epiphyseal growth plate.
    - Associated with Down syndrome.
    - Mainly an aesthetic problem, so surgical correction is not done unless there is functional impairment, needing a wedge osteotomy, or distraction.

Fig. 61.5 Clinodactyly

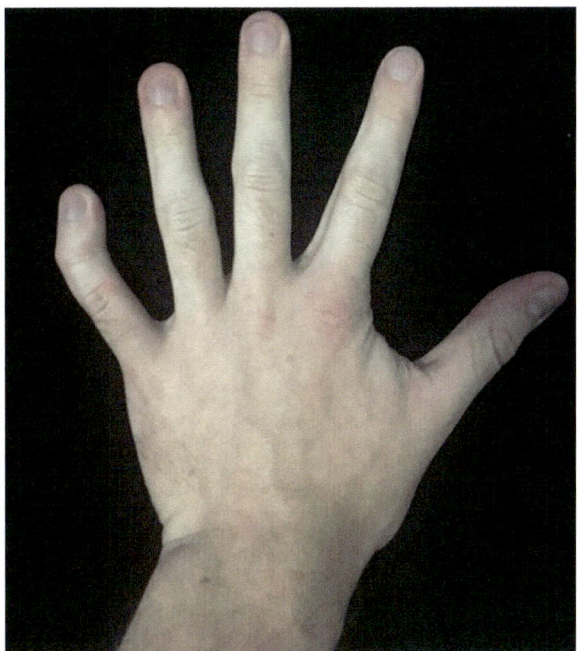

- Macrodactyly
  - Excessive growth of a singular digit.
  - Comprises about 1% of all upper extremity anomalies.
  - Often associated with lipofibromatosis or neurofibromatosis
  - Develops in the first 3 years of life, mainly in the index finger
  - Enlarged skeleton and soft tissue envelopes.
  - Management is often cosmetic with debulking and epiphysiodesis to stop digital growth.
  - Amputation is a last resort.
- Camptodactyly (Fig. 61.6)
  - Malinsertion of the lumbrical on the middle phalanx, causing progressive fixed flexion of the PIP.
  - Most often in teenage girls.
  - Treat with splinting, surgery if severe.
- Absent radius
  - Most common malformation of the forearm (1/5000).
  - Associated with many syndromes (VACTERL, Holt-Oram, TAR, Fanconi, Edward, Patau).
  - Need to watch blood counts (Fanconi, TAR) and cardiac function (Holt-Oram).
  - Absent is more common than malformed.
  - Treat with centralization of the ulna to allow a stable bony base for the wrist (Table 61.1).

Fig. 61.6 Camptodactyly

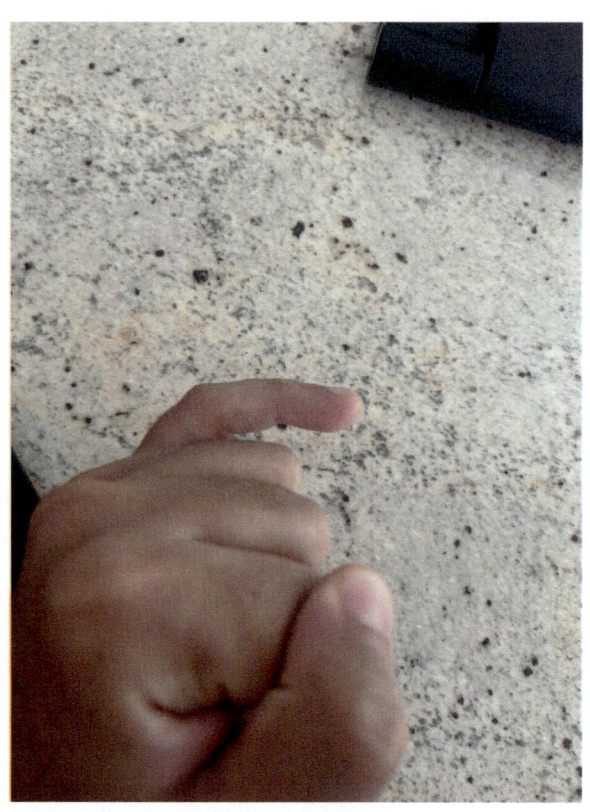

Table 61.1 Syndromes to know

Syndrome	Hand issue	Other issues
Holt-Oram	Absent radius	Heart
Thrombocytopenia absent radius (TAR)	Absent radius	Thrombocytopenia
VACTERL	Absent radius	Vertebrae, anal, cardiac, TEF, renal
Fanconi	Absent radius	Anemia
CHARGE	Absent radius	Coloboma, heart, renal
Poland	Syndactyly, symbrachydactyly	Breast, sternal head of pec
Apert	Syndactyly	Craniosynostosis
Down syndrome	Clinodactyly	Many
Klippel-Trenaunay	Macrodactyly	DVT
Maffucci	Enchondroma, macrodactyly	Venous malformation
Pfeiffer	Macrodactyly	Craniosynostosis
Muenke	Loss of middle phalanx	Craniosynostosis
Saethre-Chotzen	Syndactyly	Brachycephaly, eyelid ptosis
Orofacial digital syndrome	Polydactyly	Tessier 0 cleft
Mobius	Associated with Poland	CN VI, VII

References

1. Bamshad M, Watkins WS, Dixon ME, et al. Reconstructing the history of human limb development. Pedaitr Res. 1999;45:291.
2. Chen Y, Zhao X. Shaping limbs by apoptosis. J Exp Zool. 1998;282:691.
3. Lourie GM, Lins RE. Radial longitudinal deficiency. Hand Clin. 1998;14:85.
4. Tickle C. Genetics and limb development. Dev Genet. 1996;19:1.
5. Zaleske DJ. Development of the upper limb. Hand Clin. 1985;1:383.

Chapter 62
Rheumatoid Arthritis

Meaghan L. Barr

Background [1–3]

- Rheumatoid arthritis (RA) is a chronic inflammatory condition affecting approximately 0.5%–1% of the world's population.
- The disease is systemic, affecting the synovial joints as well as the heart, lungs, kidneys, and skin.
- Women are more frequently affected than men (F:M ratio is 2–3:1).
- Other inflammatory arthropathies to rule out include crystalline arthropathies (gout, pseudogout, calcium pyrophosphate deposition disease) and infectious arthropathies (*Neisseria gonorrhea*, Lyme disease).

Risk Factors [1, 2]

- The exact etiology of RA is unknown.
- Genetic and environmental factors contribute to RA susceptibility.
- Family history of RA elevates the risk of disease by 3–5 times baseline risk.
- Susceptibility to RA is associated with mutations on the PTPN22 gene and on the HLA-DRB1 gene.
- Environmental risk factors include smoking tobacco, exposure to silica dust, and *Porphyromonas gingivalis*, which causes periodontal disease.

M. L. Barr (✉)
Division of Plastic Surgery, Department of Surgery, University of California, Los Angeles, Los Angeles, CA, USA
e-mail: meaghanbarr@mednet.ucla.edu

Pathophysiology [1, 2]

- The exact pathophysiology of RA is unknown.
- Tissue destruction is caused by a complex interaction between T cells, B cells, macrophages, antigen presenting cells, and other immunologic cells that induces a chronic inflammatory state.
- Autoantibodies are produced against proteins including rheumatoid factor (RF) and citrulline. Antibodies against citrulline are known as anti-citrullinated protein antibodies (ACPAs).
- Inflammation of the connective tissue lining a joint capsule is known as "synovitis."
- Chronic synovitis leads to formation of a "pannus." which is enlargement of the synovial lining of a joint. Pannus formation results in bony erosion, cartilage destruction, and subsequent loss of joint function.

Diagnosis [1, 3–5]

- Patients present with pain, swelling, and redness of the joints. Small joints are more frequently affected than large joints (Fig. 62.1).
- Extra-articular manifestations include cardiovascular disease, lung disease (fibrotic and/or inflammatory), cognitive difficulties, Sjogren's syndrome, anemia, osteoporosis, and hematologic and/or renal malignancies.
- A score of ≥6 on the 2010 American College of Rheumatologic/European League Against Rheumatism classification criteria is required for definitive diagnosis of RA.
  - Large joint involvement = 0 points

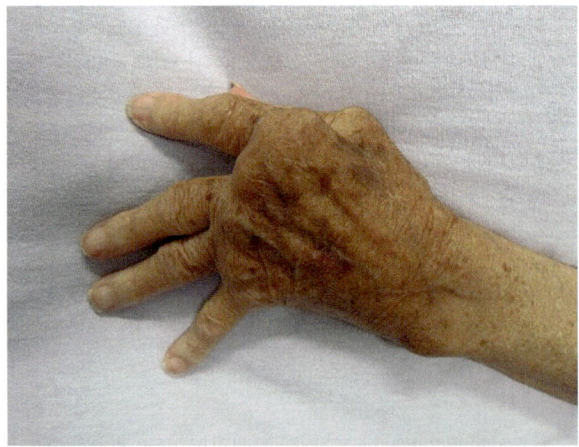

Fig. 62.1 Classical stigmata of rheumatism in the hand

- 2–10 large joints = 1 point
- 1–3 small joints (with or without involvement of large joints) = 2 points
- 4–10 small joints (with or without involvement of large joints) = 3 points
- >10 joints (at least 1 small joint) = 5 points
- Negative RF + negative ACPA = 0 points
- Low positive RF or low-positive ACPA = 2 points
- High positive or high positive ACPA = 3 points
- Normal CRP and normal ESR = 0 points
- Abnormal CRP or abnormal ESR = 1 point
- Duration of symptoms <6 weeks = 0 points
- Duration of symptoms >/6 weeks = 1 point

Treatment: Medical Management [1–3]

- NSAIDs are used to treat symptomatic RA; these drugs work by decreasing inflammation, which in turn reduces pain.
- Corticosteroids are also used to treat symptomatic RA. Due to significant side effects, use is limited to short-term courses for bridging therapy to disease-modifying antirheumatic drugs (DMARDs) or active RA refractory to DMARDs.
- Disease-modifying antirheumatic drugs (DMARDs) suppress critical pathways in the inflammatory cascade, thereby delaying or preventing joint destruction.
- Early treatment with DMARDs improves patient outcomes. While medical management is outside the scope of the hand surgeon's practice, familiarity with common agents is important for patient management and surgical planning as certain drugs may promote immunosuppression or interfere with wound healing.
- Common agents include:
  - Methotrexate (MTX)—analog of folate that inhibits nucleotide production. MTX is the first line treatment for RA. It has excellent safety and efficacy rates.
  - Leflunomide (LEF)—inhibits DNA and RNA production. It has a similar efficacy to MTX, and is useful in combination with other drugs.
  - Hydroxychloroquine (Plaquenil)—antimalarial drug with anti-inflammatory and immunomodulatory effects. Major side effects include retinal toxicity.
  - Sulfasalazine (SSZ)—considered to have both antimicrobial and anti-inflammatory effects. Significantly decreases RA symptoms compared to placebo.
  - Infliximab (Remicade)—monoclonal antibody that inhibits tumor necrosis alpha (TNF-alpha) activity. Side effects include serious infections and re-activation of latent infections (hepatitis B, tuberculosis).
  - Etanercept (Enbrel)—recombinant immunoglobulin with good efficacy.
  - Adalimumab (Humira)—monoclonal antibody that inhibits TNF-alpha. Can induce remission and prevent radiological progression.

- Other secondary biologic agents include Rituximab (monoclonal antibody that targets CD20), Abatacept (T-cell modulator), Tocilizumab (monoclonal antibody that targets IL-6), Anakinra (recombinant IL-1 receptor antagonist), and Tofacitinib (JAK inhibitor).

Treatment: Surgical Management [4, 6, 7]

- With the introduction of DMARDs, rates of significant hand pain and deformity have decreased. While hand surgeons are less likely to encounter operative RA pathology, there is still a role for surgical management to improve symptoms and function

Rheumatoid Nodules

- Subcutaneous nodules typically found at the olecranon and/or along the dorsal forearm and hand.
- Symptomatic nodules are tender, and can interfere with hand function depending on location.
- Symptomatic nodules may be resected but are prone to recurrence.

Rheumatoid Wrist (Fig. 62.2)

- The wrist is the most frequently involved joint.
- Chronic synovitis degrades ligamentous structures, resulting in a predictable pattern of disease progression.
- At the radial wrist, weakening of the scapho-lunate ligament leads to scaphoid dislocation and radial column collapse.
- At the ulnar wrist, synovitis injures the ligaments of the distal radio-ulnar joint (DRUJ), leading to caput ulna deformity.
- Caput ulna deformity describes dorsal dislocation of the ulnar head with subsequent ulnar head impaction onto the carpus.
- At the same time, the extensor carpi ulnaris (ECU) subluxates volarly, providing the wrist extensors with a mechanical advantage.
- The end result of these processes is radial deviation of the metacarpals and ulnar deviation of the metacarpophalangeal (MCP) joints.
- Surgical interventions can be preventative, reconstructive, or for salvage purposes.
- Preventative interventions include synovectomy and prophylactic tendon transfers to restore flexor/extensor balance.

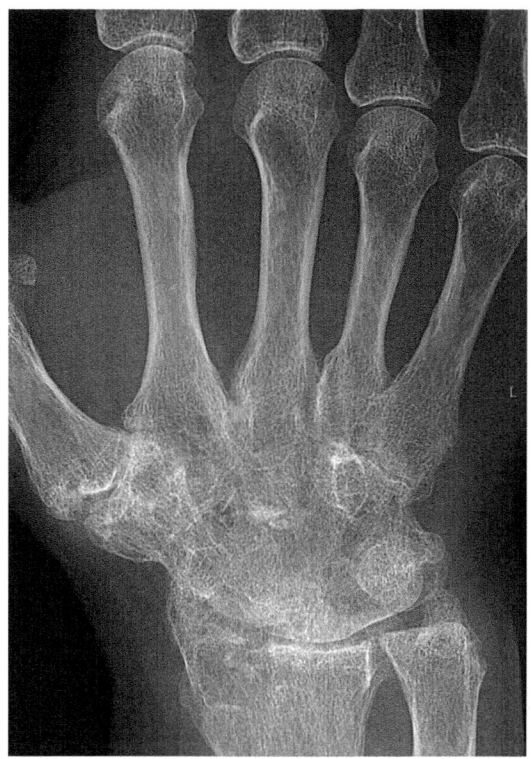

Fig. 62.2 Severe erosive arthritis of the wrist due to rheumatoid arthritis

- Reconstructive interventions include resection of the distal ulna (Darrach procedure), hemiresection arthroplasty (Bowers procedure), and DRUJ fusion with proximal ulnar resection (Suave-Kapandji procedure).
- Salvage interventions are indicated for severe pain, bony destruction, and/or unsalvageable tendon ruptures. Options include partial or complete wrist fusion.

Tenosynovitis

- Tenosynovitis is common in patients with rheumatoid arthritis. It describes chronic inflammation of the tendons and their respective sheaths.
- Tenosynovitis is most frequently encountered on the dorsal aspect of the hand and wrist.
- It generally presents as painful swelling, but can lead to tendon rupture if unaddressed.
- Synovectomy, surgical resection of the hyperplastic synovium, alleviates symptoms and helps prevent tendon rupture.

Tendon Ruptures

- Attritional tendon ruptures occur when weakened tendons are repeatedly scraped over bony prominences formed by chronic synovitis.
- Mannerfelt syndrome refers to flexor pollicis longus (FPL) rupture due to a bony spur in the carpal tunnel.
- Caput ulna syndrome (dorsal subluxation of the ulna) can cause attritional rupture of extensor tendons, specifically EDC.
- Treatment of attritional tendon ruptures requires tendon grafting versus tendon transfers.

Finger Deformities (Fig. 62.3)

- The Swan-Neck deformity describes a finger with proximal interphalangeal (PIP) joint hyperextension and distal interphalangeal (DIP) joint flexion.
- Swan-Neck deformities develop from pathology at the PIP or DIP joint level. Treatment ranges from splinting to arthroplasty depending on severity.
- The Boutonniere deformity describes a finger with PIP joint flexion and DIP joint hyperextension.
- A Boutonniere deformity is caused by central slip rupture or attenuation, leading to volar displacement of the lateral bands with subsequent contracture. Treatment ranges from splinting to arthroplasty; significant deformity is almost impossible to correct.

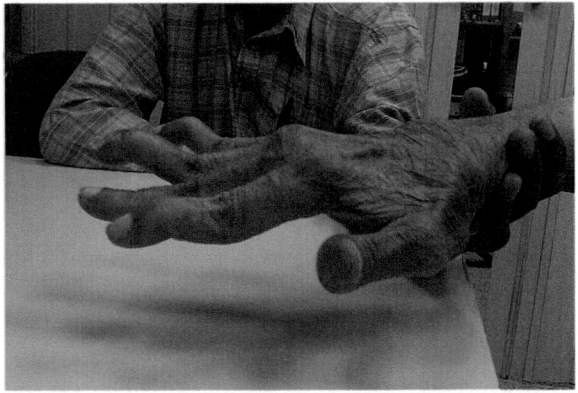

Fig. 62.3 Swan neck of the fingers

Stenosing Tenosynovitis

- Stenosing tenosynovitis ("trigger finger") refers to inflammation of the flexor tendon sheath and/or nodule formation in the vicinity of the A1 pulley that prevents smooth gliding of the tendons through the sheath.
- Stenosing tenosynovitis is commonly encountered in both RA and non-RA patients. However, management differs drastically between patient populations; A1 pulley release *should be avoided* in RA patients as it can exacerbate ulnar deviation of the digits.
  - Instead, can resect one slip of FDS to debulk the canal for trigger finger.

Metacarpophalangeal (MCP) Joints

- Synovitis of the MCP joints leads to volar subluxation and ulnar deviation of the fingers.
- Early treatment options include synovectomy and tendon transfers to address function and aesthetic concerns. For more advanced disease, arthroplasty is required.

References

1. Radu A-F, Bungau SG. Management of rheumatoid arthritis: an overview. Cells. 2021;10(11):2857. https://doi.org/10.3390/cells10112857.
2. Lin Y-J, Anzaghe M, Schülke S. Update on the pathomechanism, diagnosis, and treatment options for rheumatoid arthritis. Cells. 2020;9(4):880. https://doi.org/10.3390/cells9040880.
3. Guo Q, Wang Y, Xu D, Nossent J, Pavlos NJ, Xu J. Rheumatoid arthritis: pathological mechanisms and modern pharmacologic therapies. Bone Res. 2018;6(1):15. https://doi.org/10.1038/s41413-018-0016-9.
4. Beasley RW. Beasley's surgery of the hand. New York: Thieme Publishing Group; 2003.
5. Aletaha D, Neogi T, Silman AJ, et al. 2010 Rheumatoid arthritis classification criteria: an American College of Rheumatology/European League Against Rheumatism collaborative initiative. Arthritis Rheum. 2010;62(9):2569–81. https://doi.org/10.1002/art.27584.
6. Chung KC, Pushman AG. Current concepts in the management of the rheumatoid hand. J Hand Surg Am. 2011;36(4):736–47. https://doi.org/10.1016/j.jhsa.2011.01.019.
7. Wolfe SW, Pederson WC, Hotchkiss RN, Kozin SH. Green's operative hand surgery: 2-volume set. 6th ed. New York: Churchill Livingstone; 2010.

Chapter 63
Osteoarthritis

Carter J. Boyd and Jonathan M. Bekisz

Overview [1, 2]

- Osteoarthritis is a predominantly cartilaginous disease involving non-inflammatory degeneration of articular cartilage with subsequent reactive bone formation in the affected joint.

Demographics, Incidence, and Epidemiology [1, 2]

- Osteoarthritis is more common in females than males. Hormonal differences have been proposed as the underlying mechanism leading to ligamentous weakening and laxity.
- Older age is associated with an increased incidence of the disease. Patients are typically older than 40 years of age.
- Some have suggested genetic influences on disease development, but these associations are not well characterized [3].

Anatomy [1]

- Osteoarthritis most commonly affects the joints of the hand and wrist.
- The carpometacarpal (CMC) joint of the thumb is the most frequently affected joint

- The interphalangeal (IP) joints, both proximal and distal, are also frequently involved. The metacarpophalangeal (MP) joints can also be affected.
- In addition to the CMC joint, the intercarpal, radiocarpal, ulnocarpal, and distal radioulnar joint can all be involved.

Pathogenesis [2]

- By contrast with rheumatoid arthritis, osteoarthritis has a weaker inflammatory reaction in the affected joints.
- The visible physical manifestations of disease result from pathologic deterioration of cartilage.
  - Results in pain, stiffness, joint enlargement, angular deformity, and contracture.
- Primary osteoarthritis is idiopathic and is believed to be secondary to a possible underlying genetic predisposition in conjunction with the normal aging process from mechanical overuse.
- Secondary osteoarthritis occurs secondary to a traumatic insult, which causes joint instability and injury. It may also develop after direct cartilage injury.

Diagnosis

- History [1, 2]
  - Patients typically present with a gradual onset of pain and stiffness of the affected joints. Symptoms may interfere with work, hobbies, or activities of daily living.
  - Pain is frequently exacerbated by activity, and symptoms get worse throughout the course of the day. Patients may report avoidance of provocative activities in response.
  - CMC joint arthritis can present with weakness of pinch and grasp.
  - Often, prior to presentation to a specialist, patients present to primary care providers. Patients may have already trialed conservative therapies (see below).
  - Patients presenting with osteoarthritis of the wrist are more likely to be post-traumatic. Fractures of the region disrupt normal alignment of the joints, leading to repeated microtrauma within the joints, expediting degenerative changes responsible for the disease.
- Physical Exam [1, 2]
  - Swelling of the affected joints is commonly observed and may be accompanied by pain with palpation over the joint.

- Distinct Heberden nodes (occurring at the distal interphalangeal (DIP) joint) and Bouchard nodes (occurring at the proximal interphalangeal (PIP) joint), which involve enlargement of the joint, are often present.
- Nail deformities may occur less frequently secondary to mucous cysts at the DIP joint.
- Range of motion of the affected joints may elicit audible crepitus.
- The grind test can be performed to assess for CMC joint involvement, which involves axial loading of the thumb while simultaneously rotating the proximal phalanx. Pain or crepitus elicited in the CMC joint indicates a positive test, suggesting a diagnosis of osteoarthritis.

- Laboratory Tests [2]

    - Laboratory studies are not required to make the diagnosis but may be obtained to rule out other causes of arthritis.

- Imaging [1, 2]

    - Formal three-view radiographs of the affected hand or wrist are typically sufficient to corroborate the clinical diagnosis of osteoarthritis.
    - Radiographic findings suggestive of osteoarthritis include osteophyte formation, narrowing of the joint space, bony sclerosis known as eburnation, and subchondral cysts.
    - Importantly, symptoms experienced by the patient do not always correlate with imaging.
    - Radiographic findings have been used in the staging of thumb CMC joint arthritis.

        - Eaton Classification System [4]

            - Stage I—normal bony articulations, joint space widening, minimal subluxation
            - Stage II—joint space narrowing, minimal osteophyte/debris present measuring <2 mm, increased subluxation
            - Stage III—increased sclerosis, >2 mm osteophyte visible, subchondral cysts present
            - Stage IV—presence of significant sclerosis and cyst formation and narrowing of the scaphotrapezial (ST) joint
            - Stage V—pantrapezial arthritis

Nonsurgical Management [1, 2]

- Importantly, there is no medical cure or treatment for the degeneration of articular cartilage seen in osteoarthritis. Nonoperative management is focused on reducing symptomatology and reducing the burden of the disease on activities of daily living. Nonoperative management is the primary treatment modality,

though surgical intervention can be offered in cases of advanced or severe disease.
- Rest and heat can be beneficial.
- Patients should trial nighttime or resting splints to minimize strain on affected joints. Specifically, first opposition splints are helpful for 1st CMC arthritis.
- Occupational therapy can offer range-of-motion therapy to retain joint mobility.
- Acetaminophen and nonsteroidal anti-inflammatory drugs (NSAIDs) should be used to alleviate pain.
- Injections, including corticosteroids and hyaluronic acid, can be beneficial. Data have demonstrated improvement of thumb CMC arthritis in 80% of patients treated with a single corticosteroid injection at more than 18 months of follow-up [5]

Surgical Management [1, 2, 6]

- Indications
  - Consider age, occupation, handedness, contralateral hand and wrist involvement, and medical comorbidities.
  - Pain and functional impairment are the most common reasons to pursue surgery.
  - Should be considered in those who fail conservative treatments.
- Goals
  - Relief of pain and restoration of function are primary objectives.
  - Most procedures aim to remove diseased surfaces and either replace them via creation of a stable joint or eliminate movement at a joint surface through fusion.
- Thumb CMC (Basal) Joint
  - Isolated trapeziectomy
    - Can be done with or without K-wire fixation. Use of K-wire fixation results in similar range of motion and strength as ligament reconstruction and tendon interposition (LRTI) [7]
    - Trapeziectomy without K-wire fixation can result in the metacarpal falling proximally and into contact with the scaphoid (subsidence). Arthritis can develop between scaphoid and metacarpal, and pain and weakness may develop.
  - Trapeziectomy with soft tissue interposition
    - Trapeziectomy and LRTI are the most popular procedures and have excellent long-term outcomes [8]

- Most common variation involves using a slip of the flexor carpi radialis for both volar beak ligament reconstruction and to fill the space left behind after trapezial resection.
  - Other modifications include the use of abductor pollicis longus (APL) or extensor carpi radialis longus (ECRL) for metacarpal suspensionplasty.
- Trapeziectomy and LRTI are the most popular procedures and have excellent long-term outcomes.
- Reconstruction of the volar beak ligament
  - Uses a strip of the flexor carpi radialis (FCR) tendon to reduce an excessively mobile joint.
- Closing wedge/metacarpal extension osteotomy
  - Option in early-stage CMC arthritis.
  - Involves excision of a wedge with a 30° angle to place the metacarpal in extension.
  - Alters force distribution across the joint and shifts load dorsally [9]
- CMC arthrodesis
  - Position for fusion: 30° radial abduction, 30°–40° palmar abduction, 15° pronation [2]
  - Associated with a high complication rate, most frequently nonunion (>10%).
- CMC arthroplasty
  - Less frequently performed because of high rates of complications such as implant failure or fracture.
  - Common implant types include silicone and pyrocarbon.
- Implant suspensionplasty
  - Devices such as Arthrex Mini-Tightrope™ (Arthrex, Naples, FL) maintain metacarpal position to prevent subsidence via an implant between the thumb and index finger metacarpals.
  - Typically done in conjunction with trapeziectomy.

- Thumb MP Joint
  - Arthrodesis to provide a stable and strong pinch.
  - Utilize screw or K-wire and tension band construct to fuse joint in 0°–15° flexion and 10° pronation.
- Thumb IP Joint
  - Arthrodesis with screws is preferred method and is proven reliable with high rates of fusion [10]

- MCP Joints of Other Digits
  - Arthroplasty with silicone or pyrocarbon implants.
  - Fusion (arthrodesis) or even consideration of ray amputation if failure of other options.
- PIP Joints
  - Arthrodesis in flexion to maximize functional utility. The degree of flexion decreases with progression from radial to ulnar digits and generally ranges from 20° to 40°. Utilize screw, internal fixation, or K-wire and tension band construct.
  - Arthroplasty with silicone, pyrocarbon, or metallic/polyethylene combination implants. Requires stable soft tissue to help maintain implant position and minimize dislocation. In optimal scenario can achieve up to 75° of flexion, but primary indication for arthroplasty is relief of pain, not restoration of range of motion.
- DIP Joints
  - Should ensure excision of mucous cysts and osteophytes.
  - Arthrodesis in 0°–10° of flexion to maximize functional utility. Fusion done using screw or K-wire and tension band construct.
- Intercarpal Arthritis
  - Fusion (arthrodesis) of involved joint(s) if disease is limited. Can also consider select carpal bone excision (e.g., scaphoidectomy).
  - With involvement of multiple joints, proximal row carpectomy (PRC) and four-corner arthrodesis (limited fusion of carpal bones) are the best options.
    - PRC is more useful in low demand individuals.
    - PRC places a capitate in the lunate fossa, which may progressively develop arthritis over time due to an unnatural fit in younger patients undergoing this procedure.
  - Total wrist fusion and wrist implantation are also options.

Distal Radioulnar (DRU) Joint Arthritis

- Resection and arthroplasty of the ulnar head are recommended to allow maintenance of forearm rotation.
  - Can replace the ulnar head with a prosthetic or perform resection (Darrach)
- Sauve-Kapandji procedure is another option that involves fusion of radius and ulna at the DRU joint with limited ulnar metaphyseal resection. This procedure also preserves forearm rotation.

- Total Wrist Arthritis
  - Fusion (arthrodesis) in 20° of extension using plates or K-wires is another option.
  - Arthroplasty can be performed in patients with low degrees of functional demand.
  - Can also perform ulnar head arthroplasty or ulnar head resection (Darrach procedure).

References

1. Parker WL, Ghavami A. Osteoarthritis. In: Janis JE, editor. Essentials of plastic surgery. 2nd ed. St. Louis: Quality Medical Publishing; 2014.
2. Diaz-Garcia RJ. Rheumatoid arthritis, osteoarthritis, and Dupuytren's contracture. In: Brown DL, Borschel GH, Levi B, editors. Michigan manual of plastic surgery. 2nd ed. Philadelphia: Wolters Kluwer; 2014.
3. Wu ZY, Du G, Lin YC. Identifying hub genes and immune infiltration of osteoarthritis using comprehensive bioinformatics analysis. J Orthop Surg Res. 2021;16(1):630. https://doi.org/10.1186/s13018-021-02796-6.
4. Eaton RG, Glickel SZ. Trapeziometacarpal osteoarthritis. Staging as a rationale for treatment. Hand Clin. 1987;3(4):455–71. [Online]. Available: https://www.ncbi.nlm.nih.gov/pubmed/3693416.
5. Day CS, Gelberman R, Patel AA, Vogt MT, Ditsios K, Boyer MI. Basal joint osteoarthritis of the thumb: a prospective trial of steroid injection and splinting. J Hand Surg Am. 2004;29(2):247–51. https://doi.org/10.1016/j.jhsa.2003.12.002.
6. Bernstein RA, et al. Arthritis. In: Hammert WC, Calfee RP, Bozentka DJ, Boyer MI, editors. ASSH manual of hand surgery. 1st ed. Philadelphia: Wolters Kluwer; 2010, ch. 19.
7. Davis TR, Brady O, Dias JJ. Excision of the trapezium for osteoarthritis of the trapeziometacarpal joint: a study of the benefit of ligament reconstruction or tendon interposition. J Hand Surg Am. 2004;29(6):1069–77. https://doi.org/10.1016/j.jhsa.2004.06.017.
8. Young SD, Mikola EA. Thumb carpometacarpal arthrosis. J Am Soc Surg Hand. 2004;4(2):73–93.
9. Tomaino MM. Thumb by metacarpal extension osteotomy: rationale and efficacy for Eaton Stage I disease. Hand Clin. 2006;22(2):137–41. https://doi.org/10.1016/j.hcl.2006.02.008.
10. Cox C, Earp BE, Floyd WET, Blazar PE. Arthrodesis of the thumb interphalangeal joint and finger distal interphalangeal joints with a headless compression screw. J Hand Surg Am. 2014;39(1):24–8. https://doi.org/10.1016/j.jhsa.2013.09.040.

Chapter 64
Chest Reconstruction

Harsh Patel

1. Introduction

    Chest wounds represent a unique challenge for reconstructive surgeons, as there are both wound coverage considerations and physiological function needs. Most commonly needed for previous surgical complications, such as persistent sternal wounds or sternal osteomyelitis after median sternotomy. Ultimately, repair of these wounds should be undertaken in a multidisciplinary manner to ensure optimal coverage and restoration of physiological function.

2. Etiology

    (a) Sternal wound dehiscence usually stemming from a previous incision of the sternum (i.e., for midline access to the heart for coronary bypass surgery)
    (b) Infection such as in the case of extensive empyema (i.e., closure of previous Eloesser flap or obliteration of dead space)
    (c) Trauma leading to multiple consecutive rib fractures or penetrating injury
    (d) Tumor resection of the chest wall
    (e) Radiation-related injury

3. Goals/Workup

    (a) Restoration of chest wall stability and integrity to protect underlying structures.
    (b) Provide well-vascularized soft tissue coverage for wound closure.
    (c) Prevention of paradoxical chest wall motion.
    (d) Workup can include understanding patient goals, preoperative functional status, CTA of the chest and possible harvest sites, pulmonary function testing, nutritional labs, A1c.

H. Patel (✉)
UCLA Plastic Surgery, Los Angeles, CA, USA
e-mail: harshpatel@mednet.ucla.edu

4. Skeletal Reconstruction
    (a) In cases with significant skeletal defect, reconstruction is necessary in order to provide structural support for the overlying soft tissue, protect critical cardiopulmonary structures, and allow for appropriate physiological function.
    (b) Can be achieved with synthetic or biologic mesh placed under tension to allow for semirigid fixation.
    (c) Indications:
        (i) Defects involving >3 consecutive ribs OR defect >5 cm in diameter.
        (ii) Anterolateral and anterior defects require more stability due to greater range of physiological motion and increased bearing on respiration.
        (iii) Of note, history of radiation can lead to increased chest wall stiffness and rigid fixation may not be necessary when otherwise would.
5. Soft tissue reconstruction—choice of coverage is dependent on the location of the defect followed by available reconstructive options.
    (a) Anterior defects: pectoralis major advancement or turnover, vertical rectus abdominis in a vertical or transverse design, pedicled latissimus dorsi flap, omental flap.
    (b) Anterolateral defect: subscapular axis flap, rectus abdominis, pectoralis major.
    (c) Posterior defect: subscapularis axis flap, trapezius.
    (d) Given appropriate recipient vessels, free tissue transfer can be considered but is associated with greater chance of full flap loss than pedicled options and is therefore reserved for very select indications.
6. Workhorse Flaps
    (a) Pectoralis major advancement (Fig. 64.1)
        (i) Can be done with medialization of either one or both pectoral muscles.
        (ii) Requires freeing of the muscle from its attachment and advanced on the thoracoacromial artery.
        (iii) Previous surgery or injury to the muscles may limit how much coverage may be offered
        (iv) Inferior sternal wounds are difficult to cover with pectoralis advancement flaps due to limited reach on pedicle.
        (v) In female patients, breast tissue overlies pectoralis, which can complicate advancement.
    (b) Vertical rectus abdominis myocutaneous (VRAM) flap
        (i) Rectus muscle is isolated on the superior epigastric artery pedicle and rotated up towards the wound.
        (ii) Due to donor site morbidity, VRAM is typically done in a unilateral fashion and may be difficult to cover superior sternal wounds due to limited reach.

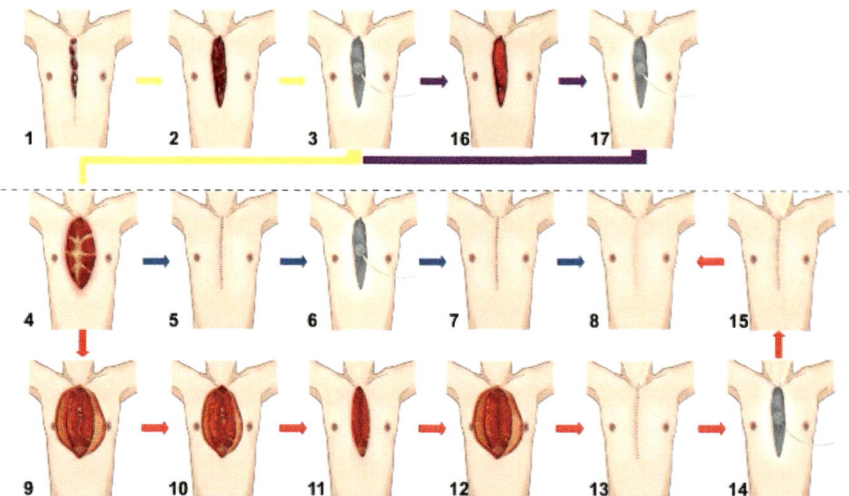

Fig. 64.1 Staging of chest reconstruction

- (iii) Previous abdominal surgery or utilization of the internal mammary arteries (i.e., for coronary artery bypass for coronary artery disease) may preclude utilization of this option.
    1. Flap swings on superior epigastric artery, which is a continuation of the internal mammary; harvest of the IMA precludes pedicled flap off of this system, but not the inferior system (type III flap) in a free tissue transfer fashion.
- (c) Latissimus dorsi flap
    - (i) Utilization of the ipsilateral flap in a pedicle fashion is typically done to cover soft tissue defects or obliterate intrathoracic dead space.
    - (ii) Primarily used for lateral defects as the muscle is delivered through the axilla to maximize reach and can be extended over the ribs or under.
    - (iii) Can be transferred with a skin paddle if required.
- (d) Omental flap
    - (i) Used often for inferior sternal wound dehiscence that cannot be covered with a pectoralis flap
    - (ii) Can be harvest open or endoscopically
    - (iii) Involves harvesting off the right gastroepiploic artery
    - (iv) Will need skin graft for coverage

7. Complications
    - (a) Persistent wounds due to flap loss, impartial closure, donor site morbidities

Chapter 65
Abdominal Wall Reconstruction

Erika Samlowski

Anatomy [1]

- *Borders of the abdominal wall*:
  - Superior: xiphoid process, costal margin
  - Inferior: pubic tubercle, inguinal ligament
  - Lateral: midaxillary line
- *Layers*:
  - Skin
  - Subcutaneous fat, Camper's fascia
  - Scarpa's fascia
  - Myofascial layer:
  - Rectus abdominis:
    - Origin: pubic ramus
    - Insertion: xiphoid process, ribs 5–7
    - Muscle fibers run vertically, three tendinous inscriptions
  - External oblique:
    - Origin: ribs 4–12
    - Insertion: Linea alba
    - Muscle fibers run inferomedially, "hands in pockets" direction

- Internal oblique
  - Origin: thoracolumbar fascia, iliac crest, inguinal ligament.
  - Insertion: costal margin, linea alba.
  - Muscle fibers run superomedially.
- Transversus abdominis
  - Origin: ribs 6–12, thoracolumbar fascia, anterior iliac crest, inguinal ligament
  - Insertion: linea alba
  - Muscle fibers run transverse
- Pyramidalis
  - Functionally insignificant
  - Not present in everyone
- Fascia:
- Linea alba:
  - Midline decussation of anterior rectus sheath
  - Runs vertically from xiphoid to pubis
- Linea semilunaris:
  - Fascial interface at lateral border of rectus
- Arcuate line:
  - Posterior rectus sheath ends at the level of anterior superior iliac spines
- Rectus sheath
  - Above the arcuate line:
    - Anterior rectus sheath: aponeurosis of external oblique, anterior leaf of internal oblique
    - Posterior rectus sheath: aponeurosis of posterior leaf of internal oblique, transversus abdominis, transversalis fascia
  - Below the arcuate line:
    - Anterior rectus sheath: aponeurosis of external oblique, anterior leaf of internal oblique
    - Posterior: transversalis fascia only
- Transversalis fascia
- Intraperitoneal fat
- Parietal peritoneum

- *Vascular*:
  - Robust blood supply with rich collateralization to the skin and subcutaneous tissue.
  - Large portions of the abdominal wall can be supplied on a single vessel—allows it to be elevated as a random flap (abdominoplasty).
  - Divided into three Huger zones.
  - Central abdomen:
    - Superior epigastric (continuation of internal mammary)
    - Deep inferior epigastric (branch of the external iliac)
    - Collateralize in the middle third near umbilicus
    - Multiple perforators to in medial and lateral rows
  - Inferior abdomen:
    - Superficial circumflex femoral artery
    - Superficial inferior epigastric artery
    - External pudendal artery (from common femoral artery)
  - Lateral abdomen:
    - Thoracic intercostal T7–12, L1 neurovascular pedicle
- *Nerves*:
  - Ventral rami of T7–L2 supplies motor and sensory innervation.
  - Nerves travel in plane between internal oblique and transversus abdominis muscles before entering posterior rectus sheath.
    - Inter-oblique plane safe for dissection.
    - Transversus abdominis plane block (TAP block) injects local anesthetic directly in this plane.
  - Iliohypogastric, ilioinguinal nerves supply suprapubic area.
- *Mechanical Forces*:
  - Abdomen is pressurized cylinder, posterior 1/3 is fixed in position.
  - Inspiration, diaphragm decent, abdominal wall contraction, arm movement all cause increased intraabdominal pressure.
  - Uniform counterpressure from abdominal wall musculature.
  - Disruption or imbalance can result in hernia or bulge (Figs. 65.1 and 65.2).

Pathology

- *Surgical Dehiscence*:
  - Opening of wound at any level superficial vs deep, dehiscence of fascia results in evisceration or exposure abdominal contents.

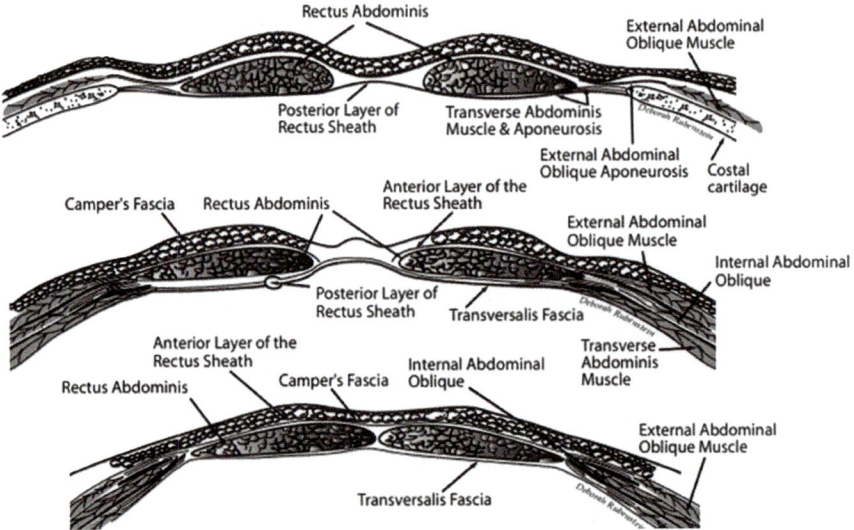

Fig. 65.1 Layers of the abdominal wall

Fig. 65.2 Huger zones

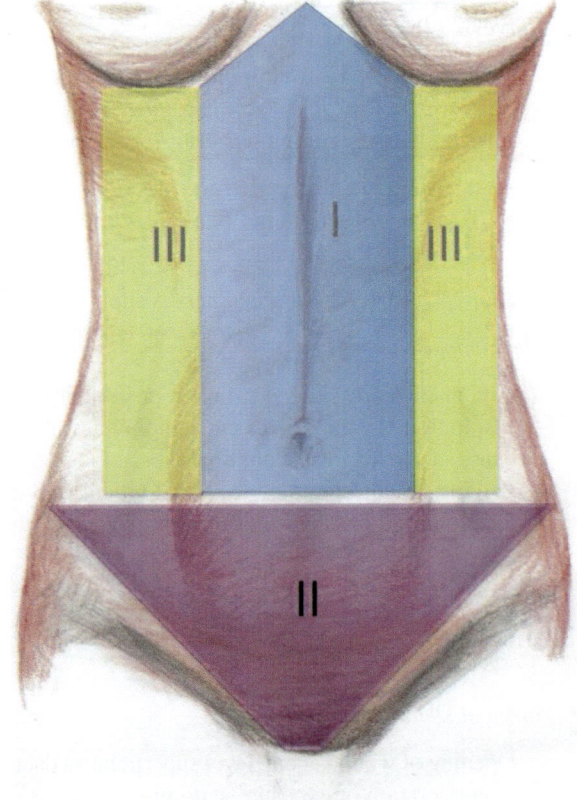

- If clean can close surgically.
- Delay closure if tissue infected or devitalized.
  - Wet to dry dressing, abdominal wound vac to delay closure
  - Can skin graft directly onto exposed bowel once granulation tissue present if unable to close
- Fistula management: decrease output, optimize nutrition, wait 3–6 months for closure.

- *Hernia*: abnormal exit of tissue or an organ, such as the bowel, through the wall of the cavity in which it normally resides
- *Ventral Hernia Etiology*:
  - Multifactorial, loss of integrity of abdominal wall and inability to resist changes in intra-abdominal pressure results in hernia formation
  - Due to multilayered anatomy of the abdominal wall, commonly occurs at areas of weakness (linea alba, semilunar line, below the arcuate line, lumbar triangle) or surgical incisions
  - Prior surgery, prior hernia repair: 3%–20% after midline laparotomy, doubles if operation associated with surgical site infection.
  - Traumatic
  - Infection: superficial, deep, organ space
  - Congenital: gastroschisis, omphalocele, umbilical defect
  - Genetic factors: connective tissue disorders (Ehlers-Danlos syndrome)
  - Diastasis recti: not a true hernia, no fascia defect
- *Risk Factors for Hernia Recurrence*:
  - Patient factors:
    - Increased intraabdominal pressure: e.g., COPD, truncal obesity, ascites, pregnancy
    - Compromised tissue integrity: steroids, infection, multiple surgeries, microvascular disease (smoking, diabetes), connective tissue disorders (Ehlers-Danlos)
    - Comorbidities: smoking, diabetes, COPD, CAD, malnutrition (albumin <2), obesity, advanced age, immunosuppression, chemotherapy, chronic steroid use
    - Wound factors:
      - Acute vs chronic
      - Prior surgery or hernia repair
      - Size and location of defect
      - Anatomic areas involved

- Ostomy
- Enterocutaneous fistula
- Infection
- Loss of domain: abdominal contents no longer fit inside the abdominal cavity

Abdominal Wall Repair [1–5]

- *Principles*:
  - Patient optimization:
    - Nutritional status—albumin >3, prealbumin >20
    - Blood sugar optimization—Hgb A1c <7
    - Smoking cessation—at least 4 weeks
    - Cardiopulmonary optimization
    - Weight loss—BMI >35 risk factor for complication, recurrence
    - Ascites control—medical management, paracentesis
  - Preparation of the wound:
    - Control of infection, fistula prior to definitive repair
    - Lysis of adhesions
    - Fistula takedown
  - Tension free repair
    - Direct repair if small (<2 cm) and no tension (small umbilical hernias).
    - Reapproximation and centralization of rectus muscles.
    - 5 mm fascial bites with 5 mm advancement, non-strangulating tension
    - Component separation if necessary (see below).
    - Mesh reinforcement.
- *Timing*:
  - Immediate: acute traumatic, at time of tumor resection, hernia repair
  - Delayed: patient instability, injury not fully declared, active infection or gross contamination, enterocutaneous fistula
- *Goals*:
  - Prevent herniation of viscera
  - Tension free closure with soft tissue coverage
  - Restoration of ability of the myofascial system to resist intraabdominal pressure

- *Mesh*:
  - Synthetic
    - Pore size: macro- vs microporous: size of pores allows variable tissue incorporation, fluid drainage, tensile strength, foreign body reaction
    - Dissolvable: polygalactin (Vicryl)
    - Non-dissolvable: polypropylene (Prolene), PTFE (Gore-Tex)
    - Composite: nonstick coating to prevent bowel adhesions
    - Pros: cheap, wide variety of sizes/weights available
    - Cons: risk of infection or extrusion requiring removal
  - Biologic:
    - Non-synthetic, made of biologic tissue
    - Human acellular dermal matrix (AlloDerm)
    - Porcine or bovine acellular dermal matrix (Strattice)
    - Porcine small intestine mucosa (Surgisis)
    - Biologic mesh (Phasix)
    - Pros: can be used in contaminated or infected field, incorporates into tissues, no foreign material present in wound long term
    - Cons: expensive, decreased strength, higher rates of recurrence, higher seroma rates
  - Placement (Fig. 65.3):
    - Goal 3–5 cm overlap between mesh and fascia
    - Underlay or sublay: deep to the anterior rectus sheath fascia, best repair due to increased intra-abdominal pressure pushing the mesh into attached muscles
    - Retrorectus or Rives-Stoppa: in the rectus sheath, posterior to rectus muscle, limited laterally by rectus sheath
    - Intraperitoneal placement of mesh (IPOM): wide intraperitoneal underlay, laparoscopic or robotic placement of mesh
    - Onlay: superficial to anterior rectus sheath, susceptible to increased intra-abdominal pressure pushing mesh away from attached muscles
  - Inlay or Bridging: bridge between fascial edges, high rates of recurrence
- *Component separation*:
  - Myofascial advancement flaps, separation of the abdominal wall layers to allow for tension free ventral hernia repair.
  - Anterior release:
    - Division of external oblique fascia lateral to the linea semilunaris.
    - Amount of advancement depends on location (doubled for bilateral).
      - 5 cm per side epigastrium
      - 10 cm per side waist
      - 3 cm per side suprapubic

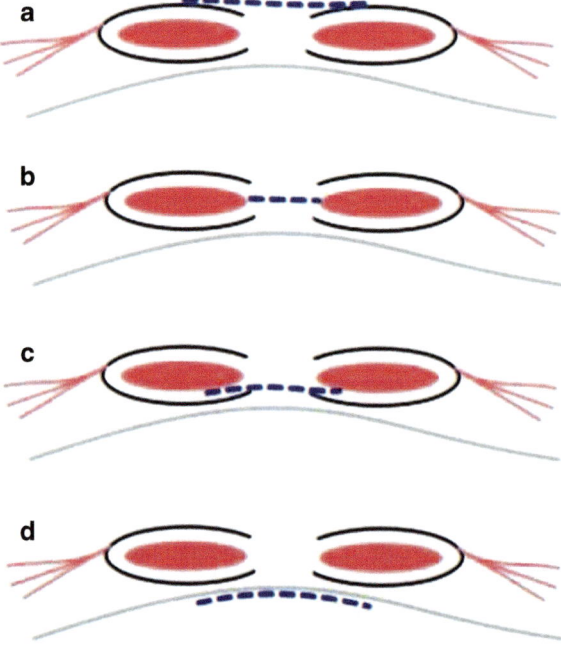

Fig. 65.3 Various placements of mesh. (**a**) Onlay. (**b**) Inlay. (**c**) Retrorectus. (**d**) Underlay

- Requires large subcutaneous flaps to be raised which can disrupt blood supply to skin.
- Preserve periumbilical perforator vessels to reduce risk of skin flap ischemia/wound healing problems.
- Can be done minimally invasively (endoscopic or robotic) to limit dead space, preserve blood supply to overlying skin flaps.

  – Posterior release:
  - Division of the posterior rectus sheath medial to the linea semilunaris
  - Done as part of a retrorectus repair

  – Transversus abdominis release
  - Division of posterior rectus sheath 1 cm medial to neurovascular bundles.
  - Can be done in combination with retrorectus repair large space for mesh.
  - Don't combine with anterior release.

- *Adjuncts*:
  – Tissue expansion can help with skin deficiency.
  – Free tissue transfer: consider with large area of tissue loss (trauma, cancer resection), radiation.
    - Innervated tensor fascia lata.
    - Anterolateral thigh.
    - Consider with large area of tissue loss (trauma, cancer resection), radiation.

- *Post-op care*:
  - Abdominal binder to provide support
  - Drains to decrease dead space, minimize seroma
  - Early ambulation
  - Multimodal pain control, consider transversus abdominis plane block, epidural
  - Aggressive pulmonary hygiene: increased intraabdominal pressure will cause atelectasis
  - No heavy lifting or strenuous exercise for 6–8 weeks because increases intra-abdominal pressure
- *Complications*:
  - Infection
  - Seroma
  - Hematoma
  - Cardiac, pulmonary, or end-organ dysfunction
  - Enterocutaneous fistula
  - Abdominal compartment syndrome
  - Hernia recurrence

References

1. Janis J. Essential of plastic surgery. 2nd ed. St. Louis: QMP/CRC Press; 2014.
2. Brown DL. Michigan manual of plastic surgery. 2nd ed. Philadelphia: Lippincott Williams & Wilkins; 2014.
3. Chung K. Grabb and Smith's plastic surgery. 8th ed. Philadelphia: Wolters Kluwer; 2019.
4. Mulholland MW. Greenfield's surgery. 6th ed. Philadelphia: Wolters Kluwer; 2016.
5. Townsend C. Sabiston textbook of surgery: the biological basis of modern surgical practice. 21st ed. St. Louis: Elsevier; 2021.

Chapter 66
Lower Extremity Reconstruction

Harsh Patel

1. Introduction [1, 2, 3]

    Lower extremity reconstruction is often required after traumatic injuries or oncologic ablation. When a functional reconstruction is possible, attempts should be made at limb salvage. Reconstruction becomes progressively more challenging for distal injuries, particularly inferior to the knee, due to the paucity of local soft tissue. Providing robust soft tissue coverage of exposed bone and hardware is a critical consideration for lower extremity reconstruction. Additionally, a reconstructive plan needs to ensure a functional outcome for the patient, given the dynamic role of the lower extremity.

2. Anatomy [4–7]

    (a) Upper leg

        (i) Can be thought of as the part of the leg spanning the femur.
        (ii) Musculature can be compartmentalized into three groups (Table 66.1):

    (b) Lower leg

        (i) Can be thought of as the portion of the leg spanning the length of the tibia to the bottom of the foot.
        (ii) Musculature is primarily posterior and can be thought of in terms of four individual compartments (Table 66.2):
        (iii) Arterial supply is from the popliteal artery, with gives off the anterior and posterior tibial arteries along with the peroneal artery, though branching patterns can be variable.

3. Upper leg reconstruction

H. Patel (✉)
UCLA Plastic Surgery, Los Angeles, CA, USA
e-mail: harshpatel@mednet.ucla.edu

Table 66.1 Anatomy of the thigh

Compartment	Muscles	Nerves	Vessels
Posterior (hamstring)	*Biceps femoris* *Semitendinosus* *Semimembranosus*	Sciatic	Profunda
Anterior (quadriceps)	*Rectus femoris* *Vastus lateralis* *Vastus intermedius* *Vastus medialis*	Femoral	Superficial femoral
Medial (adductors)	*Gracilis* *Obturator externus* *Adductor brevis* *Adductor longus* *Adductor magnus*	Obturator	

Table 66.2 Anatomy of the lower leg

Compartment	Muscles	Nerves	Vessels
Anterior	*Tibialis anterior* *Extensor hallucis longus* *Extensor digitorum longus*	Deep peroneal	Anterior tibial
Lateral	*Peroneus longus* *Peroneus brevis*	Superficial peroneal	
Superficial posterior	*Gastrocnemius* *Plantaris* *Soleus*		
Deep posterior	*Tibialis posterior* *Flexor hallucis longus* *Flexor digitorum longus* *Popliteus*	Tibial	Posterior tibial Peroneal

    (a) Due to the abundance of musculature and soft tissue in the upper leg, reconstruction of defects can primarily be achieved through primary closure or local tissue rearrangement.

    (b) Lower extremity reconstruction for the knee and below is typically more complex.

4. Lower leg reconstruction [6, 8–11]—can be separately considered in terms of soft tissue versus bony involvement. Ideal reconstructive approach depends on the size and location of the defect as well as the exposed structures.

    (a) Extent of injury: The Gustilo-Anderson classification system for open fractures is currently the gold standard (Table 66.3).

        (i) Grade I: small wound size (<1 cm) with minimal soft tissue damage, with local soft tissue coverage for reconstruction.

        (ii) Grade II: moderate wound size (>1 cm) with moderate soft tissue damage with local soft tissue coverage for reconstruction

        (iii) Grade III: separated into three subcategories (A, B, C), in which B and C require flap coverage for reconstruction, and 3C includes vascular injury that requires surgical repair.

Table 66.3 Gustilo classification

Grade	Energy	Size	Soft tissue	Fracture	Vascular	Antibiotics
I	Low	<1 cm	Low	Simple	None	Cefazolin
II	Moderate	1–10 cm	Moderate	Moderate	None	Cefazolin
IIIA	High	>10 cm	High	Complex	None	Cefazolin/gentamicin
IIIB	High	>10 cm	Periosteal stripping requiring soft tissue coverage	Complex	None	Cefazolin/gentamicin
IIIC	High	>10 cm	Periosteal stripping requiring soft tissue coverage	Complex	Need to be reconstructed	Cefazolin/gentamicin

   (iv) With every major lower extremity, discussion with the patient is vital to review reconstructive options, as well as long term outlook.
  (b) Location of injury: injuries to the lower limb below the knee are identified by location in the proximal to distal thirds. The thirds are important because of the type and availability of tissues in each third.
   (i) Zone 1—From the knee to one-third of the way down the tibia. Typically, pedicled gastrocnemius muscle flaps can be used and can cover defects as proximal as the knee. Free tissue transfer is also an option for larger defects (Fig. 66.1).
   (ii) Zone 2—Middle third of the lower leg. Pedicle gastrocnemius may have sufficient length and volume for small defects but standard is hemi-soleus flaps, pedicled perforator flaps, and free flaps. Cross-leg flaps, where tissue is borrowed from the contralateral leg in a delayed fashion is a viable option, and utilized more in the past prior to free tissue transfer.
   (iii) Zone 3—includes the distal third of the leg and foot. Due to the high amount of tendons and limited muscle volume, the majority of reconstruction is done via free tissue transfers (gracilis, anterolateral thigh, latissimus dorsi, etc) with few locoregional perforator flaps (i.e., reverse sural artery, propellor flap) for specific soft tissue defects. Free tissue transfer recipient vessels often prefer posterior tibial, but depend on patient anatomy. Preoperative imaging is helpful to determine vascular pattern and available options - end to side anastamosis may be required if concerns about remaining vascularity to foot. Again, cross-leg flaps can be utilized in this zone as well (Figs. 66.2 and 66.3).
5. Challenge/complications [9, 12, 13]
  (a) The goal of lower extremity reconstruction is aimed at limb salvage, but soft tissue coverage, especially of the lower half of the leg, is complicated by the mechanism and extent of the underlying soft tissue injury.
  (b) Gravity and venous congestion—Concerns for venous outflow issues due to forces of gravity in free flap reconstruction. It is typical for patients to

Fig. 66.1 Gastrocnemius flap

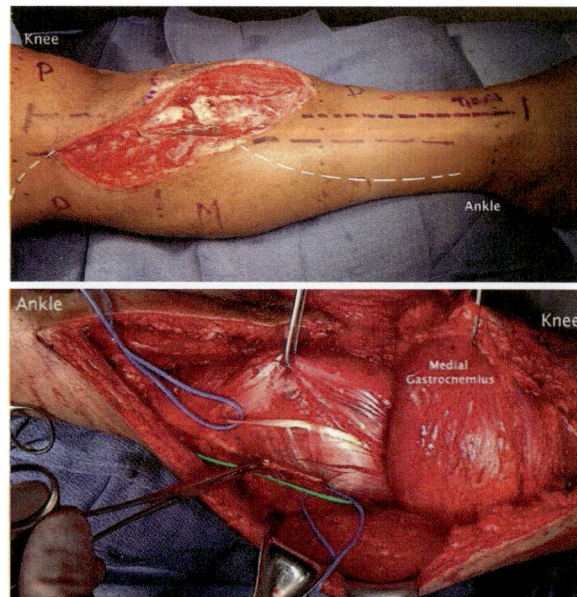

Fig. 66.2 Reversal sural flap

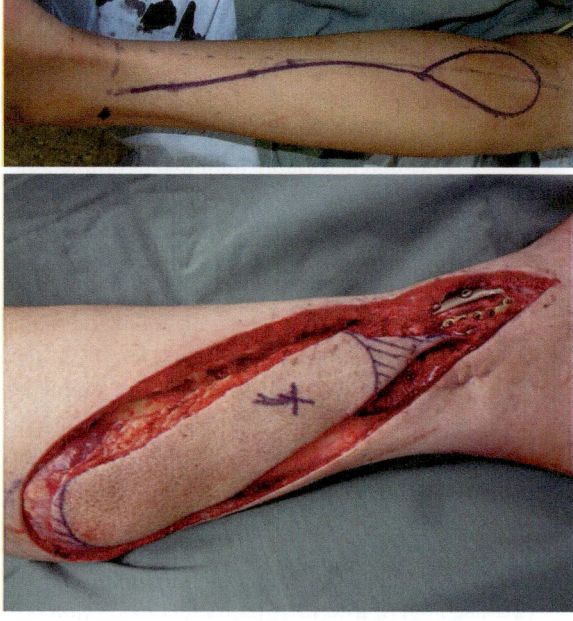

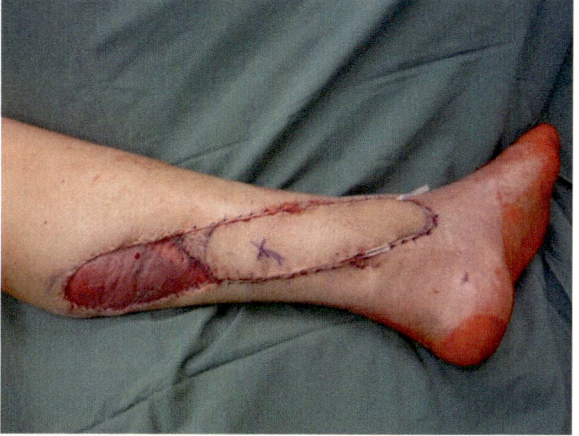

Fig. 66.3 Propeller flap after inset

undergo process of constant elevation with gradual "dangling" over time after surgery.

(c) The lower third of the leg has limited musculature with little to no soft tissue laxity, which makes tissue rearrangement for coverage a poor to nonviable option. Other options exist, but the free flap is typically considered "gold standard."

(d) Involvement of bony injury further complicates reconstruction due to the need for hardware, which adds additional bulk and the need for coverage, and increases the risk of complications such as osteomyelitis and hardware infection.

   (i) Historically, Godina in the 1980s described a need to cover injuries within 3 days; recently delayed reconstruction has been shown to have similar outcomes, likely due to advances in wound care, such as wound vac.

   (ii) Historical data (LEAP STUDY) shows patients with bony injury have poorer outcomes contingent on the extent of bony injury, with more extensive bony injury leading to poor quality of life and functional outcomes, with increased rate of chronic osteomyelitis.

   (iii) Osteomyelitis is a common complication of open bony injuries, with a large subset of patients failing limb salvage attempts.

      1. Often treated with removal of hardware and debridement, placement of antibiotic beads, and a prolonged period of systemic antibiotics, followed by a repeat attempt at fixation

   (iv) Need for reoperation further complicates reconstruction, as each reoperation further challenges the reconstructed site and poses another nidus for wound breakdown.

(e) Although free tissue transfers provide coverage to even distal injuries, these can create lifestyle limitations for the patient (i.e., an ALT for a foot wound can be bulky and limit the patient's ability to wear shoes).
(f) As improvements in medicine (i.e., surgical technique and antibiotics) have been made, outcomes for limb salvage have also improved. To that end, improvements in prosthetics have also been made, which makes it vital for providers to have a detailed discussion on patient goals and outcomes prior to committing a patient to a specific therapeutic path. Amputation with a myoelectric prosthesis is becoming an increasingly important option for limb reconstruction.

References

1. Higgins TF, Klatt JB, Beals TC. Lower Extremity Assessment Project (LEAP)—the best available evidence on limb-threatening lower extremity trauma. Orthop Clin North Am. 2010;41(2):233–9.
2. Melvin JS, Dombroski DG, Torbert JT, Kovach SJ, Esterhai JL, Mehta S. Open tibial shaft fractures: II. Definitive management and limb salvage. J Am Acad Orthop Surg. 2010;18(2):108–17.
3. Godina M. Early microsurgical reconstruction of complex trauma of the extremities. Plast Reconstr Surg. 1986;78(3):285–92.
4. Gustilo RB, Mendoza RM, Williams DN. Problems in the management of type III (severe) open fractures: a new classification of type III open fractures. J Trauma. 1984;24(8):742–6.
5. Gustilo RB, Anderson JT. Prevention of infection in the treatment of one thousand and twenty-five open fractures of long bones: retrospective and prospective analyses. J Bone Joint Surg Am. 1976;58(4):453–8.
6. Qiu E, Kurlander DE, Ghaznavi AM. Godina revisited: a systematic review of traumatic lower extremity wound reconstruction timing. J Plast Surg Hand Surg. 2018;52(5):259–64.
7. Bosse MJ, MacKenzie EJ, Kellam JF, Burgess AR, Webb LX, Swiontkowski MF, Sanders RW, Jones AL, McAndrew MP, Patterson BM, et al. An analysis of outcomes of reconstruction or amputation after leg-threatening injuries. N Engl J Med. 2002;347(24):1924–31.
8. Suda AJ, Cieslik A, Grutzner PA, Munzberg M, Heppert V. Flaps for closure of soft tissue defects in infected revision knee arthroplasty. Int Orthop. 2014;38(7):1387–92.
9. Cetrulo CL Jr, Shiba T, Friel MT, Davis B, Buntic RF, Buncke GM, Brooks D. Management of exposed total knee prostheses with microvascular tissue transfer. Microsurgery. 2008;28(8):617–22.
10. Salgado CJ, Mardini S, Jamali AA, Ortiz J, Gonzales R, Chen HC. Muscle versus non-muscle flaps in the reconstruction of chronic osteomyelitis defects. Plast Reconstr Surg. 2006;118(6):1401–11.
11. Chummun S, Wigglesworth TA, Young K, Healey B, Wright TC, Chapman TW, Khan U. Does vascular injury affect the outcome of open tibial fractures? Plast Reconstr Surg. 2013;131(2):303–9.
12. Burtt KE, Rounds AD, Leland HA, Alluri RK, Patel KM, Carey JN. Patient and surgical factors contributing to perioperative infection in complex lower extremity trauma. Am Surg. 2016;82(10):940–3.
13. Mathes SJ, Alpert BS, Chang N. Use of the muscle flap in chronic osteomyelitis: experimental and clinical correlation. Plast Reconstr Surg. 1982;69(5):815–29.

Chapter 67
Perineal Reconstruction

Andi J. Cummins

Overview

The perineum can be a challenging area for reconstructive surgeons due to the presence of structures integral to micturition, defecation, and sexual function. The goal of this chapter is to provide a basic understanding of perineal anatomy, types of injuries/illnesses requiring reconstruction, as well as a brief algorithm for various options for reconstruction. The scope of this chapter will neither include gender affirmation surgery nor pressure wound reconstruction, as those topics will be covered in more extensive detail in separate chapters.

Basic Perineal Anatomy [1–3]

- Perineum can be considered the diamond extending between the pubic symphysis and coccyx (A-P) and the 2 ischial tuberosities (lateral).
- Can be divided into anterior and posterior triangles separated by the perineal membrane:
  - Anterior triangle contains urogenital structures.
    - Male
      - Penis

A. J. Cummins (✉)
University of Texas Medical Branch, Department of Surgery, Division of Plastic Surgery, Galveston, TX, USA
e-mail: andcummi@utmb.edu

- Contains two corpora cavernosa, allowing for erectile and sexual function
- Bulbous portion of the male urethra in the corpus spongiosum allows for urination.
- Glans penis is the penile mucosa that contains distal nerve endings important for sexual function and erogenous sensation.
  - Scrotum
    - Thin-skinned, with Dartos fascia and cremaster muscle from abdominal origin
    - Contains male gonads and allows for sperm production at a lower-than-body temperature.
- Female
  - Vulva
    - Labia majora contains hair-bearing skin.
    - Labia minora are non-hair-bearing mucosa, fuse to form the clitoral hood anteriorly, and surround the introitus.
  - Clitoris
    - Analog to glans penis, collection of erectile tissue and nerves serving sexual function
  - Urethral meatus
  - Introitus and vaginal opening
- Posterior contains anorectal structures and pelvic floor muscles (levator ani).
- Blood Supply
  - External pudendal artery (external perineal structures)
    - Originates from the superficial femoral artery
  - Internal pudendal artery
    - Arises as a terminal branch from the internal iliac system and anastomoses with the external pudendal.
    - Dorsal penile and clitoral arteries arise from the internal pudendal artery.
    - Supplies external anal sphincter through inferior rectal vessels.
- Innervation
  - Genitofemoral nerve
    - Arises from the lumbar plexus and provides sensation to the anterior scrotum/mons pubis and the upper thigh

- Pudendal nerve
  - Supplies dorsal nerve of penis and clitoris
  - Motor nerve (levator ani and external anal sphincter) = deep perineal branch
- Ilioinguinal nerve
  - Course under inguinal ligament to supply root of penis/mons pubis

Common Causes of Perineal Defects [4, 5]

- Congenital
  - Female: vaginal agenesis, Mayer-Rokitansky-Kuster-Hauser syndrome
    - Vaginal agenesis with or without uterine anomalies
    - May have normal-appearing vulva/labia and blind vaginal introitus
  - Male: hypospadias, epispadias
    - Altered placement of the urethra (typically centrally placed meatus on the tip of the glans)
      - Hypospadias meatus is more ventral (hypo or toward the floor).
      - Epispadias meatus is more dorsal (epi or on top).
      - Classic mnemonic—"epi" has a "P" and "I," and if you have epispadias, you pee in your eye.
    - Typically repaired by pediatric or urologic surgeons
- Burn
  - Isolated injuries are uncommon, usually associated with massive injury.
    - Typically protected by groin and thigh folds
  - Burn to the genitals is a sufficient criterion for referral to a burn center.
  - Pediatric injuries, especially isolated ones, should raise concern for physical abuse (immersion), or sexual abuse.
- Trauma
  - Blunt trauma—straddle injuries, motor vehicle/motorcycle collisions
  - Sharp trauma—penile amputation or stab wounds
  - Explosive trauma—common in military combat due to the use of IEDs
- Infectious
  - Necrotizing infection of the perineum is called Fournier's gangrene.
    - Risk factors include diabetes mellitus, obesity, recent perineal surgery, and immunocompromised patients.

- Most important considerations are early fluid resuscitation and broad-spectrum antibiotics, and immediate surgical intervention for debridement
  - Many patients will require multiple debridements and "second look" procedures.
  - If testicles are not involved but are exposed, they can temporarily be implanted into thigh flap pockets to prevent desiccation.
- Hidradenitis Suppurativa
  - AKA "acne inversus," chronic development of draining sinus tracts and suppurative drainage.
  - Pathophysiology is not definitive, but thought to be a partially autoimmune reaction to naturally occurring bacteria in apocrine gland-bearing regions.
  - Risk factors include obesity, diabetes mellitus, a history of other autoimmune disorder, and history of other skin conditions.
    - Common locations—axillae, groin folds, perineum, gluteal cleft region
  - Medical management—topical clindamycin, oral prophylactic antibiotic regimen, immunosuppressive medications (TNF-a inhibitors like Humira)
  - If patient presents with acute infection or abscess in the region of HS, most typically managed with acute incision and drainage to relieve pressure and infection, should be started on prophylactic antibiotics after.
  - Surgery is the only definitive cure; however, recurrence after excision can occur.
    - Commonly employ wide local excision with subsequent skin grafting, or healing by secondary intention.
- Skin grafting may be performed in stages with interim wound care to ensure the wound is clean.
  - These patients are understanding of having large areas of draining dressings, so the goal is to replace a chronically draining wound with a clean healing wound.
- Neoplastic
  - Vulvar and penile cancers
    - Most commonly squamous cell carcinoma
    - Associated with HPV exposure and HIV/AIDS
    - Amenable to local tissue rearrangements or pedicle fasciocutaneous flaps
  - Vaginal and cervical cancers
    - May be primary cancers or invasive/metastatic
    - Require reconstructive options that can recreate hollow structures and potentially mucosal reconstruction

- Distal colorectal cancers
  - May require radical surgeries such as abdominoperineal resection or total pelvic exenteration.
    - Consideration for filling large amount of dead space
  - Areas of reconstruction may be within zone of previous radiation.
  - Consideration must be given to creation of any stoma for urinary or fecal diversion when selecting donor flap.

Reconstructive Options for Perineal Defects [6] (Table 67.1)

- Vulva/external female genitalia
  - Size of defect and desire for cosmesis and functionality will affect reconstructive options
    - Split thickness skin graft (sheet)
    - Local fasciocutaneous flaps (V-Y medial thigh, pudendal/groin flap)
    - Lotus flap
    - Pedicle fasciocutaneous flap (ALT, PAP, TUG)
- Vaginal defects
  - Partial defects (type I)
    - Anterior or lateral wall (type 1A)
      - Singapore flaps
    - Posterior wall
      - Rectus abdominis
  - Circumferential defects (type II)
    - Upper 2/3 (type IIA)
      - Rolled rectus abdominis flap
      - Colon transfer
    - Total defect (type IIB)
      - Bilateral gracilis myocutaneous flap
      - Colon mucosa (Fig. 67.1)

Table 67.1 Summary of Local and Pedicle Flap options, blood supply and defects that may be reconstructed

Flap name	Flap type	Blood supply	Potential Defects
Lotus petal flap	Transposition fasciocutaneous	Subdermal plexus, pudendal and perineal arteries	Vulva, labia
Singapore (pudendal) flap	Rotational and transposition fasciocutaneous	Posterior Labial Artery	Vulva, scrotum, anterior/lateral vaginal wall
Gluteal fold flap	Pedicle fasciocutaneous	Internal Pudendal Arteries	Vulva, perineum
Posterior thigh/gluteal V-Y flap	Advancement fasciocutaneous	Superior and inferior gluteal arteries	Perianal defects
Anterolateral thigh (ALT) flap	Pedicle fasciocutaneous	Descending branch of lateral femoral circumflex artery	Vulva, scrotum, penis
Superficial circumflex iliac perforator (SCIP) flap	Pedicle fasciocutaneous	Superficial circumflex iliac artery	Scrotum, penis
Rectus abdominus myocutaneous flap (VRAM, ORAM, TRAM)	Myocutaneous (vertical, oblique or transverse orientation) (Mathes-Nahai type III)	Deep inferior epigastric arteries	Posterior or upper 2/3 vagina, deep perineum
Deep inferior epigastric perforator (DIEP) or superficial inferior epigastric artery (SIEA) flap	Pedicle or free fasciocutaneous	Deep inferior epigastric artery	Posterior or upper 2/3 vagina, deep perineum
Gracilis flap	Muscle or myocutaneous flap (Mathes-Nahai type II)	Medial femoral circumflex artery	Total vaginal defect (bilateral), Lateral vaginal defect (unilateral), perineum
Omental flap	Omentum pedicle flap	Right and left gastroepiploic arteries	Pelvic defect (dead space)

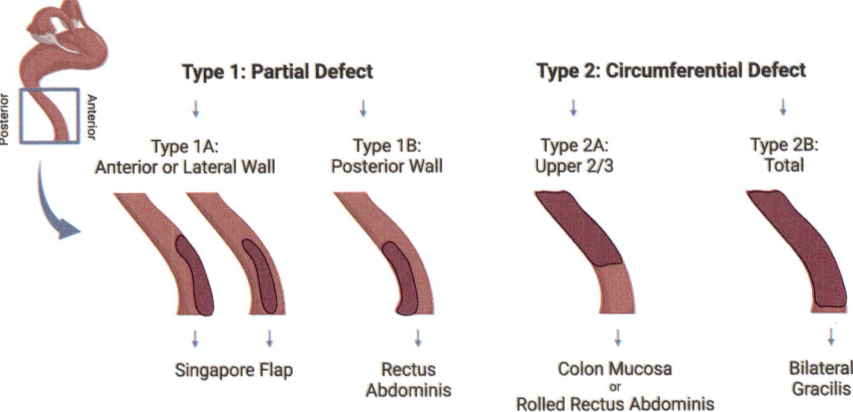

Fig. 67.1 Algorithm for reconstruction of vaginal defects based on anatomic location

- Penis
  - It is very difficult to replicate the aesthetics and sexual function of a subtotal penile defect.
    - Skin-only defects may heal well with a skin graft.
    - Pedicled fasciocutaneous flaps may have adequate reach, but may cause unwanted contracture.
  - Total defects
    - For sharp traumatic defects, microvascular replant should be attempted if the part is intact/available.
      - Critical structures for anastomosis are the deep dorsal artery, vein, and penile nerves.
    - Cancer-related or gender affirmation surgery:
      - Free flap reconstruction is the mainstay.
      - Radial forearm free flap provides adequate pedicle length, thin, hairless skin (usually), and adequate bulk when rolled.
      - Urethral reconstruction with folded region of flap "tube within a tube" design.
      - ALT flap can be pedicled to reconstruct the phallus.
    - Most free flaps will require a penile prosthesis for sexual function.
- Scrotum
  - Due to elastic and redundant skin, many defects may be closed primarily.
  - If long-term testicular exposure is planned, may bury testes in medial thigh pockets.
  - Reconstruction for large defects.
    - Split or full thickness skin graft
      - Tight tissue apposition needed for graft take, cannot replicate the hanging appearance of a native scrotum
    - Medial or superomedial thigh flaps
    - Pedicled thigh flaps (gracilis + STSG, ALT)
- Total perineal defects
  - Most important goal will not be recreating the function of any GI or urogenital organs, but filling the dead space.
  - Often requires a bulky flap with a long arc of rotation to allow tension-free closure
  - Flap types:
    - Omental flap—excellent for additional immune tissue and delivery of antibiotics

- Vertical rectus abdominis myocutaneous flap (VRAM)
    - Important to consider leaving placement of the ostomy if performing the abdominal flap
- Bilateral gracilis flap with a large skin island
- Free tissue transfer
    - Less frequently used due to the large availability of local tissue and often radiated recipient vessels

Patient Counseling and Common Concerns

- Important to understand the goals of surgery, as stated above
    - In superficial reconstructions, the primary goal is cosmetic and to maintain the external anatomy and function.
        - Patients requiring skin grafts should be counseled to expect pain and scarring at the donor site.
        - Any superficial reconstruction can lead to scar contracture and may distort the anatomy of the operative site.
    - In deep reconstructions, the most important goal will not be recreating the function of any GI or urogenital organs, but filling the dead space.
        - With isolated vaginal reconstruction, patient goals may include penetrative sexual intercourse
        - May lead to vaginal stenosis requiring regular use of dilators.
        - Unless colonic mucosa is used, may lead to vaginal dryness.
        - Patients should expect at least 6 weeks of healing before being able to insert anything into the reconstructed vagina.
- Complications:
    - Loss of function of micturition, defecation, and sexual sensation. This should be especially emphasized in cancer patients.
    - Hematoma, seroma:
        - Within a flap or rapidly expansile will require a procedure for evacuation
    - Infection.
    - Wound healing complications.
    - Dehiscence.
    - Scar contracture.

Acknowledgments Karen Lu, MD

Melanie Connolly, MS

References

1. Hansen JT. Netter's clinical anatomy. 5th ed. Philadelphia: Elsevier – Health Sciences Division; 2022.
2. Park J. Perineal reconstruction. In: Chung K, editor. Grabb and Smith's plastic surgery. 8th ed. Philadelphia: Wolters Kluwer; 2020. p. 991–9.
3. Butz DS, Fuller S, Crosby MA. Genitourinary reconstruction. In: Janis J, editor. Essentials of plastic surgery. 2nd ed. Boca Raton: Taylor & Francis; 2014. p. 632–8.
4. Garvey P. Trunk reconstruction and pressure sores. In: Buck D, editor. Review of plastic surgery. 1st ed. Toronto: Elsevier; 2016. p. 99–112.
5. Mericli AF, Martin JP, Campbell CA. An algorithmic, anatomical subunit approach to pelvic wound reconstruction. Plast Reconstr Surg. 2016;137(3):1004–17.
6. Larson JD, Altman AM, Bentz ML, Larson DL. Pressure ulcers and perineal reconstruction. Plast Reconstr Surg [Internet]. 2014;133(1):39e–48e.

Chapter 68
Lymphedema

Irene A. Chang and Michael W. Wells

Definition

Lymphedema is the accumulation of protein-rich fluid and fibroadipose tissue within the interstitial soft tissue compartment caused by dysfunction in lymphatic transport. It is a chronic disease that progresses from soft, pitting edema to regional enlargement, resulting in permanent fibrosis and lymphatic obstruction.

Demographics

- Primary lymphedema affects 1 in 100,000 people; secondary lymphedema affects 1 in 1000 Americans
  - Most commonly [1]
    - Lower extremity (90%)
    - Upper extremity (10%)
    - Genitalia (<1%)
  - Incidence
    - After lumpectomy: 4%–28% [2, 3]
    - After axillary dissection: 19%–24% [4]
    - After sentinel lymph node biopsy: 5%–7% [2, 5]

I. A. Chang (✉)
Division of Plastic and Reconstructive Surgery, UC Davis, Sacramento, USA
e-mail: irechang@health.ucdavis.edu

M. W. Wells
Division of Plastic and Reconstructive Surgery, UCLA, Los Angeles, USA

- Can occur after treatment of other malignancies [5]
    - Melanoma: 16%
    - Gynecologic malignancy: 20%
    - Genitourinary cancer: 10%
    - Head and neck cancer: 4%
    - Sarcoma: 30%

Pathophysiology

- The lymphatic system removes proteins and lipids from the interstitium through transportation into the lymphatics based on a differential pressure system (Fig. 68.1) [6].
  - Plays a critical role in the immune system [7]
- Lymphatic dysfunction causes an accumulation of macromolecules, which increases colloid osmotic pressure and leads to abnormal fluid distribution within the interstitium.
  - Predisposes to bacterial infections and malignancies [8, 9]
  - Continued lymphatic stasis results in a proinflammatory state with irreversible fibrosis, a decrease in functional lymphatic channels, and an increase in subcutaneous adipose tissue [4]
- A significant latent period can occur before symptoms (1–5 years after surgery) [12].
- Initial mild soft edema becomes irreversibly fibrotic over time.

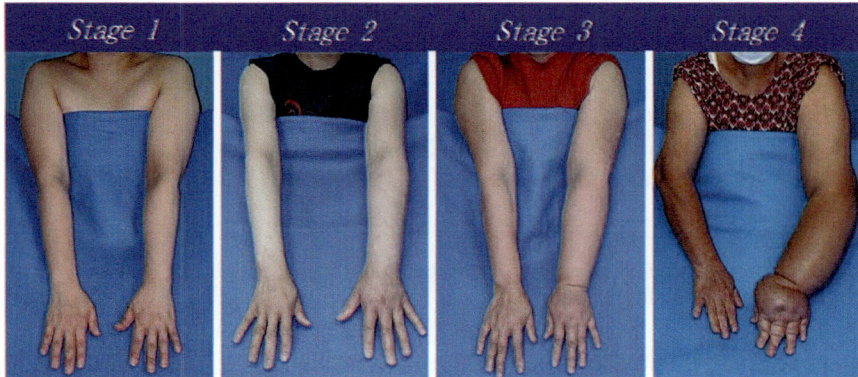

Fig. 68.1 Lymphedema in its various stages

Staging

- Four-stage system by the International Society of Lymphology [10]
  - Stage 0: latent or subclinical condition. No edema is evident, but lymph transport is impaired.
    - Can occur months or years before overt edema
    - Changes only visible on imaging
  - Stage I: early accumulation of proteinaceous fluid with edema that resolves with limb elevation. Pitting edema can occur.
  - Stage II: pitting edema may or may not be present, but tissue fibrosis develops along with nonpitting edema.
  - Stage III: lymphostatic elephantiasis with absent pitting. Fat deposits, acanthosis, and other skin changes develop.

Classification

Primary Lymphedema

- Lymphedema praecox
  - Most common form of primary lymphedema
  - Autosomal dominant inheritance
  - Presents during puberty
  - Unilateral, typically affecting the foot and calf
  - Associated with congenital anomalies: vertebral, cerebrovascular malformations, hearing loss, and distichiasis [3]
- Congenital lymphedema
  - Isolated and sporadic
  - Occurs within the first 2 years of life
  - Presents as bilateral lower extremity edema
- Lymphedema tarda
  - Lymphatic system is tortuous, hyperplastic with no competent valves
  - Usually occurs after 35 years old
  - Rare (<10% of primary lymphedema cases) [3]

Secondary Lymphedema

- Caused by obstruction or injury of the normal lymphatic system due to a diseased process
    - Filariasis: caused by the nematode *Wuchereria bancrofti*; most common cause worldwide
    - Secondary malignancy: most common cause in the United States
        - Axillary lymph node dissection and radiation increases risk [4, 8]
        - Risk factors: trauma, infection, obesity

Diagnosis

- Differential diagnosis includes [3]
    - Cardiac failure
    - Renal failure
    - Protein-losing conditions
    - Lipedema
    - Deep vein thrombosis
    - Chronic venous insufficiency
    - Myxedema
    - Cyclical or idiopathic edema.
- History
    - Family history, recent surgery, infections, travel, and prior episodes
- Physical examination
    - Soft, pitting edema (early stage)
    - Fibrosis and induration (late stage)
    - Stemmer's sign [10] inability to grasp the skin of the dorsum of the second digit of the foot
    - *Peau d'orange* skin changes
    - Blunting of the involved digits
    - Cellulitis
    - Circumferential limb measurements with a difference of 2 cm [12]
- Diagnostic studies [13]
    - Contrast lymphography
        - Direct injection of patent blue dye into lymphatic channels
        - Rarely used today due to technical difficulty and is associated with adverse reactions [12]

- Indirect lymphangiography
  - Intradermal injection of water-soluble iodinated contrast visualized with xeroradiography to evaluate lymphatics
- Isotopic or indocyanine green lymphoscintigraphy
  - Most common diagnostic study to evaluate lymphedema
  - Injection of nonionizing contrast agent (Tc 99m, Tc 99m-HAS, or Tc 99m dextran) or indocyanine green fluorescent dye into the interstitial space
  - Provides static and dynamic assessments of lymph flow
- MRI
  - Provides details about lymphatic trunks and nodes
  - Chronic lymphedema has a characteristic "honeycombing" pattern in the epifascial compartment [14]
- CT
  - Shows honeycombing and location of edema
  - Not as precise as MRI [14, 15]
- Noninvasive techniques
  - Bioelectric impedance analysis, tonometry, ultrasound, and perometry [3]

Treatment

Conservative Treatment

- Mainstay is multilayer inelastic lymphedema bandaging or controlled compression therapy [16].
  - Administered by a certified lymphedema therapist
  - Initial reductive phase, then maintenance phase
- Pneumatic compression devices.
- Elevation with proper skin hygiene.
  - Low pH solutions and water-based products
- Weight loss.

Surgical Treatment

- Indications
    - Significant loss of function
    - Frequent infection
    - Failure of conservative/medical management
    - Significant psychological morbidity
- Ablative [17]
    - Debulk areas of lymphedema to reduce morbidity
    - Improves comfort through excision of redundant tissue
    - Does not address lymphatic vessel dysfunction
    - Charles operation
        - Surgical excision of subcutaneous tissue to the level of the muscle with skin grafting using skin from excised tissue for coverage
        - Uncommon today
    - Staged subcutaneous excision
        - Only subcutaneous tissue is excised; skin flaps are spared.
        - Most performed excisional technique.
    - Suction-assisted protein lipectomy (SAPL) [18]
        - Removal of subcutaneous tissue and possibly skin flaps
        - Effective in upper extremity and later stages of lymphedema
- Physiologic [17]
    - Improves anterograde lymphatic flow by increasing the number of patent lymphatic pathways
    - Microsurgical techniques
    - Vascularized lymph node transfer (VLNT)
        - Donor sites vary, but typically from superficial inguinal (Fig. 68.2), omentum, or supraclavicular lymph nodes.
        - Effective after lymphadenectomy or radiation therapy.
    - Lymphaticovenous anastomoses (LVA)
        - Bypass operation to redirect excess lymphatic fluid into the venous circulation
        - Superficial lymphatic vessels traveling deep to the dermis are identified and anastomosed to nearby venules using microsurgical technique
        - Better results when performed in lymphatic systems with less damage

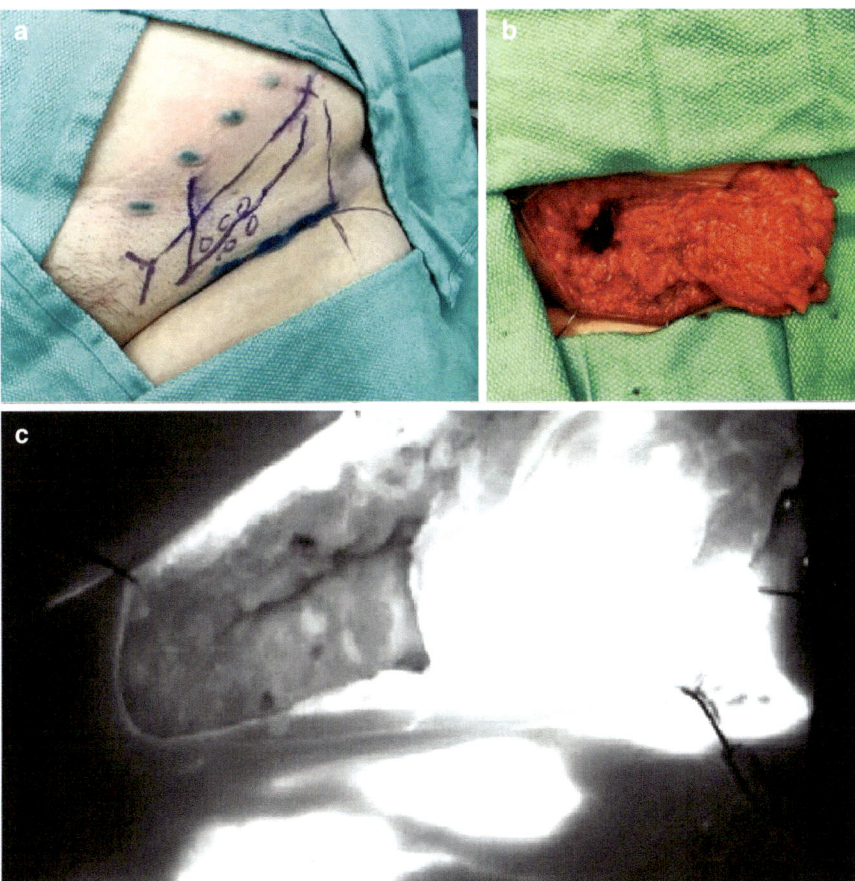

Fig. 68.2 Donor sites for VLNT demonstrating (**a**) the combined deep inferior epigastric artery perforator and VLNT flap and (**b**) the inguinal and superficial circumflex iliac artery perforator flap [19] (**c**) Indocyanine green angiography of harvested flap

Complications

- Sequelae of lymphedema
    - Erysipelas: streptococcal dermal infection
    - Lymphangitis: infection of the lymphatic vessels that starts distal to the channel
    - Lymphangiosarcoma: rare malignant tumor associated with chronic lymphedema
- Secondary to surgical procedures
    - Resection procedures
        - Wound dehiscence
        - Lymphocele

- Infection
- Hematoma

– Microsurgical techniques

- Lymphocele
- Local infection and wound breakdown
- Hematoma
- Vascular thrombosis (2% risk)

– Suction lipectomy

- Abrasion of superficial nerves
- Disruption of skin vascularity
- Damage to vital structures from sharp cannulas

Conflicts of Interest All Authors have no conflicts of interest or sources of funding to disclose.

References

1. Lee B-B, Rockson SG, Bergan J. Lymphedema: a concise compendium of theory and practice. Cham: Springer; 2018.
2. DiSipio T, et al. Incidence of unilateral arm lymphoedema after breast cancer: a systematic review and meta-analysis. Lancet Oncol. 2013;14(6):500–15.
3. Warren AG, et al. Lymphedema: a comprehensive review. Ann Plast Surg. 2007;59(4):464–72.
4. Hara Y, Otsubo R, Shinohara S, et al. Lymphedema after axillary lymph node dissection in breast cancer: prevalence and risk factors-a single-center retrospective study. Lymphat Res Biol. 2022;20:600–6.
5. Kissin MW, et al. Risk of lymphoedema following the treatment of breast cancer. Br J Surg. 1986;73(7):580–4.
6. Wheeler ES, et al. Familial lymphedema praecox: Meige's disease. Plast Reconstr Surg. 1981;67(3):362–4.
7. Szuba A, et al. The third circulation: radionuclide lymphoscintigraphy in the evaluation of lymphedema. J Nucl Med. 2003;44(1):43–57.
8. Borud LJ, Cooper JS, Slavin SA. New management algorithm for lymphocele following medial thigh lift. Plast Reconstr Surg. 2008;121(4):1450–5.
9. Coen JJ, et al. Risk of lymphedema after regional nodal irradiation with breast conservation therapy. Int J Radiat Oncol Biol Phys. 2003;55(5):1209–15.
10. International Society of Lymphology. The diagnosis and treatment of peripheral lymphedema. Consensus document of the International Society of Lymphology. Lymphology. 2003;36(2):84–91.
11. Stemmer R. A clinical symptom for the early and differential diagnosis of lymphedema. Vasa. 1976;5(3):261–2.
12. Beahm E, Walton R, Lohman R. Vascular insufficiency of the lower extremity: lymphatic, venous and arterial. Plast Surg. 2006;6:1455–90.
13. Greene AK, Goss JA. Diagnosis and staging of lymphedema. Semin Plast Surg. 2018;32(1):12–6.
14. Haaverstad R, et al. The use of MRI in the diagnosis of chronic lymphedema of the lower extremity. Int Angiol. 1994;13(2):115–8.

15. Hadjis NS, et al. The role of CT in the diagnosis of primary lymphedema of the lower limb. AJR Am J Roentgenol. 1985;144(2):361–4.
16. Badger CM, Peacock JL, Mortimer PS. A randomized, controlled, parallel-group clinical trial comparing multilayer bandaging followed by hosiery versus hosiery alone in the treatment of patients with lymphedema of the limb. Cancer. 2000;88(12):2832–7.
17. Granzow JW. Lymphedema surgery: the current state of the art. Clin Exp Metastasis. 2018;35(5–6):553–8.
18. Lee M, Perry L, Granzow J. Suction assisted protein lipectomy (SAPL) even for the treatment of chronic fibrotic and scarified lower extremity lymphedema. Lymphology. 2016;49(1):36–41.
19. Chang IA, Swanson MA, Rajan M, Schwarz GS. Dual fluorescent tracers for surgical guidance: preventing donor-site lymphedema in vascularized lymph node transfer. Plast Reconstr Surg Glob Open. 2022;10(6):e4390.

Chapter 69
Gender Affirming Surgery

Alexis L. Boson

Overview

- Gender dysphoria is defined as an incongruence of sex assigned at birth and self-identified gender leading to distress [1].
- Multidisciplinary approach is best when caring for this patient population.
  - Team includes social services, psychologist/psychiatrist, endocrinologist/hormone provider, gynecologist, urologist, plastic surgeon, and ENT.
  - Key to establishing a patient provider relationship is to begin by asking preferred pronouns.
- WPATH (World Professional Association for Transgender Health) has developed guidelines for standardized care, which should be met prior to performing any gender confirmation procedure. Also known as the WPATH criteria.
  - Latest WPATH version 8 published September 2022
- Of note, standard of care does not dictate the order or number of procedures involved in gender affirmation.

Criteria for Gender Surgery in Adults

1. Gender incongruence is marked and sustained over time.
2. Meets diagnostic criteria of gender incongruence.
3. Demonstrates capacity to provide informed consent.
4. Understands the effect of surgical affirmation on reproduction and has explored reproductive options.

A. L. Boson (✉)
Division of Plastic Surgery, Department of Surgery, University of Texas Medical Branch, Galveston, TX, USA
e-mail: alboson@UTMB.EDU

5. Other possible causes of apparent gender incongruence have been identified and excluded.
6. Possible mental health concerns have been addressed.
7. At least 6 months of gender-affirming hormone therapy unless medically contraindicated or not desired.

Criteria for Gender Surgery in Adolescents

1. Gender diversity/incongruence is marked and sustained over time.
2. Meets diagnostic criteria of gender incongruence.
3. Demonstrates emotional and cognitive maturity to provide informed consent.
4. Possible mental health concerns have been addressed.
5. Informed of the reproductive effects of surgical intervention.
6. At least 12 months of gender-affirming hormone therapy unless medically contraindicated or not desired.

Surgical Techniques and Complications

Male to Female

Genital surgery "bottom surgery." Goal: creation of functional vagina, preserve sexual sensation, and good cosmesis

- Orchiectomy
- Penectomy
- Vaginoplasty (Fig. 69.1)
    - Techniques
        - Penile inversion vaginoplasty
            - Use glans of penis as neoclitoris
            - Typically, full thickness skin graft taken from scrotum to surface inside of vagina—preoperative hair removal often recommended
        - Pedicled intestinal vaginoplasty
            - Usually performed if a limited amount of penoscrotal skin available or failed penile inversion vaginoplasty
            - Has increased risk of HIV transmission due to use of sigmoid mucosa
            - Increased risk complications due to need for intraabdominal surgery [2]
- Clitoroplasty
- Labiaplasty
- Complications [3–5]
    - Necrosis of neovagina/neolabia

Fig. 69.1 Vaginoplasty outcomes

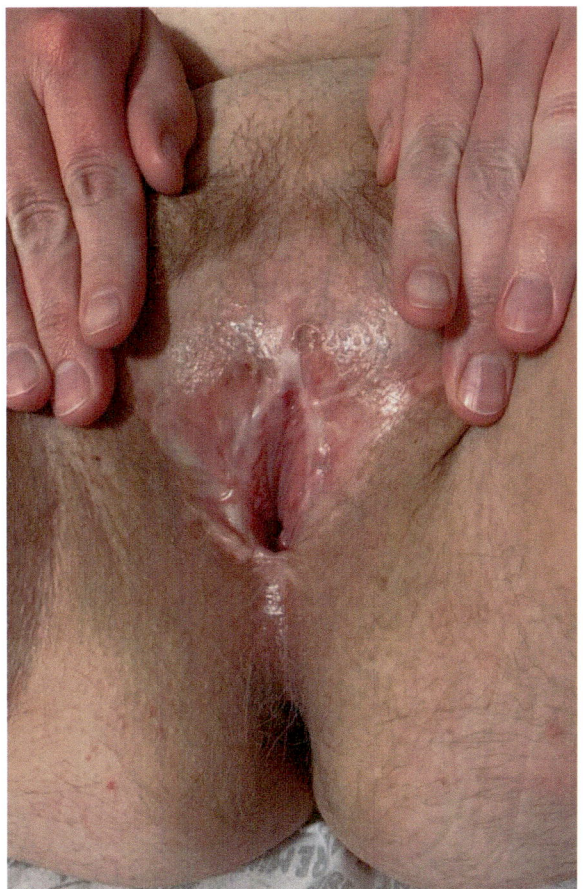

- Bladder/bowel fistula into vagina
- Urethral stenosis
- Anorgasmia
- Short/small vagina
  - Vaginal stenosis is prevented by periodic dilation by patient.
- Use of exogenous estrogen increases breast growth, decreases testicular volume, decreases body hair, softens skin and increases risk of DVT
- Nongenital surgery
  - Breast augmentation "Top Surgery": similar technique as in *cis* female
    - Silicone or saline implant may be used and placement can be dual plane, submuscular or subglandular (if pinch test >2 cm).
    - Exogenous estrogen therapy preoperatively will aid in breast development

- Complications: infection, capsular fibrosis, malposition, animation deformity, *etc* [6]
- Facial feminization [7–11] (Fig. 69.2)
  - Common procedures include: forehead reduction (both bony bossing and length from brow to hairline), hair transplant, rhinoplasty, lip lift, malar augmentation, jaw contouring, genioplasty, tracheal cartilage prominence
  - Males and females have distinct facial characteristics.
    - Masculine features are an angular hairline, marked forehead bossing, increased vertical height of chin, and mandible wider with a pronounced angle.
    - Feminine features include rounded or heart shaped hairline, shorter forehead length, higher eyebrows, "open orbit" in which upper lid is more exposed, reduced size of nose overall, smooth transition from forehead and nose, short upper lip, fullness of malar region, short rounded chin, and rounded angle of jaw.
- Liposuction, lipofilling
- Voice surgery (tightening vocal cords to increase pitch)
- Thyroid cartilage reduction (Adam's apple reduction)
- Gluteal augmentation

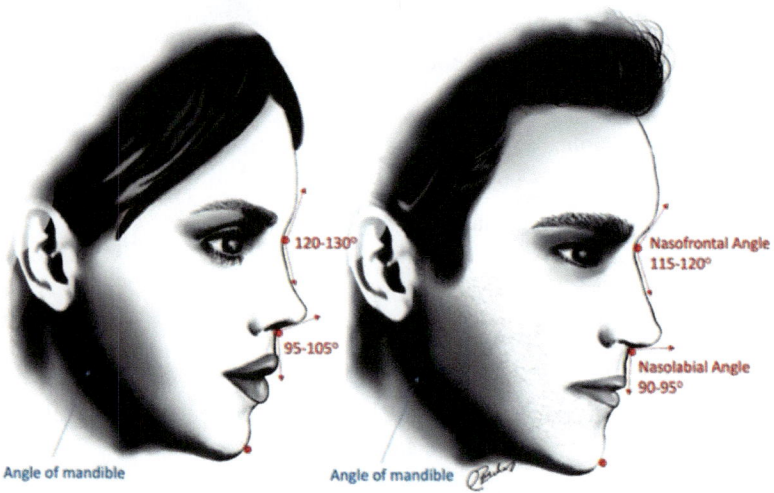

The nasolabial angle on lateral view, formed between lines along the nasal columella and the upper lip, defines nasal tip rotation and is generally more obtuse in the feminized face. The masculine nasofrontal angle measured between the nasal dorsum and forehead is typically more acute due to greater glabellar and frontal bone prominence

Fig. 69.2 Facial differences

Female to Male

- Genital surgery, also known as "bottom surgery." Goal: good cosmesis, ability to perform micturition while standing, preserve sexual sensation, ability to perform sexual intercourse [12]
    - Hysterectomy
    - Salpingo-oophorectomy
    - Vaginectomy
    - Metoidioplasty—allows for standing micturition
        - Small phallus created from clitoris in a single stage procedure
        - Testosterone therapy and vacuum pump use prior for enlargement of clitoris [13]
    - Scrotoplasty
    - Urethroplasty
    - Testicular prosthesis placement
    - Phalloplasty [13, 14] (Fig. 69.3)
        - Adult-sized phallus with the ability to perform penetrative intercourse via multistage procedure and placement of an inflatable implant
        - Technique
            - Gold standard: free tissue transfer with fasciocutaneous radial forearm flap
                - Different designs but core concept is to create a urethra within the phallus (tube within a tube).
                - Typically requires skin graft to forearm donor site which leaves characteristic scar
            - Pedicle flaps: anterolateral thigh flap, groin flap
            - Free flaps: radial forearm, anterolateral thigh flap, latissimus dorsi flap, thoracodorsal artery perforator flap
    - Complications [14]
        - Urinary tract stenosis
        - Urinary tract fistula
        - Necrosis of neophallus
        - Micropenis
        - Inability to perform penetrative intercourse
        - Extrusion of inflatable implant
- Nongenital surgery
    - Chest reconstruction "top surgery": Typically, a mastectomy is performed
        - Elliptical incision approach

Fig. 69.3 Phalloplasty

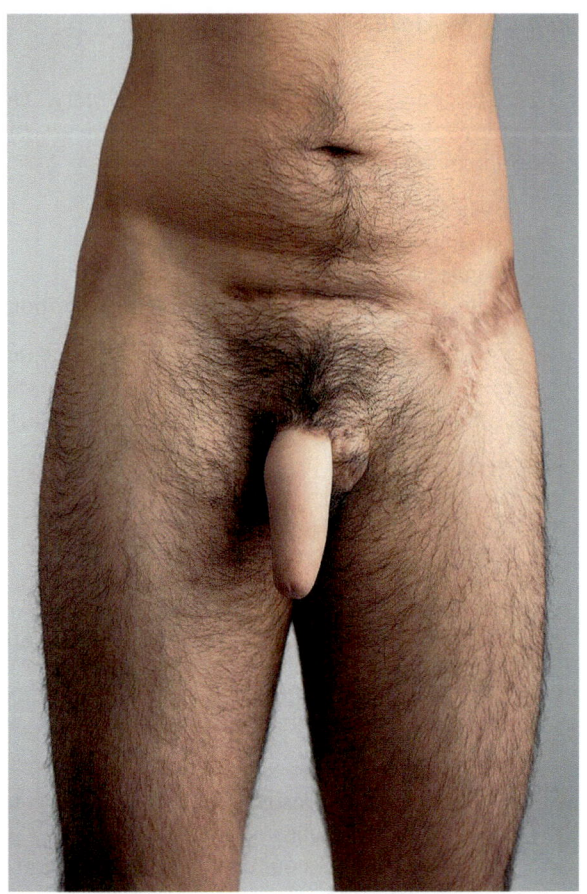

- In comparison to technique in *cis* females, incisions are camouflaged at the inferior border of the pectoralis muscle.
- Free nipple grafts usually needed. It is important to note male nipples are oval shaped in contrast to round female nipples. Ideally, the FNG is placed between the 4th and 5th intercostal space along the inferior margin of the pectoralis muscle [15].
- Periareolar approach
  - For patients with small breasts and relatively elastic skin, a small incision periareolar mastectomy may be possible.
- Liposuction
  - In rare cases with small breasts, liposuction alone can sufficiently reduce the breasts, similar to gynecomastia.

- Complications: nipple necrosis or depigmentation (particularly for free graft), contour irregularities, scarring, decreased nipple sensation [16]
- Important to note that gender affirmation mastectomies are not oncologic mastectomies, and some breast tissue may be left behind for appropriate contour; breast cancer screening guidelines have not been established for this patient population.
- Pectoral implants may be used to further shape the pectoralis contour.

– Osseous genioplasty—increase vertical height and square chin [8].

References

1. Coleman E, Radix AE, Bouman WP, Brown GR, de Vries ALC, Deutsch MB, Ettner R, Fraser L, Goodman M, Green J, Hancock AB, Johnson TW, Karasic DH, Knudson GA, Leibowitz SF, Meyer-Bahlburg HFL, Monstrey SJ, Motmans J, Nahata L, Nieder TO, Reisner SL, Richards C, Schechter LS, Tangpricha V, Tishelman AC, Van Trotsenburg MAA, Winter S, Ducheny K, Adams NJ, Adrián TM, Allen LR, Azul D, Bagga H, Başar K, Bathory DS, Belinky JJ, Berg DR, Berli JU, Bluebond-Langner RO, Bouman M-B, Bowers ML, Brassard PJ, Byrne J, Capitán L, Cargill CJ, Carswell JM, Chang SC, Chelvakumar G, Corneil T, Dalke KB, De Cuypere G, de Vries E, Den Heijer M, Devor AH, Dhejne C, D'Marco A, Edmiston EK, Edwards-Leeper L, Ehrbar R, Ehrensaft D, Eisfeld J, Elaut E, Erickson-Schroth L, Feldman JL, Fisher AD, Garcia MM, Gijs L, Green SE, Hall BP, Hardy TLD, Irwig MS, Jacobs LA, Janssen AC, Johnson K, Klink DT, Kreukels BPC, Kuper LE, Kvach EJ, Malouf MA, Massey R, Mazur T, McLachlan C, Morrison SD, Mosser SW, Neira PM, Nygren U, Oates JM, Obedin-Maliver J, Pagkalos G, Patton J, Phanuphak N, Rachlin K, Reed T, Rider GN, Ristori J, Robbins-Cherry S, Roberts SA, Rodriguez-Wallberg KA, Rosenthal SM, Sabir K, Safer JD, Scheim AI, Seal LJ, Sehoole TJ, Spencer K, St. Amand C, Steensma TD, Strang JF, Taylor GB, Tilleman K, T'Sjoen GG, Vala LN, Van Mello NM, Veale JF, Vencill JA, Vincent B, Wesp LM, West MA, Arcelus J. Standards of care for the health of transgender and gender diverse people, version 8. Int J Transgender Health. 2022;23(sup1):S1–S259. https://doi.org/10.1080/26895269.2022.2100644.
2. Claes KEY, Pattyn P, D'Arpa S, Robbens C, Monstrey SJ. Male-to-female gender confirmation surgery: intestinal vaginoplasty. Clin Plast Surg. 2018;45(3):351–60.
3. Klein C, Gorzalka BB. Sexual functioning in transsexuals following hormone therapy and genital surgery: a review. J Sex Med. 2009;6(11):2922–39; quiz 40–1.
4. Buncamper ME, van der Sluis WB, van der Pas RSD, Özer M, Smit JM, Witte BI, et al. Surgical outcome after penile inversion vaginoplasty: a retrospective study of 475 transgender women. Plast Reconstr Surg. 2016;138(5):999–1007.
5. Lawrence AA. Patient-reported complications and functional outcomes of male-to-female sex reassignment surgery. Arch Sex Behav. 2006;35(6):717–27.
6. Kanhai RC, Hage JJ, Karim RB, Mulder JW. Exceptional presenting conditions and outcome of augmentation mammaplasty in male-to-female transsexuals. Ann Plast Surg. 1999;43(5):476–83.
7. Spiegel JH. Facial feminization for the transgender patient. J Craniofac Surg. 2019;30(5):1399–402.
8. Morrison SD, Satterwhite T. Lower jaw recontouring in facial gender-affirming surgery. Facial Plast Surg Clin North Am. 2019;27(2):233–42.
9. Pittman TA, Economides JM. Preparing for facial feminization surgery: timing. Facial Plast Surg Clin North Am. 2019;27(2):191–7.

10. Berli JU, Loyo M. Gender-confirming rhinoplasty. Facial Plast Surg Clin North Am. 2019;27(2):251–60.
11. Deschamps-Braly JC. Facial gender confirmation surgery: facial feminization surgery and facial masculinization surgery. Clin Plast Surg. 2018;45(3):323–31.
12. Monstrey S, Hoebeke P, Selvaggi G, Ceulemans P, Van Landuyt K, Blondeel P, et al. Penile reconstruction: is the radial forearm flap really the standard technique? Plast Reconstr Surg. 2009;124(2):510–8.
13. Bizic MR, Stojanovic B, Djordjevic ML. Genital reconstruction for the transgendered individual. J Pediatr Urol. 2017;13(5):446–52.
14. Hage JJ, De Graaf FH. Addressing the ideal requirements by free flap phalloplasty: some reflections on refinements of technique. Microsurgery. 1993;14(9):592–8.
15. Maas M, Howell AC, Gould DJ, Ray EC. The ideal male nipple-areola complex: a critical review of the literature and discussion of surgical techniques for female-to-male gender-confirming surgery. Ann Plast Surg. 2020;84(3):334–40.
16. Monstrey S, Selvaggi G, Ceulemans P, Van Landuyt K, Bowman C, Blondeel P, et al. Chest-wall contouring surgery in female-to-male transsexuals: a new algorithm. Plast Reconstr Surg. 2008;121(3):849–59.

Index

A
Abdominal wall
  evaluation
    history, 329, 330
    patient selection, 328
    physical examination, 330, 331
  layers of, 327
  muscles of, 327
  sensory innervation, 328
Abdominal wall reconstruction
  anatomy, 567–569
  mechanical forces, 569
  nerves, 569
  surgical dehiscence, 569
Abdominal wall repair, 572
Abdominoplasty, 332
Abducens nerve, 107
Acellular dermal matrix, 315
Acrochordon, 72
Acrosyndactyly, 539
Acute paronychia, 434
Acute rejection, 52
Acute skin failure, 95
Adipose tissue of trunk, 337, 338
Adiposity, 330
Adjuvant radiation therapy, 268
Age-related fat atrophy, 365
Aging face, 349
  See also Facial aging
Alar rim graft, 377
Alloplastic materials, 273, 315, 316
Alloplastic reconstruction, 315, 316
American Joint Committee on Cancer (AJCC), 262

American Society of Plastic Surgery Practice Parameters, 295–296
Amide-linked local anesthetics, 55, 56
Amniotic Band Syndrome, 542
Anaplastic large cell lymphoma (ALCL), 317
Aneurysmal bone cysts (ABCs), 526
Angiosome theory, 26
Angle's classification of malocclusion, 177
Anotia, 205–207
Anterior division of retromandibular vein, 104
Anterolateral thigh (ALT) flap, 274
Antia-Buch helical advancement flap, 204
Antibiotics, 255
Arterial anastomoses, 43
Arterial injury, 534
Arterial puncture, 534
Arteriovenous (AV) loop, 271–273
Arteriovenous malformations, 166
Artery repair, 498
ATLS (Advanced Trauma Life Support) protocol, 496
Auricle, 197, 199
Auriculocephalic angle, 200
Auriculotemporal nerve, 199, 218
Autogenous graft, 249
Autologous breast reconstruction
  benefits of, 319–320
  DIEP flap, 322, 324
  disadvantages of, 320
  imaging, 321
  latissimus Dorsi flap, 321, 322
  lumbar artery perforator Flap, 325
  medical history, 320
  oncologic history, 320, 321

Autologous breast reconstruction (*cont.*)
  pedicled TRAM flap, 322, 323
  physical examination, 321
  profunda artery perforator flap, 325
  SGAP flap, 324
  social history, 321
  timing, 320
Autologous calvarial reconstruction, 273, 320
Avulsions, 203

B
Bags under the eyes, 381
Bariatric surgery, 329
Basal cell carcinoma (BCC), 79–80, 520
Baux score, 85
Bell palsy, 284, 285
  facial paralysis, 282
Belt lipectomy, 331
Benelli technique, 310
Benign Juvenile melanoma, 75
Benign nevi, 74
Benign skin lesions
  acrochordon or skin tag, 72
  cherry angioma, 73
  dermatofibroma, 76, 77
  dermoid cyst, 78
  epidermal inclusion cyst, 77
  lipoma, 77, 78
  melanocytic nevus, 74–75
  Nevus of Ota and Ito, 73
  nevus sebaceous of Jadassohn, 75, 76
  pilomatricoma, 76, 77
  pyogenic granuloma, 78, 79
  seborrheic keratosis, 72
  Spitz nevus, 75
Beta-blockers, 340
Bilateral cleft lip repair, 132
Bilateral postaxial finger duplication, 540
Bilateral sagittal split osteotomy
    (BSSO), 182–184
Bilobed flaps, 212
Blepharoplasty
  complications, 384
  incisions, 382
  patient evaluation, 381, 382
Body contouring, 409
  complications, 335
  patient selection, 328
  types, 332–335
Bone reconstruction, 276
Bony fixation, 497
Bony tumors, 523

Bottom surgery, 604, 607
Botulinum toxin, 285, 355
  complications, 403
  dynamic rhytides, 397
  facial palsy, 403
  facial rejuvenation, 397, 400
  FDA Approvals, 398
  patient comfort, 403
  patient evaluation, 398–399
  sample dilutions, 398
  side effects, 403
  spastic cerebral palsy, 403
Boutonniere deformity, 552
Box osteotomy, 195
Brachial plexus, 457
Brachioplasty, 334–335
Brachydactyly, 541
Brazilian butt lift
  complications, 417–418
  evaluation, 413–414
  fat harvest & processing, 414
  mortality rate, 409, 417
  outcomes, 417–418
  post-operative care, 417
  ultrasound image of the buttock, 417
Breast, 333
  anatomy (*see* Breast anatomy)
  mastopexy, 309, 310
Breast anatomy, 305
  arterial supply, 289
  blood supply, 313
  landmarks, 313
  innervation, 291
  lymphatics, 291
  structure, 289, 290
  venous drainage, 291
Breast augmentation
  complications, 308, 309
  contraindications, 306
  implants, 306, 307
  incisions, 307, 308
  indications, 306
  plane of implant insertion, 308
  postoperative management, 308
Breast implant associated anaplastic large cell
    lymphoma (BIA-ALCL), 307
Breast reconstruction, 36
  prosthetic based, 313–318
Breast reduction
  central mound, 300
  free nipple grafting, 303
  inferior pedicle, 300
  lateral pedicle, 301

Index 613

liposuction, 300
pathophysiology, 299
post-operative care, 303
preoperative workup, 299–300
skin resection patterns, 302
superomedial pedicle, 301
symptoms, 299
Breast tissue expander, 315
Brent techniques, 206
Brow aesthetics, 387
Brow lift
  anterior hairline incision, 392
  complications, 394
  coronal, modified coronal or anterior hairline incision, 391
  direct, 393
  dissection plane, 393–394
  endoscopic, 392
  facelift incision over temporalis muscle, 392
  indications and patient assessment, 391
  innervation, 389
  muscle weakening, 394
  preoperative evaluation, 390–391
  sentinel vein, 390
  surgical approach, 387
Brow ptosis, 391, 394
Brow retaining ligaments, 390
Buccal mucosal advancement flap, 238
Bunny lines, 399
Burn
  complications, 90
  delayed burn reconstruction, 90
  depth and histology, 87
  epidemiology, 85
  initial assessment, 87, 88
  pathophysiology, 86
  treatment, 87, 89, 90
  zones of, 86
Buttock danger zone, 413

C

Calcifying epithelioma, 76–77
Calcium hydroxylapatite, 357
Calvaria, 220
Camptodactyly, 543, 544
Cancer recurrence, 279
Cannula choice, 341
Canthal procedures, 383
Canthal tendons, 227
Canthopexy, 232
Canthoplasty, 231, 383
Capsular contracture, 308
Carpal bones, 420
Carpal tunnel syndrome, 442
Carpometacarpal (CMC) joint of thumb, 555
  arthrodesis, 559
  arthroplasty, 559
Cauliflower ear deformity, 202
Central mound, 300
Central polydactyly, 541
Cephalometrics, 178, 180
Champy's ideal lines of osteosynthesis, 256
Cheeks, 245
Chemical peels, 354, 355, 383
Chemosis, 384
Cherry angioma, 73
Chest reconstruction, 563–565
  staging, 565
Chest wall deformity, 207
Chest wounds, 563
Chondrodermatitis nodularis chronica helicis, 202
Chondrosarcomas, 526
Chorda tympani nerve, 108
Chromophore, 63, 65–68
Chronic paronychia, 434
Chronic rejection, 52
Chronic synovitis, 548
Cleft hand, 541
Cleft lip and palate (CLP)
  anatomy, 122–125
  and classifications, 125–127
  complications, 136
  embryology, 121, 122
  epidemiology, 119, 120
  management principles, 127
  pathogenesis, 120
  resulting from failed fusion of facial structures, 122
  sequence and timing of surgical interventions, 129
  spectrum of, 126
  techniques, 133
    bilateral, 131, 132
    hard palate techniques, 133–135
    soft palate techniques, 135–136
    unilateral, 129–131
  timing of procedures, 129
  treatment algorithm, 136
Cleft lip nasal deformity, 126
Clinodactyly, 542, 543
Clostridium histolyticum, 96, 514
Cocaine, 57
Collagen, 13
  injections, 357
Collagenase injections, 514

Collar button abscess, 436
Columellar Strut, 376
Combined augmentation mastopexy, 310
Common facial vein, 104
Compartment syndrome, 88, 447, 535
Complex/large lacerations, 203
Composite tissue allotransplantation, 2
Compression, 254
    neuropathies, 441–442
    therapy, 597
Computed tomography angiography (CTA), 263
Computerized surgical planning (CSP), 263
Conchal cartilage graft, 204
Conchal defects, 205
Conchal resection, 201
Cone beam computed tomography (CBCT), 178
Congenital craniofacial clefts, 187
Congenital hand anomalies
    axes of development of upper extremity, 538
    classification systems, 539
    embryologic development, 537–539
    incomplete simple syndactyly, 540
    patterns of, 539
    syndromes, 544
Congenital hemangioma, 164
Congenital lymphedema, 595
Congenital melanocytic nevi
    categorization, 155
    characteristics of, 156
    clinical presentation, 157
    epidemiology, 156
    neurocutaneous melanosis, 158
    pathophysiology, 156
    treatment
        indications, 159
        non-invasive, 159
        rationale, 158
        surgical management, 159
Constricted ear, 201
Contour deformity, 343
Contrast lymphography, 596
Corrugator supercilii muscle, 388
Costochondral rib graft, 153
Cottle test, 372
Cranial clefts, 187
Cranialization, 247
Cranial nerves, 117
Cranial vault remodeling, 172
Craniofacial clefts
    deficiencies, 188
    excess, 189
    management, 195, 196
    skeletal, 189–194
    soft tissue, 189–195
    Tessier classification, 188
Craniofacial microsomia, 150, 191
    background and epidemiology, 147
    clinical features, 148–152
    etiology, 148
    management, 152, 153
    preoperative workup, 152
Craniosynostosis
    classification, 169
    evaluation, 170, 171
    imaging, 172
    overview, 169
    pathogenesis, 170
    treatment, 172
    types, 171
Cross-facial nerve grafting, 287
Cross-finger flap, 505
Cryptotia, 202
Cubital tunnel syndrome, 444
"Cup" or "Lop" ear deformity, 201
Cutaneoconjuctival flap, 230
Cutaneous lesions, 61
Cutaneous melanoma, 157
Cutler beard flap, 230, 231
Cytomegalovirus (CMV), 51

D

Deep (Scarpa's) adipose tissue, 337
Deep inferior epigastric artery perforator flap (DIEP) flap reconstruction, 30, 322–324
Deep peels, 355
Deep plane (aka sub-SMAS) facelift, 364
Deep space infection, 435
Dental malocclusions, 175
Dentofacial deformities, 175, 179, 182
Depressor supercilii muscle, 388
Dermabrasion, 354
Dermal regeneration templates, 220
Dermatochalasis, 381
Dermatofibroma, 76, 77
Dermatofibrosarcoma protuberans, 82
Dermis, 35
Dermoid cyst, 78
DiGeorge syndrome, 120
Dimpled chin, 401
Direct to implant (DTI), 315
Dislocation, 470
Distal and proximal interphalangeal joint injuries, 489–490
Distal radioulnar (DRU) joint arthritis, 560–561

Index 615

Distal radius fracture with radial impaction and dorsal tilt, wrist, 473
Distal tuft fractures, 466
Distraction osteogenesis, 153
Diver test, 331
Donor site morbidity, 320
Dorsal nasal flap, 212
Dorsal onlay graft, 376
Dorsal spanning plate, 471
Doxycycline, 285
Dupuytren's disease, 511, 513
　pathophysiology, 511–513
Dynamic nasal tip ptosis, 401
Dynamic rhytids, 352
Dysport, 398
Dystopia, 196

E
Ear deformities
　acquired
　　conchal defects, 205
　　epidemiology, 202–205
　　full thickness defects of middle third, 204
　　full thickness defects of upper third, 203
　　lobe, 205
　　partial thickness, 203
　congenital
　　constricted ear, 201
　　Cryptotia, 202
　　ear molding, 202
　　macrotia, 201
　　prominent ear, 200, 201
　　Stahl's ear, 201
　microtia/anotia, 205–207
Ear molding, 202
Ear reconstruction
　embryology
　　auricle, 197
　　EAC, 197
　　tympanic membrane, 197
Ears, 245
　anatomy, 199
　　auricular branch of vagus nerve, 199
　　auriculotemporal nerve, 199
　　blood supply, 200
　　clinical measurements and angles, 200
　　greater auricular nerve, 198
　　lesser occipital nerve, 199
　　lymphatics, 200
　　topography, 198
　development, 198
Ectropion, 382, 384

Edema of the conjunctivae, 384
Encephalocele, 193
Enchondromas, 523, 524
End-to-side technique, 43
Enophthalmos, 248
Entrapment, 248
Epidermal inclusion cyst (EIC), 77, 517
Epidermis, 35
Epinephrine, 56, 57
Epstein-Barr virus (EBV), 51
Esophagus, 116
Ester-linked local anesthetics, 55
Estlander flap, 239
Eutectic Mixture of Anesthetics (EMLA), 57
Ewing sarcomas, 527, 528
Exfoliant, 354
Expansion vibration lipofilling, 415, 416
Extensor compartments, 478
Extensors at wrist, 477
Extensor tendon injuries, 481–482
External auditory canal (EAC), 197
External carotid, 216
　branches, 228
External carotid artery (ECA), 114, 270
External jugular vein, 104
External nasal valve, 370
External nose, 369
External valve collapse, 372
Eyelids, 379
　anatomy, 227
　　blood supply, 227
　　dimensions, 225
　　lacrimal system, 228
　　muscle and connective tissue, 226, 227
　defects, 228
Eyelids reconstruction
　complications, 232
　evaluation, 228
　techniques, 229–232
Eyes, 245
　cross section, 226

F
Face, fascial planes of, 116, 117
Face lift
　hematoma, 365
　incision, 362
　operative techniques
　　deep plane (aka sub-SMAS) facelift, 364
　　SMAS, 364
　　subcutaneous, 364
　patient evaluation, 362
Facial aesthetic subunits, 346

Facial aging, 347, 349
　causes of, 351
　dermabrasion, 354
　microdermabrasion, 354
　patient evaluation, 352
　treatment
　　Botulinum toxin, 355
　　chemical peels, 354, 355
　　IPL, 353
　　laser, 352, 353
　　volume restoration, 356, 357
Facial analysis
　anatomic considerations, 346, 347
　effects of aging on face, 349
　ethnic enhancement, 349
　facial aesthetic analysis, 345, 346
　facial aesthetic enhancement, 348
　imaging, 347, 348
　soft tissue and skeletal, 345
　symmetry, 345
Facial artery, 102, 270
Facial artery myomucosal (FAMM) flap, 239
Facial bipartition, 195
Facial clefts, 187
Facial fat pads, 361
Facial feminization, 606
Facial fractures
　emergency department evaluation
　　diagnostic imaging, 246
　　focused CF exam, 245
　　history, 244, 245
　　primary and secondary survey, 244
　frontal bone
　　anatomy/epidemiology, 246
　　management, 247
　　presentation, 246
　mandible, 254, 255, 257
　maxilla
　　anatomy, 256
　　classification, 258
　　management, 259
　nasal bone
　　anatomy/epidemiology, 251
　　management, 252
　　presentation, 252
　naso-orbital-ethmoidal) fractures
　　anatomy/epidemiology, 249
　　management, 251
　　Markowitz classification, 251
　　presentation, 250
　orbital fractures
　　anatomy/epidemiology, 247
　　associated syndromes, 249
　　management, 249
　　presentation, 248

　pan-facial fractures, 259
　ZMC fractures, 252, 253
　zygomatic arch, 253, 254
Facial mimetic muscles, 360
Facial nerve, 105, 115, 117, 366
　anatomy, 281
　motor and sensory nerves, 359, 360
Facial palsy, 403
Facial paralysis
　adjunctive studies, 284
　etiology, 284, 285
　examination, 282, 283
　history, 282
　nonsurgical treatment, 285
　surgical management, 285–287
Facial profiles, 180
Facial reconstruction, 348
Facial skeleton/bones, 243
　buttresses of, 244
Facial therapy, 285
Facial transplantation (FT), 49
Fascial layers, 359
Fascial release and BR tendon excision, 447
Fasciocutaneous flaps, 222
Fasciocutaneous free flaps, 275
Fasciocutaneous plexus, 26
Fat embolism, 344
Fat grafting, 238, 365
Fat pads, 380
Favorable fracture, 254
Felon, 434
Female thigh and buttock contour, 409–410
Female to male, 607–609
Fibrous histiocytoma, 76
Filler, 403
　complications, 406
Finger deformities, 552–553
First dorsal metacarpal artery (FDMA) island flap, 506, 507
Fitzpatrick (FP) skin types, 64, 352
Flaps, 26
　adjunctive maneuvers for, 30, 31
　axial flaps, 28, 30
　failure, 278
　monitoring and aftercare, 31
　random pattern flaps, 26–29
　theories for, 26
　types, 30
Fleur-de-Lis (FDL) abdominoplasty, 333
Flexor tendon injuries, 480–481
Flexor zones, 480
Floor of mouth, 109
Forehead and Glabellar Lines, 399
Forehead flap, 212
Forehead rejuvenation, 387

Index 617

Four-corner fusion (4CF), 472
Fractional Resurfacing, 353
Free flaps, 28, 212, 213, 222, 274, 278
  reconstruction, 579
Free functional muscle transfers, 455, 460
Free nipple grafting, 303
Free tissue transfer, 40, 159
Frontal bone
  anatomy/epidemiology, 246
  management, 247
  presentation, 246
Frontalis muscle, 387
Frontal nerve, 107
Full-thickness defects, 238
Full-thickness scalp flaps (FTSF), 220
Full thickness skin graft (FTSG), 24, 25, 231
Functional stabilization, 256
Furlow palatoplasty, 135, 143
Furnas concho-mastoidal sutures, 201

G
Galea, 219
  flaps, 221
Ganglion cysts, 516, 517
Gastrocnemius flap, 580
Gender affirmation, 603
  mastectomies, 609
Gender confirmation, 603
Gender dysphoria
  defined, 603
  multidisciplinary approach, 603
Gender incongruence, 603
Gender reassignment, 603
Genital surgery, 604, 607
  in adolescents, 604
  in adults, 603, 604
Genitofemoral nerve, 584
Giant cell tumor of bone (GCTB), 525, 526
Giant cell tumor of tendon sheath
  (GCTTS), 517
Giant congenital melanocytic nevi, 156
Gillies approach, 254
Gilula's lines, 421
Glabellar flap, 231
Glomus tumor, 519
Glossopharyngeal nerve, 108
Gluteal augmentation fat grafting (GFG), 409
Gluteal muscular and neurovascular
  anatomy, 412
Goldenhar syndrome, 147, 152
Graft, skin graft, *see* Skin graft
Greater and lesser occipital nerves, 218

Greater auricular nerve (GAN), 198, 360
Gruss sign, 245
Gummy smile, 401
Gustilo classification, 579
Gynecomastia, 293
  classification
    American Society of Plastic Surgery
      Practice Parameters, 295
    Rohrich et al, 296
    Simon, Hoffman, and Kahn, 295
  clinical evaluation, 295
  definitions, 293
  idiopathic, 295
  pathologic causes, 294
  pharmacologic causes, 294
  physiologic causes, 294
  surgical treatment, 297
  treatment, 297

H
Hand fractures
  anatomy, 463
  treatment principles, 463–464
Hand infections
  debridement of necrotic tissue, 437
  evaluation, 433
  treatment, 433–434
  types, 434–437
Hand surgery
  innervation patterns, 427
  lumbricals, 426
  principles, 419
  sensory and motor findings, 430
  terminology, 419
  testing flexors, 428
  ulnar, 431
  vascular supply, 423
  wrist at carpal tunnel, 424
Hand transplantation (HT), 49
Hard palate techniques, 108, 133–135
Hardware exposure, 279
Head and neck anatomy/function, 360
  cranial nerves, 117
  face, 101–106
    fascial planes, 116
  floor of mouth, 109
  general principles, 101
  glands, 105, 106
  hard palate, 108
  hypopharynx, 110
  lateral nasal wall, 112
  lateral pharyngeal wall of oropharynx, 110

Head and neck anatomy/function (*cont.*)
  muscles of tongue, 108
  nasal cavity, 111
  neck, 112–116
  nose, 111
  oral cavity, 108
  orbit, 106, 107
  oropharynx, 109
  palatine tonsils, 110
  paranasal sinuses, 112
  soft palate, 110
Head and neck cancer (HNC)
  classification, 261, 262
  demographics, 261
  diagnosis, 263
  epidemiology, 261
  head and neck surgical anatomy, 263, 264
  incidence, 261
  staging, 262
  treatments, 267
    LND, 267, 268
    radiotherapy, 268
Head and neck reconstruction
  complications, 278, 279
  mandibular reconstruction, 275
    bone reconstruction, 276
    soft tissue reconstruction, 275
    virtual surgical planning, 276
  patient evaluation, 268
    physical examination, 269
    preoperative planning, 269
  pharyngeal reconstruction, 277, 278
  recipient vessels, 269
    artery, 271
    AV loops, 271, 273
    interpositional vein graft, 271
    vein, 271
  scalp reconstruction, 273
    autologous reconstruction, 273
    cranioplasty, 273
    soft tissue reconstruction, 274
  tongue reconstruction, 274
    reconstructive algorithm, 274
    tongue defects classification, 274
Helical advancement, 203
Helical crus, 201
Hematoma, 202, 207, 297, 365
Hemifacial microsomia, 152
Hemiglossectomy, 274
Hemitransfixion, 374
Hernias, 329, 330, 571
  adjuncts, 574
  biologic mesh, 573
  complications, 575
  component separation, 573
  Onlay mesh placement, 574
  patient factors, 571
  post-op care, 575
  synthetic mesh, 573
Herniation, 381
Heterodigital flap, 505
Hidradenitis Suppurativa, 586
Holoprosencephaly, 194
Horizontal mattress suture technique, 8
Horseshoe abscess, 435
House-Brackmann scale, 283
House-Brackmann scoring system, 105
Huger zones, 570
Hugger zones, vascular supply of abdomen, 328
Hughes tarsoconjunctival flap, 230
Hyaluronic acid, 356, 403
Hyperhidrosis (excessive sweating), 402
Hypertelorism, 194
Hypertrophic scarring, 17, 18
Hypoglossal nerve, 108, 117
Hypopharynx, 110, 262
Hypoplasia, 148
Hypoplastic thumb, grade IV, 542
Hypotelorism, 194

I

Idiopathic gynecomastia, 295
Immunology, 50
Implant rupture, 309
Implant suspension plasty, 559
Index finger after replantation, 500
Indirect lymphangiography, 597
Infantile hemangioma, 163
Infection, 51, 207, 284
Inferior pedicle, 300
Inferior tarsal muscle, 227
Infrahyoid strap muscles, 114
Inframammary fold (IMF), 307
Infraorbital groove, 248
Inhalational injury, 85
Injection techniques, 404, 414–417
Integra, 220
Intense pulsed light (IPL), 353
Intercarpal arthritis, 560
Internal carotid artery, 115
Internal carotid branches, 227
Internal jugular vein, 104
Internal nasal valve, 370
Internal valve collapse, 372

Index 619

Interpositional vein graft, 271
Interrupted suture technique, 6
Intraperitoneal placement of mesh (IPOM), 573
Intravelar veloplasty (IVV), 135
Inverted T-scar technique, 310
Ipsilateral nerve transfers, 286
Ischemia
   etiology, 532
   traumatic Injury, 533
   types, 533–535
Ischemic injury, 495
Isolated trapeziectomy, 558
Isotopic or indocyanine green lymphoscintigraphy, 597

J
Jugular veins, 271
Juncturae tendinum, 477

K
Kaposiform hemangioepithelioma, 164
Karapandzic flap, 239
Keloids, 17–19
Keystone region, 369
Killian, 374
Klinefelter syndrome, 294
Klippel-Trenaunay syndrome, 166, 167

L
Lacerations, 203
Lacrimal duct system, 230
Lacrimal nerve, 107
Lactiferous ducts, 289
Lagophthalmos, 384
Laissez faire method, 231
Large FT defects, 239, 240
Larynx, 116, 262
Laser-assisted liposuction (LAL), 342
Lasers, 352–353
Laser safety, 65
Lasers in plastic surgery
   "C's" of laser properties, 62
   chromophores and treatment options, 65–68
   interaction with tissues, 62, 63
   parameters, 63
   patient selection criteria, 64
   post-operative care, 68, 69
   Q-Switching, 63

   safety, 65
   steps, 61
   summary, 69
Lateral canthal lines (Crow's feet), 399
Lateral canthus, 232
Lateral crural strut graft, 376
Lateral nasal wall, 112
Lateral pedicle, 301
Lateral pharyngeal wall of oropharynx, 110
Lateral thigh-to-buttock ratio, 410, 411
Latissimus dorsi or anterolateral thigh flaps, 222, 274, 321, 322, 565
Le Fort I, 185
   osteotomy, 182–185
   transverse, 258
Le Fort II–pyramidal, 258
Le Fort III–craniofacial disjunction, 258
Le Fort-type fractures, 258
LEAP study, 581
Leser-Treélat sign, 72
Lesser occipital nerve, 199
Levator labii superioris, 122
Levator palpebrae superioris, 227, 379
Lidocaine toxicity, 343
Ligamentous injuries, 490, 492
Ligament tear, 489
Limb development, 537
Lingual nerve, 108
Lip augmentation with filler, 404
Lipomas, 77–78, 517
Liposuction, 300, 335, 337
   evaluation
      history, 339
      physical examination, 339, 340
      outcomes and complications, 343, 344
   treatment
      fluid management, 343
      general technique, 340, 341
      post-operative care, 343
      preoperative considerations, 340
      wetting solutions, 341, 342
Lips, 245
   anatomy, 236
      aesthetic subunits, 236
      blood supply, 237
      innervation, 237
      landmarks, 235–236
      layers, 235–236
   defects
      classification of, 237
      etiology, 237
      treatment, 238–240
Lips reconstruction, *see* Lips

Lip switch, 238
Liquid rhinoplasty, 405
Lobe, 205
Lobular Capillary Hemangioma, 78–79
Local anesthetics (LA), 56, 57
   additives, 56, 57
   characteristics and dosages, 58
   cocaine, 57
   EMLA, 57
   maximum safety dose, 57
   mechanism of action, 55
   toxicity, 58–59
      treatment, 59
   types, 55, 56
   uses and timing, 56
Local flaps, 212, 215, 220, 221
Local muscle transfers, 286
Local skin flaps, 203
Locoregional scalp flaps, 274
Lower extremity reconstruction, 337, 338
   anatomy, 578
      lower leg, 578
      thigh, 577
   gravity and venous congestion, 579
   traumatic injuries or oncologic ablation, 577
Lower eyelid
   anatomy, 380
   patient evaluation, 381
   treatment procedures, 382
Lower leg reconstruction, 578
Lower lid distraction test, 381
Lumbar artery perforator flap, 325
Lyme disease, 285
Lymphangioma, 165
Lymphatic drainage, 305
Lymphatic dysfunction, 594
Lymphaticovenous anastomoses (LVA), 46, 598
Lymphatics, 291
Lymphedema
   classification, 595–596
   complications, 599–600
   conservative treatment, 597
   differential diagnosis, 596, 597
   incidence, 593
   latent period, 594
   pathophysiology, 594
   primary, 595
   protein-rich fluid and fibroadipose tissue accumulation, 593
   secondary, 596
   stage system, 594, 595
   surgical treatment, 598–599
   treatment, 594
Lymphedema praecox, 595
Lymphedema tarda, 595
Lymph node dissections (LND), 267
Lymphoscintigraphy, 597

M

Macrodactyly, 543
Macro-fat embolism, 417
Macrotia, 201
Maffucci syndrome, 167
Malabsorptive, 329
Malar augmentation with filler, 405
Male to female, 604–607
Malignant skin lesions
   BCC, 79, 80
   dermatofibrosarcoma protuberans, 82
   melanoma, 81
   Merkel cell carcinoma, 82
   SCC, 80
Mandible biomechanics, 254
Mandible fracture, 254, 255, 257
Mandibular deformity, 148, 149
Mandibular reconstruction, 275, 276
   bone reconstruction, 276
   soft tissue reconstruction, 275
   virtual surgical planning, 276
Marionette lines, 401
Markowitz classification of NOE fractures, 250, 251
Masseter hypertrophy, 402
Mastopexy, 309, 310, 335
Mathes and Nahai Classification System, 30, 31
Maxilla, 182
   anatomy, 256
   classification, 258
   management, 259
Maxillary retrusion, 181
Maxillomandibular fixation, 255
Mcburney incisions, 330
McKinney's point, 360
MCPJ (Thumb), 491–492
Meatuses, 112
Medial canthal tendon (MCT), 230
Medial femoral condyle (MFC) free flap, 472
Median cleft of lower jaw, 194
Median nerve compression, 442–445, 448
Medium depth peels, 355
MedPor (porous polyethylene), 207
Melanin, 64

Index 621

Melanocytic nevus, 74–75, 155
Melanoma, 81–82, 157, 521, 522
Melomental folds (Marionette lines), 401
Merkel cell carcinoma (MCC), 82, 83, 522
Metacarpal shaft fractures, 464, 465
Metacarpophalangeal (MCP) joints, 553
   of fingers, 490
Metallo-endoproteinase, 96
"Meurman" classification, 151
Microdermabrasion, 354
Micro-fat embolism, 418
Micrognathia, 147
Microsurgical techniques, 26, 600
   anastomosis, 42, 43
   contraindications, 40
   end-to-side technique, 43
   equipment, 40
   evaluation, 39, 40
   flap compromise, 45
   lymphatics, 46
   monitoring, 44
   nerve repair, 45, 46
   operative steps, 41
   planning, 40, 41
   post-operative monitoring, 45
   systemic anticoagulation, 45
   vessel preparation, 41, 42
Microtia/anotia, 205–207
   classification, 151
Microvascular anastomoses, 500
Midface, 245
Midfacial aging, 405
Midline facial cleft, 188
Mid space infections, 435
Migraine therapy, 402
Mirror hand, 541
Moberg flap with advancement, 504, 505
Modified radical neck dissection, 268
Mohs micrographic surgery, 79, 80
Motor and sensory nerves, 359, 360
Mouth, 245
Mucosectomy, 274
Mucous cyst, 516, 517
Mueller's muscle, 380
Multidisciplinary approach, 269
Multi-view videofluoroscopy, 141
Muscle of velum, 138
Muscle scoring, 394
Muscles of facial expression, 101, 103
Muscles of mastication, 102, 149
Muscles of tongue, 108, 109
Muscles of velum, 124, 139, 140
Muscle-sparing TRAM, 324

Musculature, 305
Musculocutaneous flaps, 222
Musculomucosal posterior pharyngeal flap, 144
Mustarde cheek rotation flap, 229
Mustarde lid switch flap, 230
Mycophenolate mofetil (MMF), 50
Myocutaneous flap, 229
Myofascial advancement flaps, 573
Myomucosal V-Y advancement flap, 238
Myovermillion advancement flap, 238

N

NAC, *see* Nipple-areolar complex
Nagata techniques, 206
Nager syndromes, 191
Nasal bone fractures, 373
   anatomy/epidemiology, 251
   management, 252
   presentation, 252
Nasal breathing, 370
Nasal cavity, 111
Nasal reconstruction
   complications, 213
   pre-operative evaluation for, 211
   surgical approaches, 211–213
Nasociliary nerve, 107
Nasofrontal duct obstruction, 246, 247
Nasolabial flap, 212
Nasolabial folds, 405
Nasometry, 141
Naso-orbital-ethmoidal (NOE) fractures
   anatomy/epidemiology, 249
   management, 251
   Markowitz classification, 251
   presentation, 250
Nasopharynx, 111
National Comprehensive Cancer Network
   (NCCN), 262
National Pressure Injury Advisory Panel, 95
National Pressure Ulcer Advisory Panel
   (NPAUP), 93
Neck, 112
   highlighted muscles, 114
   lymph node basins of, 114
   nerves of, 115, 116
   triangles, 112, 113
   vasculature, 114
Neck dissection levels, 113
Neck lift
   incision, 362
   operative techniques, 365
   patient evaluation, 362

Needle aponeurotomy (NA), 514
Neoplasm, 284
Nerve allograft or autologous nerve
    grafts, 499
Nerve-based injuries
    anatomy, 451–452
    classification, 453–454
    electrodiagnostics, 452–453
    EMG patterns, 453
    physiology, 451–452
Nerve-based surgical options, primary repair/
    grafting, 460
Nerve compression physiology, 441
Nerve injury, 366, 457
Nerve management during upper or lower
    extremity amputation, 456
Nerve repair methods, 454–455, 499
Nerves of orbit, 107
Nerve transfer, 455, 460
Nerve tumors, 516–518
Neurilemomas, 518
Neurocutaneous melanosis, 158
Neurofibromas, 518
Neurovascular Island Pedicle Flap, 507
Neurovasculature, 264
Nevus of Ito, 73
Nevus of Ota, 73, 74
Nevus Sebaceous of Jadassohn, 75, 76
Nipple-areolar complex (NAC), 290
Nipple reconstruction, 316
Non-cutaneous melanoma, 157
Nongenital surgery, 605, 607
Non-nerve-based surgery, 460–461
Nonsurgical facial rejuvenation, 351
    botulinum toxin, 355
    chemical peels, 354, 355
    dermabrasion, 354
    IPL, 353
    laser, 352, 353
    microdermabrasion, 354
    volume restoration, 356, 357
Nonvascularized bone grafts, 276
Nose, 111, 245
    analysis, 371
        aesthetic components, 370
        alar base width, 372
        dorsal aesthetic lines, 371
        nasal tip projection, 372
        nasal tip rotation, 372
        tip defining points, 372
    anatomy, 209, 210, 369–371

O
Oberg, Manske, Tonkin (OMT), 539
Occipital artery, 102
Occlusal relationships, 175–178
Oculo-auriculo-vertebral syndrome, 152
Oculomotor nerve, 107
Omental flaps, 222, 565
Optic canal/foramen, 248
Optic nerve, 107
Oral cavity, 108, 262
Oral vestibule, 108
Orbicularis, 125
Orbicularis oculi, 226, 379, 389
Orbicularis oris, 122
Orbicularis sandwich flap, 230
Orbital anatomy, 226, 248
Orbital apex syndrome, 249
Orbital dystopia, 195
Orbital fractures
    anatomy/epidemiology, 247
    associated syndromes, 249
    management, 249
    presentation, 248
Orbital hypertelorism, 194
ORIF, 253, 255
    indications, 249
Orocutaneous fistulas, 279
Oronasal-ocular cleft, 190
Oropharynx., 109, 111, 262
Orthodontic decompensation, 181
Orthognathic surgery
    evaluation, 180–181
    imaging, 178, 180
    occlusal relationships, 175–178
    procedures, 182–185
Orticochea flap, 222
Osseous genioplasty, 609
Osteoarthritis
    anatomy, 555–556
    demographics, 555
    diagnosis, 556–557
    epidemiology, 555
    hormonal differences, 555
    incidence, 555
    non-inflammatory degeneration of articular
        cartilage, 555
    nonsurgical management, 557–558
    pathogenesis, 556
    physical manifestations, 556
    surgical management, 558–560
Osteochondromas (Exostoses), 525

Osteocutaneous pedicle flap, 29
Osteoid osteoma, 524
Osteomyelitis, 581
Osteosarcoma, 527
Otoplasty, 201

P
Palatal obturators and lift devices, 143
Palatine Tonsils, 110
Palpation, 245
Palpebral, 226
Pan-facial fractures, 259
Panniculectomy, 331
Pan-plexus injury, 460
Paranasal sinuses, 112
Parathyroids, 116
Parenchyma, 290
Parkes-Weber syndrome, 167
Parotid gland, 105
Parotidomasseteric fascia, 359
Partial flaps, 221
Partial glossectomy, 274
Partial-thickness defects, 238
Pathologic scarring, 17–19
Pectoralis major advancement, 564
Pedicled flaps, 28
    reconstruction, 588
Pedicled intestinal vaginoplasty, 604
Pedicled pectoralis major, 275
Pedicled subcutaneous flaps, 222
Pedicled TRAM flap, 322, 323
Pelvic reconstruction, 584
Penile inversion vaginoplasty, 604
Periareolar incision, 297, 307
Periareolar or circumareolar technique, 309
Pericranial flaps, 221
Pericranium, 220
Perineal anatomy
    blood supply and defects, 588
    female, 584
    local and pedicle flap, 588
    local tissue rearrangements, 586
    male, 583
    patient counseling, 590
    penis, 589
    scrotum, 589
Perineal defects
    causes, 585–587
    reconstructive options, 587
Perineal reconstruction, 583–585, 587–590
Perioral rhytides (Smoker's Lines), 401
Periosteal chondromas, 524
PHACES, 167
Phalangeal fractures, 465

Phalloplasty, 608
Pharyngeal reconstruction, 277, 278
Pharyngoesophageal reconstruction, 278
Pharynx, 277
Pilomatricoma, 76–77
Pitanguy's ligament, 370
Plastic surgery
    3 A's of surgery, 10
    closure methods, 5, 6
        primary closure techniques, 6, 7
        sutures and needles, 7–9
    operating room etiquette and expectations, 10
    overview, 1
    principles of, 3, 4
    procedures, 2
    reconstructive ladder of, 3
    scope of practice, 1, 2
    wound closure and sutures, 4, 5
Platysma, 114
Platysmaplasty, 365
Pneumatic compression devices, 597
Pneumocystis carinii (PCP), 51
Pneumothorax, 207
Poisseuille's law, 42
Polydactyly, 540
Poly-L-lactic acid (PLLA), 357
Polymethyl methacrylate (PMMA), 273, 357
Port-wine stain, 165
Postaxial polydactyly, 540
Posterior auricular artery, 102, 200
Posterior auricular vein, 104
Posterior division of retromandibular vein, 104
Posterior pharyngeal flap, 144
Posterior pharyngeal wall augmentation, 146
Posterior thigh-buttock angles, 411
Post-operative laser care, 68, 69
Power-assisted liposuction, 342
Preauricular incision, 362
Preaxial Polydactyly, 541
Precise injection technique (PIT) method, 414, 415
Pressure injury, 95
Pressure ulcers
    diagnosis, 95
    etiology, 94
    incidence, 93
    presentation, 95–96
    prevalence, 93
    prevention and treatment, 96–97
    stages of, 95
        prevention, 98
        risk factors for recurrence, 97
        stages I and II, 96
        stages III and IV, 96–97
    wet to dry and wet to moist dressings, 96

Primary closure techniques, 6
Primary lymphedema, 593, 595
Primary rhinoplasty, 375
Procerus muscle, 388
Profunda artery perforator flap, 325
Prognathia, 181
Propeller flap after inset, 581
Prophylactic antibiotics, 89
Prosthetic based breast reconstruction, 313
　alloplastic reconstruction, methodology for, 315, 316
　alternatives, 317
　complications, 317
　considerations, 317
　decisions on, 314
　history and physical examination, 314
　nipple reconstruction, 316
　options for alloplastic materials, 315
Prosthetics, 510
Proximal row carpectomy (PRC), 472
Pruzansky classification, 148, 149
Pseudomonas aeruginosa, 96
Pulmonary embolism, 344
Pyogenic flexor tenosynovitis, 434, 435
Pyogenic granuloma, 78–79, 164

R

Radial forearm flap, 275
Radial nerve compression, 445–447
Radial tunnel syndrome, 447
Radical neck dissection, 268
Radiocarpal joint, 420
Radiofrequency-assisted liposuction, 342
Radiotherapy, 268
Ramsay Hunt syndrome, 285
Rashes, 331
Raynaud phenomenon, 534
Reconstructive elevator, 40
Reconstructive surgery, 3
Rectus diastasis, 330
Recurrent laryngeal nerve (RLN), 116, 117
Regenerative peripheral nerve interface, 456
Regional flaps, 221, 222
Regional neurovascular anatomy, 410–413
Repaired nerves, 455
Reperfusion Injury, 495
Replantation
　absolute contraindications, 496
　indications, 496
　postoperative care, 500
　preoperative care, 497
　relative contraindications, 496

Resection procedures, 599
Resorption of cartilage graft, 207
Retro-auricular skin flap, 366
Retrobulbar hematoma, 384
Retrognathia, 181
Retromandibular vein, 102
Reversal sural flap, 580
Revision rhinoplasty, 375
Rheumatoid arthritis
　autoantibodies, 548
　chronic inflammatory condition, 547
　classical stigmata, 548
　diagnosis, 548–549
　environmental risk factors, 547
　etiology, 547
　genetic and environmental factors, 547
　medical management, 549–550
　pathophysiology, 548
　severe erosive arthritis of the wrist, 551
　surgical management, 550–553
　susceptibility, 547
　treatment, 549–553
Rheumatoid nodules, 550
Rheumatoid wrist, 550–551
Rhinoplasty, 371
　complication, 377
　goals, 374
　grafts, 375–377
　incision, 374, 375
　transcolumellar incision, 374
Rhytidectomy, 366
Rigid fixation techniques, 182, 255
Rolando fracture, 468
ROOF (retro-orbicularis oculi fat), 380
Rotation advancement flaps, 222

S

SAFElipo technique, 341
Sagittal closure patterns with LARGE defects, 144
Saline implants, 306, 307
Salivary glands, 262
Sausage digit, 435
Scalp, 245
　galea, 219
　hair and hairline, 218
　layers, 215–216
　neurological, 217
　oncologic reconstruction, 219
　sensory, 218
　territories, 216, 217
　trauma, 218

Index 625

Scalp reconstruction, 273
  autologous reconstruction, 273
  cranioplasty, 273
  dermal regeneration templates, 220
  general guidelines, 222
  local flaps, 220, 221
  primary closure, 219
  regional flaps, 221, 222
  replantation, 222
  secondary closure, 219
  soft tissue reconstruction, 274
  STSG, 219
  tissue expansion, 221
Scalp trauma, 215
Scaphoconchal angle, 200
Scaphoconchal sutures, 201
Scaphoid lunate advanced collapse (SLAC) wrist with severe radiocarpal erosion, 493
Scar formation
  hypertrophic scarring, 17, 18
  keloids, 18, 19
  pathologic scarring, 17–19
  principles of, 17
Scarpa's fascia, 338
Schnur scale, 300
Schwannoma ex vivo, 518
Schwannomas, 518
Scope of practice, 1, 2
Scroll ligament, 369
Seborrheic Keratosis, 72
Secondary lymphedema, 596
Second metacarpal head fracture, 465
Selective neck dissection, 268
Selective photothermolysis, 64
Septal deviation, 372
Septal extension graft, 376
Septal harvest pearls, 375
Septum, 370, 375
Silicone implants, 306, 307
Simple lacerations, 203
Skate technique, 316
Skeletal deficiencies, 189
Skeletal reconstruction, 564
Skin cancer, 520
Skin grafting, 159
  stages of, 25, 26
  stratification, 24, 25
  types of, 24
Skin lesions
  benign skin lesions (*see* Benign skin lesions)
  evaluation, 71
  malignant skin Lesions (*see* Malignant skin lesions)
Skin necrosis, 207, 366
Skin resection patterns, 302
Skin resurfacing, 68
Skin tag, 72
Small FT defects, 239
SMAS, *see* Superficial musculoaponeurotic system
Snapback test, 381, 383
Sodium bicarbonate, 57
Soft palate techniques, 109, 135–136
Soft tissue coverage, 499
Soft tissue defect, 504
Soft tissue reconstruction, 274, 275, 564
Soft tissue sarcomas, 522
SOOF (suborbicularis oculi fat), 380
Spastic cerebral palsy, 403
Speech therapy, 143
Sphincter pharyngoplasty, 145
Spina bifida occulta, 167
Spinal accessory nerve, 117
Spinal cord transfers, 455
Spitz Nevus, 75
Splinting, 489
Split calvarial bone grafts, 273
Split thickness calvarial graft, 273
Split thickness skin graft (STSG), 24, 25, 219
Spock ear, 201
Spreader grafts, 376
Squamous cell carcinoma (SCC), 80–81, 202, 521
SSRI, 340
Standard Z-plasty, 508
Staphylococcus aureus, 96
Static rhytids, 352
Stenosing tenosynovitis ("trigger finger"), 553
Stenson's duct, 106
Stenstrom technique, 201
Sternal wound dehiscence, 563
Sternocleidomastoid muscle (SCM), 114, 360
Stria, 330
Sturge-Weber syndrome, 167
Subclavian artery, 115
Subclavian vein, 104
Subcutaneous adipofascial layers of trunk, 338
Subcutaneous adipose tissue, 337
Subcutaneous face lift, 364
Subcutaneous fat with pinch test, 331
Subcuticular suture technique, 7
Sublingual gland, 106
Submandibular gland (SMG), 106
Submental flap, 239

Subtotal amputation with possible adequate length, 507–508
Suction-assisted lipectomy, 297, 337, 600
Suction-assisted liposuction (SAL), 342
Sunderland I (neuropraxia), 453
Sunderland II (axonotmesis), 453
Sunderland III (axonotmesis), 453
Sunderland IV (axonotmesis), 454
Sunderland V (neurotmesis), 454
Sunderland VI (neuroma in continuity), 454
Superficial (Camper's) adipose tissue, 337
Superficial musculoaponeurotic system (SMAS), 264, 359, 364
Superficial peels, 354
Superficial temporal artery, 102, 200, 271
Superior gluteal artery and vein, greater sciatic foramen, 411
Superior gluteal artery perforator flap (SGAP), 324
Superior laryngeal nerve (SLN), 116, 117
Superior orbital fissure syndrome, 248, 249
Superior thyroid artery, 271
Supermicrosurgery, 46
Superomedial Pedicle, 301
Supraorbital nerve, 218
Supratrochlear nerve, 218
Surgical sutures, 4, 5
Swan neck of the fingers, 552
Swan-neck deformity, 552
Symbrachydactyly, 542
Syndactyly, 539
Syndromic craniosynostosis, 170
Synkinesis, 283
Synostosis, 171
Synovectomy, 551
Syringe-based techniques, 414
Systemic therapies, 80

T
Tabletop test, 513
Tacrolimus, 50
Tanzer classification, 151
Targeted muscle reinnervation, 456
Tarsal plate, 227
Tarsoconjunctival flap, 229, 230
Tear trough deformity, 381, 405
Telecanthus (soft tissue), 194
Temporal branch, 217
Temporoparietal fascia, 359, 360
Tendon injuries
  anatomy, 477–479
  repair, 479–480

Tendon repair technique, 498
Tendon ruptures, 552
Tendon transfer, 460, 461, 477, 479
  indications, 485
  injury patterns, 486–487
  principles, 485–486
Tenosynovitis, 551
Tension free repair, 572
Teratogen, 148
Tessier classification, 187, 188
Tessier clefts, 195
Thighplasty, 335
Thoracic outlet syndrome, 447
Thoracodorsal artery and vein, 321, 322
Thoracodorsal artery perforator flap, 321
3-D tattooing, 316
Thumb amputation, 509
Thumb CMC (basal) joint, 558, 559
Thumb fractures, 467, 468
Thumb reconstruction, 503–505, 507, 508
Thyrocervical trunk, 115
Thyroid gland, 115
Tip graft, 377
Tissue expansion, 159
  applications, 36
  biologic creep, 35
  complications, 36
  contraindications, 36
  mechanical creep, 35
  physiology, 35
Tissue flaps, 319
Tissue injury, 86
Tissue revascularization, 495
Toe-to-thumb reconstruction, 508–510
Tongue anatomy, 275
Tongue defects classification, 274
Tongue flap, 238
Tongue reconstruction, 274
  reconstructive algorithm, 274
  tongue defects classification, 274
Topical Anesthesia, 57
Top surgery, 605, 607
Total amputation with destruction of CMCJ, 510
Total amputation with preservation of CMCJ, 508
Total glossectomy, 274
Total wrist arthritis, 561
Traction injury, 458
Transaxillary incision, 307
Transcolumellar incision, 374
Transcutaneous near infrared tissue oximetry, 45

Transhumeral amputation transfers, 456
Transpalpebral/Transblepharoplasty, 392
Transumbilical incision, 308
Transverse cervical artery, 271
Transverse rectus abdominis myocutaneous flap (TRAM), 322
Trapeziectomy with soft tissue interposition, 558
Trauma, 284–285, 448
Treacher Collin's syndrome, 147, 191
Trigeminal nerve, 104, 117
Trochlear nerve, 107
Tubed retroauricular graft, 204
Turbinates, 371, 373
Two flap palatoplasty, 134
Tympanic membrane, 197
Tyndall effect, 75

U

UCL tear with associated fracture, 491
Ulnar impaction syndrome, 471
Ulnar nerve compression, 444–445
Ulnar tunnel (Guyon canal), 444
Ultrasound-assisted liposuction, 342
Ultrasound-assisted technique, 416
Umbilicus, 328
Unfavorable fracture, 254
Unilateral cleft lip nasal deformity, 126
Unilateral cleft lip repair, 130
Unilateral or bilateral reconstructions, 322
Upper body lift, 335
Upper extremity nerves, 443
Upper eyelid
  anatomy, 379–380
  patient evaluation, 381
  treatment procedures, 382
Upper leg reconstruction, 577
Upper motor v lower motor neuron injury, 283
Urine or blood nicotine test, 331

V

Vaginal defect reconstruction, 588
Vaginoplasty, 605
Vagus nerve, 108, 115, 117
Vascular disease, 533
Vascular insult theory, 148
Vascularized bone free flaps, 276
Vascularized composite allograft (VCA), 2
Vascularized composite allotransplantation (VCA)
  anatomy, 50

definition, 49
demographics, incidence, and epidemiology, 50
ethical considerations, 52
facial transplantation, 49
future directions, 52
hand transplantation, 49
history of, 49
immunosuppression, 50
patient selection, 50
postoperative care, 51–52
surgical technique, 51
Vascularized lymph node transfer (VLNT), 598, 599
Vascular lesions, 65
Vascular malformations (VMs), 164–167, 519, 520
  classification and specific anomalies, 162–166
  commonly associated syndromes, 167
  evaluation, 161
    patient history, 162
    radiologic, 162
  pathogenesis, 161
  treatment, 167
Vascular supply transfer, 23
Vascular tumors, 163–164, 516
Vasculature, 108, 305
  of hand, 531–532
Vasculogenesis, 161
Vasospastic disorders, 402, 533
Veau classification, 127, 128
Veins, 102
  grafts, 46
  injury, 531
  repair, 498, 499
Velopharyngeal competence, 133, 137
Velopharyngeal dysfunction, 137
  anatomy, 138
  clinical presentation, 138–139
  diagnosis, 140–143
  etiologies of, 138
  management
    non-operative, 143
    operative, 143–146
Velopharyngeal insufficiency (VPI), 136, 138, 140
Velopharyngeal port, 142
Venous anastomosis, 42
Venous thromboembolism, 344
Ventral hernia, 571
Vermillion, 238
Vertical mattress suture technique, 7

Vertical maxillary deficiency, 181
Vertical maxillary excess, 181
Vertical rectus abdominis myocutaneous (VRAM) flap, 564
Vertical technique, 310
Vessel blowout, 279
Video nasopharyngeal endoscopy, 140
VLNT, *see* Vascularized lymph node transfer
Volume restoration, 356, 357
Von Hippel-Lindau, 167
Von-Langenbeck palatoplasty, 134
VPI, *see* Velopharyngeal insufficiency
V-Y pushback (with intravelar veloplasty), 144, 222

W

Wartenberg syndrome, 447
Water-assisted liposuction, 342
Wetting Solutions, 341, 342
Wharton's duct, 106
Wound closure, 509
    types of
        primary, 4
        secondary, 5
        tertiary, 5
Wound healing, 87
    care, principles of, 19–20
    failures of, 16
    management, 20–22
    principles of, 14–16
    surgical procedures, 21–22
    tissue anatomy and structure, 13–14
WPATH (World Professional Association for Transgender Health), 603
Wrist
    articulation, function and anatomy, 469
    physical examination, 469–470
Wrist fractures
    Injury patterns and management, 470–475
    radial inclination, 471
    types, 470
    vasculature of a scaphoid, 474
    volar (or dorsal) tilt, 472
Würinger's septum, 291

Z

ZMC fractures, 252, 253
Zone of coagulation, 86
Zone of hyperemia, 86
Zone of stasis, 86
Zones of adherence, 339
Z-plasty, 143, 508
Zygoma, 252
Zygomatic arch, 253, 254
Zygomaticotemporal nerve, 218

GPSR Compliance

The European Union's (EU) General Product Safety Regulation (GPSR) is a set of rules that requires consumer products to be safe and our obligations to ensure this.

If you have any concerns about our products, you can contact us on ProductSafety@springernature.com

In case Publisher is established outside the EU, the EU authorized representative is:

Springer Nature Customer Service Center GmbH
Europaplatz 3
69115 Heidelberg, Germany

Batch number: 09727458

Printed by Printforce, the Netherlands